Caesarean Birth in Britain

REVISED AND UPDATED

A book for health professionals and parents

Caesarean Birth in Britain

REVISED AND UPDATED

A book for health professionals and parents

HELEN CHURCHILL

WENDY SAVAGE

COLIN FRANCOME

Middlesex
University
PRESS

First published in 2006 by Middlesex University Press

Copyright © Helen Churchill, Wendy Savage and Colin Francome

ISBN 1 904750 17 6

A CIP catalogue record for this book is available from The British Library

Illustrations, with the exception of those on pages 19 and 24, by Helen Chown

Book design by Helen Taylor

Printed in the UK by Hobbs the Printers, Hampshire

Middlesex University Press, Queensway, Enfield, Middlesex EN4 3SF

Tel: +44 (0)20 8411 5734: +44 (0)20 8880 4262 Fax: +44 (0)20 8411 5736
www.mupress.co.uk

Contents

Biographies

Dr HELEN CHURCHILL is Senior Lecturer and Health Studies Subject Leader at Manchester Metropolitan University. She has completed extensive research on the history of caesarean birth, current practice, women's experiences of and reactions to caesarean birth, and informed choice in maternity services. Her publications include a number of papers on women's health issues and the books *Caesarean Birth in Britain* (1993) and *Caesarean Birth: Experience, Practice and History* (1997).

Professor WENDY SAVAGE qualified as a doctor in 1960. She worked in the USA, Nigeria, Kenya and New Zealand and in 1977 became Senior Lecturer in Obstetrics and Gynaecology and Honorary Consultant at the London Hospital Medical College. She was suspended from her post in 1985 accused of incompetence in the management of five obstetric cases, four delivered by Caesarean section. The subsequent debate and public inquiry became a cause célèbre. The allegations were not upheld and she was reinstated in 1986 and retired in 2000. She wrote about this experience in *A Savage Enquiry: Who controls childbirth?* and is the author and co-author over forty-five papers on a number of topics including induced abortion, sexually transmitted disease, childbirth and caesarean section. She was an elected member of General Medical Council 1989-2005.

Dr COLIN FRANCOME is emeritus professor in the Sociology of Health at Middlesex University and editor of the health series for Middlesex University Press. He formerly headed the Master's Programme in deviancy theory and his first published article was in the *British Journal of Criminology*. He has published studies about Hindu, Sikh and Muslim students in Britain and widely in the area of health, including writing an editorial for *British Medical Journal*.

Acknowledgements

Helen Churchill would like to thank Kate and Leah for their support. She would also like to thank the hundreds of women who participated in the studies and the consultants, midwives and care managers who organised the distribution and collection of questionnaires without whose help and the goodwill of their staff the research would not have been possible.

Wendy Savage would like to thank Drs Susan Bewley, Gavin Young, Mike Robson and midwife Deb Hughes who made useful comments on some chapters.

The authors would all like to thank all the women who took the time to write up their VBAC stories for this book. Also the RCOG who provided us with a list of Clinical Directors in Obstetrics and Gynaecology and those doctors who responded to our questionnaire and took time to record thoughtful comments. The computer department of the Royal London Hospital especially Deidre Gillon who maintained the obstetric database, and were always willing to do analyses. Robert Kyffin who analysed the data using the Robson groups and those obstetricians who shared their hospital data.

We are grateful to the NCT for commenting on a draft; however, the responsibility for the final text lies entirely with the authors.

1 Introduction

The differences in caesarean rates between countries and regions cannot be explained by the physical characteristics of the women and they therefore raise serious ethical and economic considerations.

WOMEN ARE OVER FOUR TIMES MORE LIKELY to have a caesarean birth now than they were thirty years ago and eight times more likely than they were fifty years ago. In the 1950s around 3 per cent of births were by caesarean.[1] By 1973 the estimated caesarean rate for England and Wales was 5.3 per cent and latest data shows a rate for Britain in 2004 of 22.9 per cent.

When a caesarean is necessary it can be life saving for mother and baby. However, we have written this book because we are of the opinion that many caesareans are being performed unnecessarily. At the beginning of the twentieth century, some obstetricians were concerned about the then rising rates and brought up the same issues that we deal with here. By the beginning of the twenty-first century, rates had risen much higher. When we wrote the first edition of this book, in 1993, there was little public debate about rising rates and a worrying lack of concern in many quarters. Since that time there has been a move to audit caesarean section rates in NHS hospitals and a level of demonstrable concern from some professional bodies,[2] culminating in the first national audit of caesarean section rates in England, Wales and Northern Ireland.[3]

In 1992, the Winterton Committee reported on its investigation into Maternity Services and for the first time MPs listened to women. They emphasised that women should be at the centre of care and that communication, continuity of carer, cooperation and choice should replace the fragmented system of care

---

1 POST, 2002
2 See for example: National Childbirth Trust, Royal College of Midwives & Royal College of Obstetricians and Gynaecologists Conference proceedings 23 November 1999, *The Rising Caesarean Rate – A Public Health Issue* (2000); and Conference proceedings 7 November 2000, *The Rising Caesarean Rate – Causes and Effects for Public Health* (2001)
3 Thomas & Paranjothy, 2001

1

given by too many people who did not always talk to each other. The government response was to set up a task force headed by Julia Cumberlege and they reported in 1993. *Changing Childbirth* provided the blueprint for a change in midwifery and obstetric practice to a more woman-centred approach. The main recommendations of the report were that women should be provided with adequate information to enable decision-making regarding care and that continuity of care is essential for the communication between professionals and their patients. However, rather than reducing the number of caesareans, it has been suggested that this document has actually led to an increase in the section rate. It is claimed that giving women choice in maternity services means that more women request caesarean section. Little research has been carried out on the practice of caesareans on demand[4] or the ethics of surgery by choice in these circumstances.[5] (See p.46 for discussion of caesareans on request.)

Our aim in updating this book is to inform and promote debate between all interested parties but particularly women, who are the ones who have to undergo the operation and its attendant risks and cope with its aftermath, in addition to caring for a new baby. We therefore hope that this book will be read by women and their families as well as health professionals and antenatal teachers.

One of our authors, Wendy Savage, has commented that as the developed world becomes more and more dependent on technology, there is a danger that people will cease to believe that women can give birth naturally.[6] There is no doubt that some doctors have seen caesarean sections as the birthing method of the future. Philip Steer (Professor of Obstetrics) has suggested that, through the process of evolution, the female pelvis is now unsuitable for vaginal birth and that caesarean birth is the only way forward.[7] Furthermore, Professor Nick Fisk and Sara Paterson Brown have argued that caesareans are the safest way to give birth.[8]

The lack of concern among many obstetricians about the after-effects of the rising caesarean rates may result from the fact that they spend little time postnatally with women who have had caesarean sections and are far removed from any physical or psychological ill-effects resulting from the operation. Two studies undertaken by one of our authors, Helen Churchill, in 1991–2 and 1996 showed that low emotional well-being and negative feelings about the baby were both associated with having had a caesarean.[9] More women were likely to have positive experiences of caesarean birth if it was performed under local anaesthesia. The risk of endometritis, need for transfusion and pneumonia are

4   Bergholt et al., 2004; Kwee et al., 2004
5   Minkoff et al., 2004
6   Savage, 1992
7   Steer, 1998
8   Fisk & Paterson Brown, 2004
9   Churchill, 1997

higher following caesarean compared to spontaneous vaginal birth.[10] One study of the post-operative morbidity associated with CS found that only 9.5 per cent of women have no recorded morbidity in the postnatal period and concluded that there was considerable postnatal morbidity associated with the operation, particularly if it is carried out as an emergency procedure.[11] This was also the finding in our recent survey of women's experiences (see chapter 7) and it is encouraging to see regional anaesthetic, spinal block in particular, being used in the majority of cases since the mid 1990s.[12]

Literature on effects of caesarean birth on the infant is limited and there appears to be little research on the long-term effects of caesarean birth on child development. The evidence available does not suggest increased use of caesareans to have reduced infant morbidity or mortality and there may be problems of iatrogenic prematurity[13] and risk of respiratory disorders in caesarean-born infants.[14] In view of the wealth of evidence pointing to negative side-effects of caesarean section for the mother and, to a certain extent the infant, it is not unreasonable to assume that these effects will have repercussions on the mother-child relationship. Caesarean mothers have reported negative effects on bonding[15] and breastfeeding.[16]

Reasons for the rise and variation in rates of caesarean section

Twenty years ago women in the United States were twice as likely to have a caesarean as women in Britain. At that time nearly a quarter of American births were performed by caesarean.[17] However, recent evidence shows that we are now catching up with our American counterparts.[18] The CSR in the US levelled out for a time in the 1990s (see p.65) which meant that by the turn of the century the CSRs in the US and the UK aligned at around 22 per cent. Subsequently the rate in the US rose to an all time high of 26 per cent in 2002. The UK rate is also rising with a CSR of almost 23 per cent in 2004.

There are some perfectly good reasons for the rise in caesarean rates. The operation is much safer than it was and improvements in anaesthetic techniques are an important factor in the increase. However, there are wide differences in practice between different countries. The caesarean section rates in the US and

---

10 Burrows et al., 2004
11 Hillan, 1995
12 Churchill, 1997
13 Churchill, 1997
14 Zanardo et al., 2004
15 Hillan, 1992c; Churchill, 1997
16 Mathur et al., 1993; Ever-Hadani et al., 1994; Menghetti et al., 1994; Churchill, 1997
17 Taffel et al., 1992
18 Ventura et al., 2000

UK are almost double those of the Netherlands or Norway (see chapter 4). There may be demographic explanations for rising caesarean section rates. For example, women are delaying childbirth and having fewer children. It is well documented that caesarean rates increase with increasing age of mothers. However, such changes have been shown to account for only a small part of overall caesarean section rate rises. Scandinavian countries, for example, have experienced similar demographic transitions but have not witnessed similar increases in caesarean rates.[19] If the differences in caesarean rates between countries and regions cannot be explained by the physical characteristics of the women or demographic changes, they therefore raise serious ethical and economic considerations.

If the high level of caesareans in some countries were due to better medical practice, more accurate diagnosis and better management of labour problems, leading to healthier mothers and babies, then there would be a strong case for increasing the caesarean rate in other countries. However, we know that both the maternal and perinatal mortality rates in the United States are higher than in Western Europe, despite the fact that the United States is materially wealthier. If, as this suggests, the US rate is high because of non-medical reasons such as doctors being frightened of being sued for negligence, it would suggest that women in the United States are undergoing a great deal of unnecessary surgery. It has been suggested that in the States about 500 women die following CS each year from infections, haemorrhaging or other complications. The maternal mortality rate associated with CS in the US is 0.02 per cent but this is still four times the death rate associated with vaginal birth.[20] In the UK between 2000 and 2002 the fatality rate for vaginal birth was 0.004 per cent, considerably less than for caesarean section at 0.17 per cent.[21] However, interpretation of mortality statistics concerning caesarean birth is always complicated as the condition that necessitated the operation may be a contributory factor in the death of the mother.

British obstetric care

In Britain, unlike in North America, most deliveries are carried out by midwives who are trained as sole practitioners in their own right. Midwives provide most of a woman's care during pregnancy, labour and in the postnatal period. However, the number of midwives practicing in Britain is reducing steadily: a decade ago there were 39,000 whereas today only 32,745[22]. It is not unusual for a midwife to assist more than six or seven women during one shift. This reduction in the number of midwives together with the corresponding increase in each midwife's case load may have an impact on the caesarean rate as other professional groups are called in to help.

19 Thomas & Paranjothy, 2001
20 Thivierge, 2002
21 DoH, 2004a, table 1.11
22 NMC, 2005

Women in Britain have the right to have a baby at home and almost 2 per cent of births are home births. However, the overall responsibility for the vast majority of births is perceived to lie with 1,384 consultant obstetricians.[23] These consultants head teams, formerly known as 'firms'. These are hierarchical groups which usually include doctors at various stages of training and experience, known as specialist registrars (SPRs) and senior house officers (SHOs). (Some hospital protocols use the phrase 'chain of command' in describing situations when appropriate medical assistance should be sought.) The SHO will be someone at the first level of their formal training. The higher-level doctors will be called in if there are any problems and will perform fetal blood sampling, assisted vaginal births and caesareans. In a typical British maternity unit there will be any number of consultants from two to ten and they will meet regularly to discuss such issues as perinatal deaths. General practitioners (GPs) can also carry out births either in conjunction with a consultant unit or independently, either at home or in a GP- or midwife-led unit. However, one of the effects of *Changing Childbirth* was to encourage midwives to use their professional skills and, along with changes in the GP workload, this has virtually removed GPs from the obstetrical field apart from a few rural areas. If a caesarean should become necessary, this will almost always be carried out under a consultant's authority and women may have to be transferred to a larger unit from a small unit or from home should the need for a caesarean arise.

Variations in caesarean rates in Britain

Reports within the countries in Britain also show some variation in rates. In 2004 there was a CSR of 22.7 per cent in England, 23.8 per cent in Wales and 24.4 per cent in Scotland. In 2002 Northern Ireland had a rate of 25.8 per cent.[24]

The National Caesarean Section audit (2001) found considerable regional variation within England and Wales, and the pattern of this is similar to that found in earlier surveys. The caesarean section rate in England ranges from 20 per cent in the North East to 26 per cent in Essex.[25]

Caesarean section rates for maternity units across the UK range from 10 to 65 per cent.[26] This size of difference cannot be justified by differences in case-mix. Women who attend teaching hospitals are more likely to have a caesarean than those in other hospitals.[27] Some hospitals have high rates because they have specialist units and so receive higher-risk pregnancies. Regional variations in factors such as height, social class and ethnic mix cannot explain all of the

23   2002 figures
24   birthchoiceuk.com, 2005
25   Thomas & Paranjothy, 2001
26   Thomas & Paranjothy, 2001
27   Savage & Francome, 1993

differences in caesarean rates. Some people believe that women should be informed before they book into a hospital for maternity care about the overall rates of intervention and those of individual consultants.

Why has the caesarean rate increased so markedly over the last thirty years in developed countries?

Sixty years ago, mortality following caesarean section was much higher than following vaginal birth, because of infection, thrombosis and anaemia. The improved safety of surgery with modern anaesthetic techniques, the availability of antibiotics and of blood transfusion has meant that caesareans are safer than they were. Thus obstetricians, when balancing the risks, have a stronger case for surgery even though there is still a significant maternal mortality and morbidity rate following caesarean section.

There is a second factor which has lowered the threshold for performing the operation in premature labour or in cases of severe high blood pressure (pre-eclampsia) or proven intra-uterine growth retardation of the pre-term infant. This is due to the success of modern neonatal intensive care in saving the lives of low-birthweight infants. The proportion of low-birthweight babies (less than 2,500g) and pre-term babies (less than thirty-seven weeks) has increased. The incidence of low birthweight was about 6 per cent in Scotland and 8 per cent in England in 1998.[28] These increases may be due to increases in multiple pregnancies (due to increased use of IVF) and increases in obstetric intervention and may explain a small proportion of the rise in caesarean rates.

The reasons for the rising caesarean rate are complex. Over twenty years ago Arney, in discussing the way that professional input into birth has developed, called the era of obstetrics the 'monitoring' period.[29] He suggested that obstetricians have surrendered their skills to a system of checks and technology. In essence, they have become the slaves of machines, not the masters. There is general agreement in the literature that continuous electronic fetal monitoring in labour of low-risk women increases caesarean rates without significantly improving perinatal mortality rates.[30]

Yet electronic fetal monitoring continues to be used on many low-risk women, often without recourse to fetal blood sampling which has been shown to keep caesarean rates down.[31]

Our position is that some increase in the caesarean rate can be justified, but by no means the entire rise that has occurred. There is a great deal of evidence for this position:

28 Thomas & Paranjothy, 2001
29 Arney, 1982
30 Thomas & Paranjothy, 2001
31 NICE, 2004

- Our evidence shows that many caesareans are conducted because of the fear of litigation in Britain, just as in the United States (see chapter 8).
- There is evidence of a convenience factor in some places. For example, a study of childbirth practices in the Campania region of Italy highlighted certain aspects of physician convenience. Sixty-three per cent of caesareans were recorded as being performed in the morning and 93 per cent on working days.[32]
- There is ample evidence that financial incentives to perform caesareans influence obstetricians' decisions about whether or not to perform a caesarean. Therefore healthier, wealthy women have on average more caesareans than less well-off women. For example, the Portland Hospital in London (private) has a section rate of 44 per cent whereas the highest rates in NHS hospitals are around 30 per cent.[33]
- Thus it appears that the relative risks and benefits to mother and baby do not appear to be the major factors in the decision to perform a caesarean.

We have been raising the issue of high caesarean rates since 1978 and are glad to see that some others are beginning to share our view. Since the publication of the first edition of this book in 1993 there have been a number of audits and guidelines produced.[34]

The report into maternal deaths 1997 to 1999 stated that:

> ...the results show, sometimes in dramatic fashion, that the routine use of national guidelines can work. In this triennium, following the routine introduction and use of guidelines... there have been significant decreases in deaths from pulmonary embolism and sepsis following caesarean section. In the very few cases where deaths occurred from these causes, guidelines do not appear to have been followed.[35]

In Britain the rates have risen as high as elsewhere and, in some cases, higher. The reasons for this rise are discussed in chapter 3.

Vaginal birth is still safer than abdominal birth

A vaginal birth has always been safer for the mother than a caesarean and this remains the case. The fatality rate for vaginal birth is significantly less than for caesarean section and other forms of operative birth. Death from caesarean section is three-times greater than for vaginal birth. For emergency caesareans this figure rises to four-times greater; for planned caesareans the rate is still more

---

32 Saporito et al., 2003
33 Thomas & Paranjothy, 2001
34 See for example Thomas & Paranjothy, 2001 & NICE, 2004
35 DoH, 2001, p.4

than twice that for vaginal birth.[36] How much of this difference is due to the problem for which the caesarean is performed, and how much is due to the risk of the surgical procedure itself, has been a matter of much debate.

Over the last fifty years, a period for which detailed analysis is available for maternal deaths in the UK, the number of maternal deaths fell to 261 in 2000-2, the last three-year period for which a report has been published, although this figure shows a slight (not significant) increase compared to the previous three-year period. The last report on maternal mortality did not include a separate chapter on caesarean birth as many of the previous reports had done. The reason for this was because of difficulties in interpreting mortality as a *consequence of* the operation and mortality from a pre-existing condition which was an *indication for* the operation. For the 2000-2 report, Gwyneth Lewis wrote:

> There were several cases in this triennium in which the caesarean section itself may well have contributed to the fatal outcome but, in these cases, the caesarean section itself was undertaken as a possible life-saving measure for the mother and/or her baby. For the large majority of deaths that followed caesarean section, however, there were serious prenatal complications or illness that, in many cases, precipitated the caesarean section.[37]

During the three-year period from 2000 to 2002 the maternal mortality rate following CS was 0.17 per cent. However the rate following emergency operations was 0.02 per cent compared to 0.013 per cent for planned sections.[38] The risks to the mother have always been higher for an emergency than an planned caesarean. This has led some obstetricians to schedule more planned operations, a trend which would almost certainly increase the caesarean rate still further.

The Confidential Enquiry into Maternal Deaths (2004) recommended:

> …that a prospective study be undertaken to help to estimate more robustly what, if any, is the degree of increased risk of maternal deaths associated with caesarean section particularly for those undertaken without a clinical indication.[39]

Although the number of caesarean-related deaths has fallen relative to the number of operations being performed, the actual number of deaths has risen as the overall rate of caesareans rose. The operation is more dangerous for women than a normal vaginal birth. Thus any further increase in the caesarean rate is likely to lead to the deaths of more women overall.

---

36 DoH, 2004a
37 Lewis, 2004, p.1 of 23
38 DoH, 2004a, table 1.11
39 Lewis, 2004, p. 22 of 23

Maternal and fetal morbidity is also higher following caesareans than vaginal birth. The increased use of operative delivery together with other interventionist techniques have had a deleterious effect on women's experience of birth and denied them the opportunity to achieve a sense of accomplishment in childbirth. Iatrogenic effects on the mother include psychological consequences such as disappointment, guilt and depression and physiological outcomes including endometritis, urinary tract infections, wound infections, longer recovery times,[40] blood transfusions and pneumonia.[41] Some women have experienced problems getting pregnant following caesarean births, although whether this is due to physiological or psycho-social issues is unclear.[42] Caesareans may also adversely affect subsequent pregnancies with complications including placenta previa and placental abruption.

For babies born by caesarean there are increased risks of neonatal respiratory distress.[43] There is a small (1.9 per cent) chance of laceration to the fetus during the operation; this risk goes up to 6 per cent if the fetus is not in cephalic presentation. There are also risks associated with iatrogenic prematurity.[44] There may also be implications for bonding and breastfeeding.[45]

The structure of this book

The next chapter shows the development of the caesarean operation in its historical context and reveals that many current issues were also contentious in the past. Some of the practices in the past were somewhat primitive, and we therefore warn pregnant women and other lay readers that they might find some of the material in chapter 2 disturbing. Chapter 3 covers caesarean birth in the twenty-first century including policy changes in the past five years and current trends in caesarean birth. We then consider caesarean birth as a global phenomenon, examining maternity services in general and caesarean practices in particular, in a number of selected countries around the world (chapter 4). In the subsequent two chapters we explain why a caesarean may be necessary (chapter 5) and then describe what a woman who needs one might expect from the operation and how she might cope and be best supported afterwards (chapter 6). We then give first-hand information from our survey of women's experiences and what they felt about the operation, whether it was planned or occurred in an emergency (chapter 7). Next, we present the results of our survey of 100 British obstetricians' views on caesareans (chapter 8). Chapter 9 contains important information about vaginal birth after caesarean. Chapter 10 aims to help women

---

40 Churchill, 1997
41 Burrows et al., 2004
42 Churchill, 1997; Mollison et al., 2005
43 Hannah, 2004; Zanardo et al., 2004
44 Hall, 1999
45 Churchill, 1997

make informed choices about their maternity care and the book concludes with a chapter suggesting constructive ways for women and health professionals to avoid unnecessary caesareans (chapter 11).

We have written this book for parents, health care professionals, antenatal teachers, childbirth support workers (doulas) and academics. As some of the information in this book is quite technical, lay readers may choose to begin with chapters 3, 5, 6 and 10 and Appendix A, before embarking on the rest. It is not necessary for lay readers to understand the statistics in the remainder of the book, but they should feel able to concentrate on those parts of the book most relevant to their needs. Antenatal teachers will, in addition to the above, find much of particular interest to them in chapter 7. Any one with an interest in medical history (including some of the more gruesome aspects) will enjoy chapter 2.

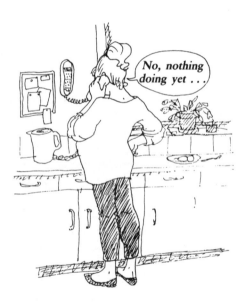

2 The history of the caesarean section

As far as the obstetrician facing a difficult labour was concerned, the crucial choice would be what gave the woman the best chance of survival.

THERE ARE EXAMPLES OF CAESAREANS BEING carried out in pre-Christian times. Very often the operation would only be performed if women died during pregnancy: for example, the ancient Hindus only carried out the operation if the mother had died and there were detectable movements of the fetus. There is also some evidence that the operation may have been known to the ancient Egyptians.[1] It is probable that the operation was well known to the early Jews, as it is mentioned in one of the oldest books of Judaism which was first published in pre-Christian times. In fact among this religious group it was carried out on living women who were expected to survive. Their law stated that women having caesareans were not required to observe days of purification as did those who had a vaginal birth. Such evidence suggests that it is extremely likely that the CS was practised long before the start of the Christian era,[2] although we do not have the history of individual cases. It is quite possible that the skills needed to carry out a successful caesarean were lost over time, for it appears that from early Christian times to the sixteenth century the CS, if it was used at

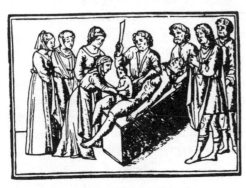

Sixteenth-century depiction of the birth of Julius Caesar

1   Delee, 1913
2   Young, 1944

all, was more often practised in cases where women had died late in pregnancy, in the hope of saving the child.

There is debate over the origin of the word 'caesarean'. James Guillimeau said it was 'in imitation of Caesar who was ripped out of his mother's wombe at the very instant she died'.[3] However, others go back to 715 BC when the king of Rome introduced a law by which it was forbidden to bury a pregnant woman until her child had been removed from her abdomen, even if there was little, if any, chance of its survival. This was so that the two could be buried separately. Newell suggests that this offers a possible explanation for the origin of the term 'caesarean'. The law, the Lex Regia, became the Lex Caesaria and thus the practice became known as the caesarean operation.[4] However, a totally different and more plausible explanation is proposed by Delee. He suggests that the word comes from the Latin 'cedere' meaning 'to cut' and that the term 'caesarean section' literally means 'cut out'.[5]

THE DEBATE: TO SECTION OR NOT TO SECTION?

Although caesareans came to be usually performed after the death of the woman, it is also likely that throughout history they have been carried out while the woman was still alive but could not give birth vaginally. We shall see from the medical literature that there have been several cases of women carrying out the operation on themselves (see the last section of this chapter) and it is also likely that there have been many unrecorded cases of women doing this and of those attending them making an attempt to end a long labour. Young suggests that the oldest authentic case of a living child being born by caesarean was that of Georgias, a celebrated orator of Sicily in 508 AD.[6]

However, there are no recorded attempts of performing a caesarean on a living woman in Europe before 1500. Some suggest that this date marks a watershed, for by the sixteenth century claims were being made that a CS with maternal and infant survival was possible. This led to a rethinking of the operation. One school of thought believed that, in the event of obstructed labour, the mother's life could be saved by surgical removal of the child. However, others took the view that chances of survival were so slim that the operation was tantamount to murder. A determined opponent of the operation was Ambrose Pare (1510–90) who condemned those who dared to perform it because 'no man can persuade me [the operation] can be done without the death of the mother'.[7]

---

3   Guillimeau, 1612, p.185
4   Newell, 1921
5   Delee, 1913
6   Young, 1944
7   Young, 1944, p.24

In 1581 Rousset wrote an important French paper which opened the debate on the relative benefits of the operation and argued the case for the possibility of performing a caesarean on a living woman.[8] In fact it was not a medical practitioner but Jacob Nufer, a hog gelder of Sigerhausen, Switzerland, who performed the first recorded successful CS as measured by maternal survival. He carried it out on his wife, Elizabeth Alespachin, during a prolonged and obstructed labour in 1588. Remarkably, reports suggest that both mother and child survived and recovered. Mrs Nufer is said to have gone on to give birth to six more children, one set of twins and four single births, and the caesarean child is said to have lived to the age of seventy-seven.[9]

There was a debate on the value of the operation and Guillimeau discussed the usefulness of performing it on a living woman. He did not advocate the practice although he tried it twice, unsuccessfully.

> I know that it may be alleged that there be some have been saved thereby: but though it should happen so, yet ought we rather to admire it rather than practice or imitate it. For 'one swallow make not a spring' neither upon one experiment only can one build a science.[10]

Mercurio became the first surgeon to advocate CS for cases of contracted pelvis in 1604.[11] This suggestion showed that birth attendants had begun to take into account the results of a prenatal examination. Once the decision to carry out a caesarean was taken before labour began, the woman would be in a better physical condition than if she had failed in an attempt at giving birth.

On 21 April 1610, Professor Sennert of Wittenberg University recorded a case of a CS being performed by Trautmann on a woman for whom a natural birth was impossible because of a large hernia.[12] According to Young this operation represents 'The first definitely authentic case of CS intentionally performed upon a living woman'. Unfortunately the woman died twenty-five days after the operation from an infection because the surgeon had not closed the wound or the uterus.[13] Such omission was common. According to accounts at the time, during the sixteenth and seventeenth centuries the caesarean operation was very rudimentary. Anaesthetics were unknown and the patient was tied down or held by assistants. The wound was not stitched but left gaping. Attempts were occasionally made to bring the abdominal walls together by a couple of crude stitches or bandages.[14]

---

8 Young, 1944
9 Hull, 1798
10 Guillimeau, 1612, p.187
11 Young, 1944
12 Newell, 1921
13 Young, 1944, p.30
14 Young, 1944

Performing the operation on a living woman therefore remained highly controversial. In 1616 William Harvey, renowned for discovering the circulation of the blood, was one of those who took the view that the caesarean operation should only be used on the death of the mother.[15]

THE ROLE OF THE CHURCH

During pre-industrial times religion played a leading role in the decision making of most aspects of life, including pregnancy and childbirth and from 1869 it proscribed abortion throughout pregnancy.

In 1733 the medical profession asked the doctors of theology at the Sorbonne whether it was religiously correct to sacrifice the woman in order to try to save the life of the baby in the case where a woman could not give birth vaginally. On 30 March they replied that if one could only save the life of one or the other, there was a conflict. Justice would imply that it was better to sacrifice the baby. However, they believed that, according to charity, it was better to save the baby because it was only at the expense of the mother's own life that the baptism of the child could be assured and eternal life therefore secured.[16] This ruling meant that craniotomy (the perforation, breaking or crushing of the fetal skull) in order to save the life of the mother was not allowable. It was their view that the child must be removed in order that it might be baptised. This would save it from having to spend eternity in 'Limbo', a place which, according to the official doctrines of the Church, was between heaven and hell. In fact, other Church authorities have in the past suggested an even worse fate. As late as 22 May 1936 the major Catholic paper *The Universe* stated: 'It is now, and always has been, the mind of the Church that unbaptised infants go to hell.'

The Church also advocated a caesarean in cases where the woman had died. This is similar to the earliest practices in ancient civilisations, but the justification was different. The rationale of the Catholic Church was that a caesarean might save the soul of the child. Guillimeau stressed the importance of the operation 'that thereby the child may be saved and receive baptism'.[17] He continued:

> Lawyers judge them worthy of death, who shall bury a great bellied woman that is dead before the child is taken forth because they seem to destroy the hope of a living creature. The chirurgion [surgeon] must be certainly assured that the woman is dead, and that her kinsfolk, friends and others that are present, do all affirm that her soul is departed.[18]

---

15 Young, 1944
16 Young, 1944
17 Guillimeau, 1612, p.224
18 Guillimeau, 1612, p.185

He proposed that, to be assured that the mother had in fact died, one should place some light feathers over her mouth for with even light breath they would fly away.[19]

In fact the practice of carrying out a caesarean if the mother had died carried on right up until the 1930s. In the fifth edition of his book *Moral Problems in Hospital Practice*, published in 1935, Finney stated:

> The canon directs that, if the mother dies during pregnancy, the fetus should be extracted by those upon whom this duty devolves... the Catholic physician is obliged to perform the caesarean operation in all stages of pregnancy beginning with the period when the embryo is distinguishable and has the form of a fetus... This fourth provision of the canon is based on the fact that the fetus often survives the mother who dies after [giving birth] and therefore nothing should be left undone to extract the fetus without delay, because, under the circumstances there is nearly always the chance to administer baptism and therefore secure eternal life for the fetus.[20]

In his book Finney stressed the importance of ensuring that the woman was in fact dead prior to the performance of the operation, as in some cases the woman had been killed by this kind of intervention.[21] Baudelocque related a case in which a birth attendant thought a woman had died and extracted the child.[22] The woman, who had apparently fainted, woke up and complained of the injury done to her and the surgeon fled. They had difficulty in persuading him to return to sew up the wound. Fortunately the woman recovered but, unfortunately for the surgeon, she developed a hernia and sued, arguing that the wrong kind of needle had been used.

It does not seem that post-mortem caesarean was often successful, although extravagant claims were sometimes made. Hyman and Lange reported 331 cases during the nineteenth century up to 1878 when only nineteen children were saved.[23]

CAESAREANS IN THE EIGHTEENTH CENTURY

From the early eighteenth century, doctors became increasingly involved in obstetric practice with a resultant increase in publications on the subject. The numbers of caesareans being performed slowly increased and successful cases were described in great detail, success still being measured in terms of maternal survival. Some earlier attempts had managed to save the child but had resulted in maternal death.

---

19 Guillimeau, 1612
20 Finney, 1935, p.46
21 Finney, 1935
22 Baudelocque, 1801
23 Young, 1944

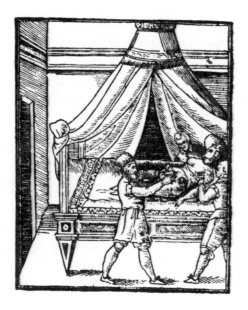

The operation was more commonly performed on the Catholic continent and, in part because it was less often the last resort, it had more success than in Britain. It was still controversial and rather dangerous for the women involved. Writing in 1788, Jacques Rene Tenon recorded only seventy-nine successful CSs in the whole of Europe since 1500.[24]

The first recorded CS performed in Great Britain was by Smith, an Edinburgh surgeon, on 29 June 1737, when summoned to a woman who had been in labour for six days. On examination he found that a normal birth was impossible and performed the CS with the approval of two other physicians and the relatives of the patient who had been warned of the risks involved. Unfortunately the child was removed dead and the woman died the following day.[25]

In the following year, the first successful CS in Ireland was recorded. It was performed by a midwife, Mary Donally, the mother was Alice O'Neale, aged 33, a farmer's wife of Charlemont and mother of several children. Alice had been in labour for twelve days, numerous midwives had attended her and attempted treatment but with no success. The child was believed to be dead after the third day. In desperation they called in Donally, a local woman famous among the community for extracting dead births. After trying to help the patient to give birth vaginally without success she performed a caesarean operation. On removing the dead infant Mary Donally held the sides of the wound together with her hands while neighbours went to fetch silk and a tailor's needle with which she stitched the wound. Alice O'Neale made a full recovery but later developed a large ventral hernia (as did many other patients of CS at that time). Donally smeared the wound with the white of eggs. Duncan Stewart, a surgeon from Dungannon, wrote:

> In about twenty-seven days the patient was able to walk a mile on foot, and came to me in a farmer's house, where she showed me the wound covered with a cicatrice, but she complained of her belly hanging outwards on the right side

24 Young, 1944
25 Young, 1944

where I ... advised to support the side of her belly with a bandage. The patient has enjoyed good health ever since, manages her family affairs, and has frequently walked to market in this town which is six miles distance from her own house.[26]

The fact that the first successful operation was done by a midwife did not please the medical profession and in the literature there was much disparagement of midwife Donally's success. As late as 1944, Young called the achievement 'a matter of good luck rather than good judgement'.[27]

It was not until 1793 that the first successful British caesarean performed by a

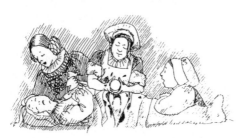

physician was carried out. James Barlow, a surgeon of Blackburn, Lancashire, was tending Jane Foster who had an extremely deformed pelvis due to being run over by a loaded cart prior to becoming pregnant. When she went into labour she understandably became very distressed and was in much pain. As normal birth was impossible, CS was suggested and the likely outcome of the operation explained to the patient. Her pain and distress being considerable by this time, Mrs Foster agreed with little hesitation. The operation was performed with no anaesthetic, the wound was stitched and the patient was then wrapped in flannel. While the mother survived, the child died.[28] During the rest of the century, however, six further attempts at caesareans failed and Radford recorded that in Britain at the end of the eighteenth century there had been nineteen CS operations and only two mothers and seven children had survived. However, he was of the opinion that this figure was remarkable considering that the operation was such a 'hazardous undertaking' at that time.[29]

The first successful caesarean performed in the United States was carried out by Dr Jesse Bennet on his own wife in 1794 in a frontier settlement in the Shenandoah Valley in Virginia. Labour was difficult owing to a contracted pelvis and Dr Alex Humphrey was called for consultation. Forceps failed and the wife did not want a craniotomy. Dr Humphrey would not perform the caesarean and so Dr Bennet did it himself. His wife was stretched out on a crude plank resting on two barrels and put under the influence of a large dose of opium. The *Journal of the American Medical Association* (vol. 115, p.1940) stated dramatically:

26 Stewart, 1747, pp.361–2
27 Young, 1944, p.54
28 Young, 1944
29 Radford, 1865, p.11

The courageous frontier surgeon by one quick stroke of the knife opened the abdomen and uterus and quickly delivered the child and placenta. At this stage he delayed long enough to remove the ovaries. The wounds were closed by a stout linen thread and contrary to the expectations of everyone present Mrs Bennet was soon well and active.

The baby daughter lived to be seventy-seven, so there were some successes with the operation. However, before 1800, CSs had largely been operations of desperation, performed as a last resort on dying mothers, in an attempt to save the baby. Those British surgeons who dared to perform it were most often treated with scorn and condemnation by their colleagues, so that few would actually attempt the operation.

One important point is that the women undergoing the operation were usually in a very bad physical condition. The length of labour before the operation is known in fourteen of the nineteen recorded cases. All but two had been in labour for longer than thirty hours, and four had laboured for a period of over five days.

Symphysiotomy as an alternative to caesarean

During the eighteenth century, surgeons began to experiment with other forms of surgical intervention to aid labour. Thus in 1777, the poor success rate of the caesarean operation meant that it was almost entirely superseded by the development of a new operative delivery technique.[30] The symphysiotomy operation was introduced by a French surgeon, M. Sigault. His earlier proposal for the operation, in which he suggested that it should be tested on animals and condemned criminals, was not favourably received. The later proposal, which was successfully tested on a patient, consisted of cutting through the skin in the direction of the pubic bone and then dividing the junction of the cartilaginous symphysis with the knife. The knees of the patient which were being held firmly by assistants could then be gently forced apart in order to separate the bones, thus making room for the birth of the child under the strength of the uterine contractions. If this failed, embryotomy was performed. 'The section of the symphysis pubis, it was thought, would banish for ever the use of crotchets, or perforators and other destructive instruments, as well as premature birth and the caesarean operation'.[31]

Subsequent to his initial attempt, Sigault operated on four other women, one of whom died. Although Sigault was the first to propose and successfully perform the operation, it was M. Le Roy, an assistant at the operation, who was the first to publish an account of it. However, opposition to the operation was strong. In 1803, Hamilton wrote: 'from the history of between 30 and 40 cases, where the

---

30 Newell, 1921
31 Baudelocque, 1801, pp.48–9

division of the symphysis pubis was performed on the continent, and one case in Great Britain, we consider ourselves authorised to condemn that operation in every view, and advise that it be had recourse to in *no case whatever*'.[32]

As time went on, Sigault became less confident about the procedure and before his death he recommended CS instead of symphysiotomy for difficult births. The operation still continues to be used in some countries and the Maternity Report of St Luke's Hospital, Anua, Nigeria, revealed that in 1991 a total of twenty symphysiotomy operations were carried out.

The debate over caesareans in Britain and France

The year 1798 was very important in deciding the future of policy for performing caesareans during the nineteenth century. This ended with doctors in Britain and France making different decisions about the operation.

In France Baudelocque presented a report to the Society of Medicine in Paris, in September 1798. In it he said that the caesarean operation was once again the subject of great controversy. He admitted that the operation was not always successful but supported it and argued that if the caesarean was not performed the woman's fate would often be worse than death.[33] He pointed out that the vaginal birth of a child alive is generally impossible when the diameter of the pelvis is only 2½ inches. He considered craniotomy to be very dangerous for the woman and also that one should not kill the child. He gave notes of seventy-three cases, of which thirty-one mothers survived and where the main indication for the operation was a distortion of the pelvis. He continued to argue: 'Far from prohibiting the caesarean operation, other laws should oblige us to perform it, if we can demonstrate that this operation is the only one which can preserve the child without being essentially fatal to the mother.'[34]

After a discussion of Baudelocque's report the Society of Medicine accepted that the operation had been a success and in some cases could lead to saving the lives of both the mother and baby. It unanimously decided that it was the duty of the physician to carry out caesareans and that 200 extra copies of Baudelocque's report should be sent to different judicial and administrative bodies.[35] There was some opposition outside the Society, notably from a colourful character called Saccombe who had studied in England under William Hunter, the best known of the contemporary British obstetricians. He called Baudelocque a 'murderer' for one of his patients had died after a caesarean and claimed that he himself could deliver any woman with his hands. In 1798 he

---

32 Hamilton, 1803, p.333
33 Baudelocque, 1801
34 Baudelocque, 1801, p.37
35 Baudelocque, 1801

formed his 'Ecole Anti-Caesarienne' but was fined 3,000 francs for the slander of Baudelocque and fled the country.

Three months after the decision in Paris, the Manchester obstetrician W. Simmons wrote his 'Reflection on the Propriety of Performing the Caesarean Operation' in which he ignored the two successful cases and argued that, in contrast to the rest of Europe, the operation was universally fatal in England.[36] Believing the rates for other countries to be of no relevance, he therefore advocated the traditional conservative use of the operation only in the event of the death of the mother. He also quoted Hunter's view that the life of the woman was more important than that of the fetus. He recommended the use of craniotomy and stated: 'the child may be extracted by the crochet whatever the distortion shall be, if in any part of the cavity there shall be a space of 1½ inches in diameter'.[37] The normal range in Britain today is 4–5¾ inches (10–14 cm), with an average of 5 inches (12 cm).

This opened up an acrimonious debate. Hull, a fellow Mancunian, took exception to Simmons's condemnation of CS. In a reply written in a paper published later that month he pointed out many discrepancies in Simmons's argument against the operation, not least his assertion that it is always fatal to the mother. He also argued that there could never be a pelvis so contracted that at some point there was not 1½ inches diameter.[38]

Hull's book, entitled *A Defence of the Caesarean Operation*, questioned whether the operation was always fatal to the mother and listed the situations in which he would recommend the use of the operation:

1. Where the Mother is dead, for the preservation of her Offspring;
2. Where the Child is dead, or supposed to be so, for the preservation of the Parent;
3. Where the Mother and Child are living, for the preservation of both.[39]

Hull quoted Simmons as saying that the caesarean 'has proved fatal in England in every instance' and is 'an operation that has proved so fatal to my country women' that it must be abandoned.[40] He went to great lengths to point out the difference between the patient 'dying *from an operation, and after an operation*'.[41] Hull went on to accuse Simmons of being 'blinded by prejudice' and suggested that he had made his judgement on cases without knowledge of the full facts and conditions of the patient in each case, and as such 'the value of the operation ought to be appreciated' for certain cases.[42]

---

36 Simmons, 1799
37 Young, 1944, p.60
38 Hull, 1798
39 Hull, 1798, p.5
40 Simmons, 1799, p.30 quoted ibid. p.7
41 Hull, 1798, p.8, emphasis in original
42 Hull, 1798, pp.8–10

Simmons responded to Hull's work following the death of a woman, Elizabeth Thompson in Manchester after a caesarean operation. The theme of Simmons's response was that to perform the operation on a living woman was tantamount to murder. Throughout his writings Simmons upheld the notion that only God is able to decide who should live and who should die.[43]

The debate that took place between Hull and Simmons is an important one in the history of CS because it highlighted the relative advantages and disadvantages of performing the operation. As Radford states, the controversy 'brought the greater part of the medical profession to entertain more clear and definite opinions'.[44] However, the balance of the view in Britain, contrary to that in France, was against the operation.

Baudelocque made an influential contribution to the CS debate in his *Two Memoirs on the Caesarean Operation* (1798 and 1799, translated by Hull in 1801). While accepting the necessity of the operation for contracted pelvis and other unusual conditions, Baudelocque added the condition of tumours of the vagina as an indication. He therefore highlighted the fact that there are some cases where vaginal birth is absolutely impossible and CS was thus the only option available to extract the fetus. Baudelocque was critical of other interventionist techniques such as the use of the crochet, symphysiotomy and induction, suggesting that laws needed to be passed obliging obstetricians to carry out CS in certain circumstances, rather than outlawing its practice as some of his predecessors had argued.[45]

In Britain the anti-caesarean school was in the ascendant and led to the difference in practice from the rest of Europe.

CAESAREANS IN THE NINETEENTH CENTURY

At the beginning of the nineteenth century the bulk of British obstetric opinion was opposed to caesareans and the textbooks of the time reflected that view. Alexander Hamilton, for example, published one entitled *Outlines of the Theory and Practice of Midwifery* in which he argued against the indications commonly used to justify the operation: 'Experience has proved, that where ready access is obtained for the admission of the necessary instruments, the head of the child may, by the operation of embryotomy, be so diminished... [that] the extraction of the mangled infant is practicable'.[46]

He gives great detail of particular cases, charting every stage of complicated labours, including one case of a woman with extreme contraction of the pelvis

---

43 Simmons, 1799
44 Radford, 1865, p.1
45 Baudelocque, 1801
46 Hamilton, 1803, pp.270–1

where the pelvic gap was so narrow that Hamilton's instruments could not be introduced into the uterus in order to extract the child. Despite the fact that the woman died after great suffering, Hamilton went on to state: 'the histories of the [caesarean] operation, hitherto on record, do not appear to me to contain the ample information which would be required by one compelled to perform it'.[47]

A royal catastrophe

A catastrophic royal birth in 1817 appears to have been the catalyst for more CSs in this country. Sir Richard Croft attended Princess Charlotte and allowed an obstructed labour to continue in preference to using forceps or dismembering the heir to the throne of England. Fearing her death from CS, Sir Richard did nothing. The infant was stillborn, the princess died, and three months later Sir Richard shot himself.[48] These events had a major historical impact. They brought Queen Victoria to the throne and marked an important turning point away from 'ultra-conservatism' in obstetrics.

Saving the women

British obstetricians were often critical of their European counterparts for carrying out caesareans unnecessarily. A French doctor in 1829 commented that when the smallest diameter of the pelvis was nearly 2¼ inches, the child must be alive and the decision had to be taken whether to follow the English and destroy the fetus or, on the other hand, to give it life while exposing the mother to great danger. The French generally took the latter position while an unnamed English doctor commented, 'Pity the poor French women we say'. However, it would be wrong to assume that the French doctors never performed embryotomy, for in 1849 several cases were reported where it was tried before a caesarean was performed.[49]

In Britain the preconditions for a caesarean were strict and, after reviewing the evidence of the years 1822–62, Young commented: 'The highest authorities in Great Britain at this time fixed the degree of pelvic Contraction in which the dimensions varied from 3–3½ inches in the long diameter as the lowest limit below which birth by embryotomy could be performed' and below which it was always necessary to perform a caesarean.[50] Instead there were three other major methods in the case of a difficult birth.

---

47 Hamilton, 1803, p.293
48 National Institutes of Health, 1982
49 Young, 1944, pp.74–8
50 Young, 1944, p.76

The alternatives to caesarean

Forceps

Forceps were in popular use as an aid to difficult deliveries during the nineteenth century. Once again there were proponents on both sides of the debate. For example, Radford claims that:

This instrument most justly takes a high position in obstetrics, because its sole employment is for the preservation of life. It is intended, within a certain range of protracted labour, to supersede craniotomy. In the hands of a discreet and judicious practitioner, it is both a safe and a very powerful instrument. Before its introduction into practice, whenever turning could not be performed, the child was doomed to destruction by craniotomy.[51]

Further, Radford stated that 'There are no statistics published which afford any truthful information either as to the frequency of the application of this instrument, or as to the mortality of those women who have been delivered by it'.[52] He claimed that he had used forceps many times and never had a death as a result of their application.

The debate over the relative benefits of forceps as opposed to CS continued through the twentieth century and the latest evidence from the 1990s showed that the use of forceps had diminished as caesareans became safer.[53]

Craniotomy

This is a difficult and upsetting procedure by which the head is crushed in the womb in order to make it small enough to pass through the vaginal canal. The procedure was a very difficult one as may be seen by some of the recorded case histories. J. Hamilton, for example, described in 1840 how, in a woman with width at the pelvic brim of only 1½ inches, he performed a craniotomy at midnight but did not completely finish with his efforts until two o'clock the next afternoon. The woman was saved and he was 'carried home in a sedan chair exhausted'.[54]

If the head was not the part of the body presenting then the operation was called an embryotomy and there was continuing debate about the rectitude of killing the child about to be delivered. Many argued that it had no sensation of feeling or pain.[55] However, the procedure was difficult and the obstetrician had to gather all the pieces together to make sure that nothing had been left inside the woman. There were strong critics. Bedford stated in 1844: 'The man who would

51 Radford, 1865, p.27
52 Radford, 1865, p.29
53 Francome, 1990b
54 Young, 1944, p.77
55 Young, 1944

wantonly thrust an instrument of death into the brain of a living foetus, would not scruple, under the mantle of night, to use the stiletto of the assassin'.[56]

Churchill in 1855 gave the mortality rate of craniotomy as about one in five. He also said that in Britain the operation occurred once in 219 deliveries compared to once in 1,205 deliveries in France, and was even more rare in Germany with one in 1,944 deliveries. To make a comparison he collected data for 321 operations since 1750 and said that the majority of women (172) had died. In 1872 Parry pointed out that the overall death rate of one in five masked the fact that women with a width at the pelvic brim of 2½ inches or below had a death rate of 38 per cent.[57] However, even such analysis did not undermine the essential fact that, at that time, maternal mortality was lower for a craniotomy than for a caesarean and was therefore the preferable British policy unless one gave high value to the fetus.

In Catholic countries theologians often gave the fetus a very high status and, as doctrine has changed so much in recent years, it is important to remember the official doctrine of the time. As late as 1935 papal authority approved the publication in London and St Louis of the fifth edition of the book *Moral Problems in Hospital Practice*. It stated:

> To preserve one's life is generally speaking duty; but it may be the plainest duty, the highest duty, to sacrifice one's life. War is full of such instances, in which it is not man's duty to live but to die... A parallel case is the situation of a woman in a difficult labour, when her life and that of her unborn child are in extreme danger. In this situation it is the mother's duty to die rather than to consent to the killing of her child.

The author Patrick Finney continued: 'The first fact in the world is that justice, law and order should be observed no matter what the cost; better that ten thousand mothers should die than one foetus be unjustly killed'.[58]

Finney's book was reviewed in the British medical literature and widely read. He balanced the life of one fetus with ten thousand women. Others went even further. A. J. Shulte, a professor of liturgy, stated: 'Even if the life of the mother is in danger, a physician has no right to destroy the child's life. I say now and with all seriousness that it is better that one million mothers die than to have one innocent little creature killed.'[59]

With such attitudes it is clear that strict Catholic doctors, nurses and mothers would not agree with craniotomy.

---

56 Young, 1944, p.80
57 Young, 1944
58 Finney, 1935, p.47
59 Shulte, 1917, p.52

Despite the dominant British view being in favour of craniotomy there were a few in Britain who also became concerned with the loss of fetal life. In 1865 Radford calculated, on the evidence available to him, that 2,861 infants were being destroyed annually by this operation and suggested that this figure was an extremely conservative estimate.[60]

A determined opponent of craniotomy, Radford argued that if craniotomy was used, certain great men [sic] would not have been born – an argument that was to be repeated later by opponents of birth control: 'Suppose the head of Shakespeare had been opened, what would have been the loss to society.' In addition he commented: 'It is one thing to deliver the woman, and another to do so safely. It is much to be deplored, that this operation is still permitted to be so unconditionally performed'.[61]

However, this minority view did not hold much appeal, and the clear view among British obstetricians was that caesarean was such a dangerous operation that it must be the last resort.

Induction

Induction of premature labour was not originally intended to supersede CS but rather to prevent craniotomy.[62] If a woman had endured a craniotomy at full term and again fell pregnant, she could then have earlier induction of labour with much greater safety. The state of contraception was so bad that one woman who could not deliver normally had eleven pregnancies between 1862 and 1885. Eight of these ended in embryotomy and in three others labour was induced halfway through pregnancy.[63]

However, according to Radford, in general, by the time induction of labour was proposed, the woman had passed the period when a caesarean could be advantageously performed. Radford objected to this situation, stating that induction was not as safe a technique as was commonly presented, and indeed sometimes caused the death of the mother;[64] he advocated CS instead.

As far as the obstetrician facing a difficult labour was concerned, the crucial choice would be what gave the woman the best chance of survival.

Safety of caesareans until the 1870s

After the first successful caesarean in England there were six other caesareans in which the mother died, until the second successful one was performed in

---

60 Radford, 1865
61 Radford, 1865, p.48
62 Radford, 1865
63 Young, 1944
64 Radford, 1865

April 1834, nearly forty years later.[65] Radford stated that 'The statistics of the results of the caesarean section, especially as concerns the mothers, are highly unfavourable.' He recorded that, of 77 British and Irish women whose cases were tabled, 66 (86 per cent) died and 11 (14 per cent) survived. From those 77 cases, 78 infants were extracted (including one case of twins), 46 (59 per cent) of the infants survived and 32 (41 per cent) died. Radford claimed that nearly all of the infants that did not survive were dead before the operation and it was his opinion that the infants might have been saved if the CS had been performed earlier.[66]

One of the best pieces of research into mortality was that of Kayser of Copenhagen. He suggested that there were many cases that were not reported 'but that of the 338 operations on record from 1750 to 1839, 38 per cent of women survived. He felt that this was an overestimate because in 67 cases in which the operation was carried out in a hospital, where concealment would be much more difficult, the success rate was only 20 per cent and he believed care would have been better than average. He may have been wrong, of course, because infections were likely to be much more common in hospitals. However, one of his findings was that the success rate was improving. During the period 1750–1800 one-third of women survived (32 per cent); from 1801 to 1832, 37 per cent survived; and from 1833 to 1839 over half (51 per cent) survived. He also found that where the woman had been in labour for seventy-two hours or more, the success rate was only 28 per cent, whereas if labour was under twenty-four hours the success rate was four out of five (80 per cent).[67]

Table 2.1 Some international rates of caesarean survival 1800–1880

Country	Period	Number of cases	% mothers survived	Source
USA	To 1877	80	48	Young (1944)
Germany	To 1872	712	47	Schroeder (1873)
France	To 1872	344	45	Schroeder (1873)
Britain	To 1879	131	18	Radford (1880)

The results show that survival rates in Britain were below half of those in the other three countries. This difference had been known throughout the nineteenth century although it had not been so clearly documented before, and in 1833 Campbell pointed out that this difference was at least in part due to the fact that

---

65 Young, 1944
66 Radford, 1865, p.7
67 Young, 1944, p.87

on the continent the operation was carried out in different circumstances. First, they often performed it when in Britain it would not have been carried out at all; and second, it was carried out earlier in the pregnancy. Other later obstetricians held a similar view.[68] However, in making comparison with the United States, Harris declared that the major reason was the poor state of the British women when they came to have the operation. They had poor nutrition and drank too much. It is, however, unlikely that the British women drank more than the French and so this is unlikely to be the real reason.

By the middle of the nineteenth century the British were taking a slightly more positive view towards caesareans. It was the influence of Radford among the medical profession that began the shift in position towards a more accepting climate for the operation.[69] Even so it was only performed occasionally on a living woman. This was usually when a craniotomy could not be performed: if, for example, ovarian cysts prevented access to the fetus. In other words, it would only be performed when everything else had been tried and had failed.[70]

NEW AGE OF CAESAREANS

The dangers of the operation meant that in Britain the caesarean was usually only carried out when a craniotomy could not be performed, possibly because ovarian cysts prevented access to the fetus. An example of this is provided by a debate in *The Lancet* in 1881. In the June edition, a Dr John Galton described a caesarean where a patient died. In the July edition he was attacked by A. C. Tweedie (25 June): 'It seems a somewhat new thing for this very formidable operation to be at all warranted where there is no pelvic deformity. I am satisfied that had I a similar case to deal with I would be able to accomplish birth without having recourse to caesarean section.' However, Galton retorted that although he had not specifically stated it in his paper, the description of the symptoms should have alerted Tweedie to the fact that the woman had cancer and that CS is indicated where there is malignant disease of the lower segment of the uterus.

In the 1880s there were new developments of technique which changed the balance of risks of the operation and led to it becoming safer than craniotomy *for women who were relatively early on in labour*. This was due to a number of improvements in general medical practice, including the introduction of the sterilisation of instruments, the use of anaesthetics and also specific improvements in technique.

A major change began in 1876, when Porro of Pavia developed his technique. In his own city no woman had ever survived the operation. Porro carried out a

---

68 Young, 1944
69 Young, 1944
70 Newell, 1921

caesarean on a young woman with a distorted pelvis due to rickets. The child lived but the mother died fifty hours later from haemorrhage and peritonitis. It appeared to him that the greatest risk to the woman came from the damaged uterus. The incision in the uterine walls allowed the escape of infected lochia into the pelvic cavity. He therefore advised amputation of the body of the uterus in order to lessen the dangers of haemorrhage and infection. The wound surface of the uterine stump would be much smaller than that of the whole uterus and he knew it was easier to control the haemorrhage from his experience of previous operations to remove ovarian tumours. Porro carried out the first successful operation on 21 May 1876. The woman had been under observation for twenty-four days and the operation was carried out seven hours into labour. Porro and his assistants washed their hands in a dilute solution of carbolic acid and administered chloroform. The child also survived.

When others tried the operation the results at first were mixed. In fact, the next three women all died but two children lived. Three out of the first four women operated on in the United States died, and four out of the first five in Britain. However, some places showed a remarkable improvement and none greater than the Vienna lying-in hospital. Here, in the previous one hundred years not a single woman had recovered. From 1877 to 1885 there were twenty-seven Porro operations with nearly half (48 per cent) of the women surviving. Then in the following three years there was a remarkable series of operations and out of twenty-seven cases, all except two of the women lived.[71]

Harris advanced a number of reasons for the improved results of the Porro operation, which included the following:

- Carrying it out as a planned operation and not as the last resort
- Operating early in labour
- Rigorous antiseptic technique
- Washing all the blood out of the abdominal cavity
- Antiseptic treatment of the stump of the uterus.

Harris said that, at that time (in 1880), there was only an average of about three caesareans a year in the United States, many women died undelivered and that to increase the number by the Porro operation might be helpful to women.[72] In a second article in the same year he collated the results of the first fifty Porro operations carried out in Europe, in which twenty-one women and forty-three children were saved.[73]

There was some opposition to the operation on the grounds that it sterilised the woman. One of the most vehement was in the *American Journal of Obstetrics*

---

71 Newell, 1921
72 Harris, 1880a
73 Harris, 1880b

in 1883, where Schlemmer argued that the operation was against religious tenets and that men should not have marital intercourse with wives who had undergone it.[74] In contrast, the English writer Dr Playfair said that many women needing caesareans suffered from rickets and came from the poorer parts of the community suffering from ill-nourishment.[75] He continued by suggesting that the sterilisation may have been of benefit to the community. Others prophetically saw Porro's method as a transitory one and this is what it became.

The caesarean operation was revolutionised in 1882 by the German Max Sanger (1853–1903). He publicised his results in the *American Journal of Obstetrics* in 1886. Sanger believed that any operation to replace craniotomy needed to save not only the woman and child but also the reproductive organs. Others had experimented with suturing the uterus and in the 1870s this technique seemed to become more widely used. Braxton Hicks used silver wire, as did Robert Barnes. However, Sanger proposed many more sutures than had been used hitherto and a procedure of closing the uterus in layers by the use of sutures or stitches. This would 'close the uterine wound by a system of deep (muscular) and superficial (peritoneal) sutures and so keep the uterine and peritoneal cavities shut off' (*The Lancet*, April 1891, p.885). The eight or ten deep sutures were made of silver and about twenty superficial ones of silk. The advantage of so many sutures was that each one had to bear less strain and so was unlikely to break. At previous autopsies a gaping wound had often been found.

Sanger did not make any grand claims about having invented a new method of operating. Rather, he painstakingly studied the developments and innovations of the operation, comparing success rates, and came to a conclusion which brought together the best of what had gone before.[76]

The first operation carried out according to Sanger's recommendations was done by G. Leopold in Leipzig on 25 May 1882, the mother and child made a smooth recovery. However, the next two operations were not successful. It is surprising that Sanger himself did not carry out the operation according to his own suggestions until 4 December 1884 when it was the tenth to be performed. The mother and child made a good recovery.

Analysis of the first fifty Sanger operations by Harris in the United States up to 1887 showed that 70 per cent were saved, compared to only 40 per cent of the first fifty Porro operations.[77] Closer analysis of the data showed that of the first fifty operations, thirty-three were done in Germany: all but one of the children and all but four of the mothers were saved. However, in seventeen operations carried out abroad, only six mothers were saved. This may be in part because, in

74 Young, 1944
75 Playfair, 1886
76 Young, 1944
77 Young, 1944

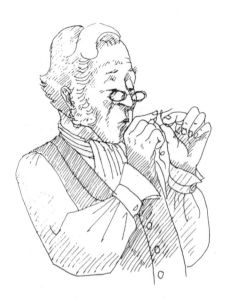

Germany, the criteria for performing the operation had been relaxed, but it is probably also indicative of greater experience and skill.

Some information that caesareans might be becoming safer was published in *The Lancet* (6 January 1886). Dr Playfair referred to the statistics of caesareans published by the French obstetrician M. Dufeilley. These showed that where the operation was performed in favourable circumstances, 80 per cent of women recovered, compared to only 17 per cent in unfavourable conditions. The Lancet commented that these were better results than had been obtained in England, but from 'the semi moribund condition in which the patients generally had been found before the operation' it was surprising that even the small success of 11 per cent maternal survival had been obtained. However, it further concluded that the statistics 'at least prove that the caesarean section need not be the almost certainly mortal operation we were generally thought to consider it'.

At the annual meeting of the British Medical Association (BMA) in 1886 there was a discussion of the relative merits of craniotomy and caesarean, the new Sanger method was not mentioned by the principal speaker. However, W. T. Lusk of New York presented evidence of the improved results with the new technique. In 1887 a death from caesarean was reported at a meeting of the Obstetrical Society of London and the comment was made that, although improved results had been obtained abroad, there had been no comparable improvement in this country (*The Lancet*, 11 June 1887).

A liberalisation of attitudes towards the operation occurred in the 1890s. An article based on a meeting appeared in *The Lancet* entitled 'Modern Methods of Caesarean Section' in April 1891. This drew attention to the improvements in the operation brought about by Sanger, whose results were originally published in the United States in 1882 but were not reported in either *The Lancet* or the *British Medical Journal (BMJ)*. However, his improvement was introduced in 1886 (*The Lancet*, 19 May 1894). The 1891 meeting also disclosed a recent mortality rate of caesarean of 23 per cent. This was above the death rate from craniotomy (at Guy's Hospital this was 16 per cent). So by these statistics craniotomy was still safer; a Dr Herman commented that 'Caesarean section should not replace craniotomy where mortality should not be above normal labour'.

In 1892 a meeting was reported in *The Lancet* where Dr Murdoch Cameron described his experience of performing caesareans. He had carried out fifteen and only two of the women had died; in neither case was their death due to the operation. He described his procedure as follows:

> If labour has not set in it should be induced, then a five or six inch incision in the abdominal wall ought to be made. The uterus is not brought out until the foetus has been extracted. Any rotation is carefully rectified, and a small incision made in the median line until the membranes (which must not be ruptured) are reached. Next the incision is enlarged upwards and downwards, and the child extracted. The uterus is now brought out and thoroughly emptied of placenta and membranes. The edges of the uterine incision are everted by an assistant and deep carbolised silk sutures inserted, with, if necessary a few cat gut ones.
> (*The Lancet*, 12 March 1892, p.594)

It was around 1890 that instruments began to be sterilised. Dr Lewers was reported in the *BMJ* in 1911 as saying 'He could remember when in surgical practice generally the instruments were not boiled; this was not much more than 20 years ago, if, indeed, it was quite so long' (4 March).

With this change and the new method of performing the operation, the CS could now be justified more readily, although there was still a great deal of debate about the operation. In 1894 the death rates following the improved techniques of 1886 were given as follows: London – twenty-two caesareans and nine deaths; Glasgow – thirty-two caesareans and five deaths; and the provinces six operations and five deaths (*The Lancet*, 19 May 1894).[78]

Thus the 1870s were a period of great improvement in the operative technique.

CAESAREANS IN THE TWENTIETH CENTURY

By the beginning of the twentieth century it was possible to have good results with CS unless women were operated on late in labour, had received repeated vaginal examinations or been subject to other techniques such as failed forceps or external cephalic version. The mortality rate was rapidly diminishing. In Glasgow it was 38 per cent in 1891, 20 per cent in 1902 and 12 per cent in 1904.

A major article appeared in the *Journal of Obstetrics and Gynaecology of the British Empire* in January 1911 by Dr Amand Routh based on a survey of over 100 consultants. It showed the increase in the use of caesareans at Queen Charlotte's Hospital. This had taken two decades, from 1890 to 1909: broadly speaking, these represent the last period before the caesarean was generally performed and the first period when it was adopted more widely. In the last decade of the nineteenth century, out of more than 10,000 deliveries only 7 were

---

78 Routh, 1911

carried out by caesarean. In the first decade of the twentieth century there were 15,222 deliveries, an increase of 50 per cent, and the numbers of caesareans increased tenfold to 74. The main switch was away from craniotomy, which declined from 28 cases in the first decade to 13 in the second.[79]

The article also drew attention to the way that mortality from the caesarean operation varied according to the condition of the woman. In favourable conditions it was 2.9 per cent, but in suspect ones it was 17.3 per cent. When the woman had previously had a vaginal examination or attempts had been made to deliver by other means, the death rate was 34.3 per cent. The message was that it was better to carry out the operation earlier rather than later, as Radford had suggested almost fifty years previously.[80] Some doctors felt that it was time for caesareans to replace destruction of the fetus. In a discussion of the subject in 1911, Hastings Tweedy said it was time that craniotomy on the living child was relegated 'to its place amongst the obsolete barbarities of the past' (BMJ, 4 March). However, the maternal mortality rate for high-risk cases of caesarean was such that craniotomy was still safer.

The changes in technique in the early part of the twentieth century meant that there was continuous debate over what the indications for CS should be. R. W. Holmes in 1915 argued that the operation had become a sort of makeshift for real obstetric practice. He pointed out that those who were carrying out caesareans for reasons such as high blood pressure must accept the responsibility for deaths in subsequent pregnancies if the uterus ruptured. He argued that such deaths should be considered in calculating the mortality rates for first caesareans.[81] In 1916 J. T. Williams advocated a caesarean for all cases where there was breech presentation for a primiparous woman, but the same year a cautionary article by F. S. Kellogg entitled 'Caesarean Section Overdone' appeared. Commentators noted that the operation was performed in America for conditions for which British obstetricians would use other methods. In the following year Whitridge Williams told the Clinical Congress of Surgeons of the United States: 'Advances in the practice of medicine and surgery are rarely attained in a thoroughly rational manner, but that a period of undue enthusiasm, or even absurd reckless abuse, usually precedes the establishment of the actual value of a given procedure'.[82]

Home birth by caesarean

On 7 September 1915 a miner's wife had been in labour for fifteen hours with no sign of the head engaging in the pelvis. Her two previous labours had resulted

79 Routh, 1911
80 Radford, 1865; Routh, 1911
81 Young, 1944
82 Young, 1944, pp.155–7, 165

in the sacrifice of the child and Dr Gordon Bell commented thus:

> As the parents were very unwilling to risk the loss of another child, and as the conditions demanded either craniotomy or caesarean section, I elected to do the latter. There was one clean room available; the removal of superfluous ornaments, hangings and furniture was followed by a cleansing with a damp cloth and the spraying of the walls, floor and ceiling with formalin; the room was then closed for two hours; this gave me the nearest approach possible in the circumstances to the surroundings of an operating room. Meantime detailed preparations were made for the sterilising of all necessary articles. Two drums of sterile dressings and masks can always be at hand but in addition I transported a small Cathcart steriliser which was placed on a gas ring and towels and gowns were steamed, sterilised, and dried in this. Instruments and gloves were easily dealt with in the small portable steriliser contained in most operating bags. The skin of the patient was prepared in the usual way, and after being thoroughly dried was coated with a 2½ per cent solution of iodine in spirit and water.

> Preparations were all completed within three hours from the time the message was received. The patient's condition was good, the pains strong and frequent, and re-examination revealed not the slightest progress. The details of the operation scarcely differed from the description in Berkeley and Bonney's 'Gynaecological Operations', and included the use of boiled silk throughout except for skin sutures. The child, a girl, weighing 8 lbs was easily removed and breathed at once. It lacked the usual frontal and occipital moulding of the ordinary baby, and therefore looked more like a child a month old. The mother made an uninterrupted recovery; the pulse never rose above 76, and the temperature was normal throughout, not having even the ordinary rise when the milk flow was established on the third day. I should much have preferred the comfort of a nursing home for this operation, but it was not possible, and I am convinced that many operations involving the transport of the patient by road could quite well be done at home.[83]

Sterilising the mother after caesarean

Sterilisation after a caesarean was recommended by Blundell in 1819 and he proposed that after the operation the woman should have a portion of her Fallopian tubes removed. In fact in 1830 he suggested that every woman known to have contracted pelvis should be sterilised before marriage.[84]

We have seen that the Porro operation entailed the sterilisation of the mother. However, this was common practice even with other kinds of caesarean operation. In 1920 the *BMJ* reported a meeting at which Dr Eardley Holland gave

83 Bell 1916, 195–6
84 Routh, 1911

details of 1,089 caesareans which had been followed up. Of these women, 610 had no further pregnancy as 42.6 per cent had been sterilised at the time of the operation. Of the 479 who had a subsequent pregnancy, 91 had not delivered and 42 had had abortions or miscarriages. There had been a total of 396 subsequent births with more than 4 out of 5 of them (82 per cent) being performed by caesarean. Eighteen of the mothers suffered a ruptured scar: this was 3.7 per cent of *all* those with a subsequent pregnancy.[85] It is not clear from his work what percentage of women undergoing a trial of labour suffered a ruptured scar. In fact some confusion arose and in the subsequent debate, Holland's figures were used to support the view that about 4 per cent of women would have a ruptured scar if they attempted a vaginal birth. This error of interpretation was not pointed out until Chassar Moir wrote to the *BMJ* about it on 9 July 1938.

Once a caesarean, always a caesarean

The *BMJ* supported this dictum in an editorial in 1922.[86] It argued that there was a very real risk of the rupture of the uterine scar which Eardley Holland's figures put at a 4 per cent risk. The main causes of this were identified as infection of the uterine wound during healing, imperfect methods of suture and improper suture material. Also it drew attention to Professor Munro Kerr's suggestion that with the lower segment operation this risk would diminish as the uterine wall was thinner and could be repaired more easily. However, British obstetricians were reluctant to adopt the new methods and it was not until 1931, when an article by J. St George Wilson of Liverpool was published in which he reported fifty cases with only one death, that their attitudes began to change and the operation came into popular usage.[87] With this development British obstetricians moved away from the policy of repeat caesareans. However, the classical caesarean with the vertical scar still remained important, especially when the emergency was such that the baby had to be extracted quickly. A study of a series of births in nineteen hospitals over the period 1943–47 showed that a classical caesarean was used in over one-fifth (22 per cent) of the operations.[88]

In the United States too, the practice developed of allowing some mothers to have a vaginal birth after a caesarean. In 1944 the *Journal of the American Medical Association* (25 November, p.855) reported that out of 496 deliveries of women with a previous caesarean, 109 were delivered vaginally and that these had lengths of labour similar to women approaching their first birth.

---

85 Holland, 1920
86 *BMJ*, 1922
87 Young, 1944
88 McIntosh-Marshall, 1949

Debate over the level of caesareans

The caesarean operation was becoming safer. Munro Kerr pointed out that, while the maternal mortality rate for women having a caesarean before going into labour was 3.6 per cent in the twenty years up to 1910, it had more than halved to 1.6 per cent in the decade 1911 to 1920.[89] Not surprisingly there were a number of obstetricians arguing for more intervention in childbirth and, in an article entitled 'A Plea for More Frequent Use of Caesarean Section', Dr Arnold Jones spoke of caesareans taking the place of other procedures and of his wish that craniotomy would become 'a relic of a barbaric past'. He continued to suggest that there was no question about the simplicity and safety of the caesarean operation and that the one drawback was the unreliability of the scar in future pregnancies, unless the woman was sterilised (*BMJ*, 16 July 1921).

Inevitably, increased intervention in childbirth led to further concerns over the possible abuse of interventionist techniques. In 1922 the *BMJ* led with a major editorial on caesareans. It commented: 'No subject in obstetrics or gynaecology is being more talked about and discussed at present than caesarean section'.[90] It stated that the increase in popularity was in large part due to the collected statistics of Dr Routh in 1911. It went on to say that there was a danger that the operation could become a panacea for all obstetric ills and quoted a Dr Blacker who said that the ease and safety of the caesarean operation was leading to its abuse.

After considering US evidence, the *BMJ* concluded that there was a temptation to perform an easy, quick and dramatic operation instead of following the safer and better, but more tedious, path of ordinary obstetric methods. It argued that the increased number of indications for the operation, which included varicose veins, abdominal pain and epilepsy, 'is enough to show that the operation is indeed being abused here and now'. It stated the view of one eminent and experienced obstetrician: 'The art and science of midwifery have either been lost by the younger generation in this country or will certainly be lost if this mad rage for caesarean section is continued'.[91]

The *BMJ* conceded that the operation often led to a better outlook for the child, but argued that the profession should not lose its sense of the proportionate value of maternal life as compared to that of the fetus. It said that only in exceptional circumstances was it justified to expose the woman to increased risk in the interests of the unborn child.

The reduced risk of the operation was reflected in a steady decline in operative mortality to 4 per cent by the 1930s. This produced not a decline in the rate of medical intervention in childbirth but rather a move away from the older-style

---

89 Kerr, 1937
90 *BMJ*, 1922, p.277
91 *BMJ*, 1922, p.278

intervention techniques to a surgical procedure that appeared to be proving itself less damaging to the mother and child.

Dame Louise McIlroy said that the operation was much favoured by young surgeons and obstetricians, but commented that giving a trial labour produced valuable information and had reduced the incidence of caesarean in some circumstances, for many women were able to deliver normally.[92]

The changes led to continual debates over the level of operations. One such occurred in 1935 when the British Medical Association had its annual meeting in Melbourne. J. Bright Banister complained that the procedure had degenerated from being a life-saving attempt into an apparently easy way of avoiding difficulties without regard to its perils. There had been an enormous increase in the incidence of the operation, often for such slender reasons as failure to progress, advanced age of the mother, breech and unwillingness to undergo the pains of labour. He argued that from the evidence of 1,763 deliveries in large maternity hospitals in England and 1,723 births in Brooklyn occurring between 1921 and 1926, it appeared that the death rate of the mother for caesarean was 6.6 per cent. For vaginal birth, it was only 0.45 per cent in England and Wales. He went on to state that in 1932 alone there had been 170 deaths after caesarean.

Dr H. A. Ridler of Sydney agreed that there were too many caesareans: 'This was the result in modern times of the love of the dramatic, of the desire to earn a big fee easily, and of the love of speed.' However, others argued that in using statistics in this way Bright Banister was not comparing like with like, because women having caesareans were often in a very difficult situation anyway. Professor J. B. Dawson said that in Britain there were not too many caesareans, but rather too many done too late. Disasters occurred not after prompt action but after undue delay.[93]

Too many caesareans in the United States

In 1921 the Massachusetts State Medical Society said that CS was the highest cause of maternal death due to puerperal infection.[94] In 1922 the rise in the number of caesareans led to a great deal of opposition. Dr Franklin Newell, Professor of Clinical Obstetrics at Harvard, said that the caesarean was the most abused obstetric operation:

> The operative indication has been a slow though normal labour which the attendant has hastened to end in the manner easiest for himself though often not best for the patient. The increased safety of abdominal surgery, combined with the fact that the operation is much easier to perform than any but the easiest

92 McIlroy, 1932
93 Bright Bannister, 1935, pp.684–5
94 Bright Bannister, 1935

obstetric operation, has caused a loss of perspective and today there is no question but that caesarean section is one of the most abused operations in surgery... I am convinced that caesarean section as performed by local operators in small communities for the indications furnished by the local practitioner of obstetrics is one of the most fatal of surgical operations.[95]

This represents the first indication that the medical profession was beginning to recognise the possible abuse of the operation in terms of its being used in the interests of the practitioner rather than of the patient. One very important contribution to the debate was that of Plass, writing in the *American Journal of Obstetrics and Gynaecology* in 1931. He stated that, in general, the death rate was 5–10 per cent. In the United States the death rate seems to have been lower, but he estimated a death list each year of 900–1,800, with three-quarters of these being unnecessary.[96]

Two years later, the *BMJ* carried a major article on the subject. It pointed out that in the United States between 1915 and 1929 the neonatal death rate had risen from 3.9 to 5.5 per 1,000 and commented 'There is little doubt that the great increase in operative deliveries, which has characterised obstetric practice generally during the last fifteen years supplies the explanation for the increased loss of infant life.' It was not just caesareans that had increased but also forceps deliveries, and the *BMJ's* informant, Professor Plass of Iowa, said that in some hospitals all deliveries were by forceps except 'precipitate delivery' where the baby was born before the obstetrician had a chance to get there (*BMJ*, 13 January, 1934).

In 1933, the New York Academy of Medicine in its report on maternal mortality concluded: 'The data reveal an excessive use of the caesarean section and as a result a great increase in mortality... a sharp reduction in the number of caesareans performed is to be recommended.'

In 1934, the White House Conference on Child Health, set up by President Hoover, produced a report which showed that the concerns about unnecessary deaths from caesareans were justified. It showed wide differences in practice. The forceps rate varied between 3.8 per cent in one hospital to 81 per cent in another. The caesarean maternal mortality rate varied a great deal, from 4.2 per cent in Los Angeles to 16.1 per cent in New Orleans. The caesarean mortality rate depended to a large degree on skill of the operator. In one series of just over 100 operations divided equally between obstetricians on the one hand and general practitioners and surgeons on the other, the obstetricians had a maternal mortality rate of 1.8 per cent whereas for the other groups it was 33 per cent. British observers noted that this finding 'illustrates the results which may ensue when men of less skill and experience attempt to follow the example set by

---

95 *BMJ*, 1922, p.277
96 Young, 1944

obstetricians'. They called for the specialist hospitals to set an example of restraint lest others should try to follow the practice to be 'up to date', with disastrous consequences (*BMJ*, 1934, p.69).

This theme was maintained in a subsequent article in the *BMJ* which discussed a report on maternal mortality in New York City. It commented: 'The data reveal an excessive use of caesarean section and, as a result, a great increase in mortality.' It recommended a sharp reduction in CS (December 1935).

This reduction did not happen and, during the Second World War, Commentators in the United States were still concerned about levels of caesareans. Cotgrove and Norton commented that CS had been frequently used for such reasons as 'primigravidity in the elderly, election by neurotic patients and high social value of the offspring, which can hardly be considered legitimate.'[97] Delee concurred with these sentiments and stated that the high level of operations was a crucial factor in the continuing high maternal mortality rates.[98]

Thus the data in the earlier part of the twentieth century showed great concern among some obstetricians about the caesarean rates which were recognised as being above those necessary for the best care of mothers and their babies; indeed the rates had reached levels where maternal mortality was being increased as a result, rather than being decreased.

Caesareans in the late twentieth century

CSRs soared in the late twentieth century, prompting concern and raising questions over the ethicacy of its use on both sides of the Atlantic. In 1980, the National Institutes of Health (NIH) in the US held a Health Consensus Development Conference to address a number of issues relating to caesarean childbirth. The main points of concern were: the increasing rates of CS and reasons for these; the effects of increased use of CS on pregnancy outcomes; the short and long term medical and psychological effects of caesarean birth on mothers, infants and families; the legal and ethical aspects of decisions to perform caesarean operations and the financial considerations of the rising caesarean rate. After considering the evidence available at that time the task force decided that the increasing rate of caesareans could not be justified in terms of maternal and infant outcomes and was therefore a cause for concern. It went on to stress that the rise could be halted and even reversed while continuing to make improvements in maternal and fetal outcomes. Writing almost a decade after the NIH statement, one report suggested that part of the NIH's message had reached some obstetricians but that much of the message had not reached the majority of obstetricians.[99]

---

97 Cotgrove & Norton, 1942, p.201
98 Delee, 1942
99 Myers & Gleicher, 1990

In 1993 the first edition of this book was published in the UK. This major text raised concerns on this side of the Atlantic over the rising caesarean rate and effects on women. While the US has had some success in stemming the rising tide of caesareans, the number of caesareans performed in this country continues to rise. The important debate over the optimum level of caesarean, absolute indication for the operation and possible effects of women and their children continues and is discussed in chapter 3.

'Sisters were doing it for themselves!'

Throughout history, many women have performed the caesarean operation on themselves. Presumably ignorant of any surgical procedure, these operations were performed out of fear and desperation. In the majority of such cases the outcome was not good for the infant. Often the child would die before or during the complicated labour, or else it would die due to mutilation from the surgery. The earliest known case of a woman performing the operation on herself was recorded in 1769 in the West Indies. It was suggested that the woman had carried out the operation because of impatience with the pain of a prolonged labour,[100] although, of course, this explanation is that of an observer and not of the woman herself.

The first recorded case in the United States was on 29 January 1822, when a fourteen-year-old girl performed the operation on herself. She was carrying twins and delivered herself lying in a snow bank. After the birth of the first baby she buried it in the snow. Doctors were called in to remove the second child and to attend to the wound. The patient survived but the fate of the other child is unknown.[101]

In 1876, Von Guggenberg reported that a woman in labour for three days performed a CS, which she had heard was possible, on herself to obtain relief from abdominal distention and violent pain. The child did not survive although it is possible that it was dead before the operation as the mother reported that fetal movements had ceased. Her wound was treated by a physician and she made a full recovery.[102]

In Turkey, in 1879, a woman cut open her abdomen and uterus with a razor after being in labour for over thirty-six hours without progressing. The wound was then sewn up by a neighbour and both mother and child apparently survived.[103] The fact that the operation was considered so dangerous meant that the case of an Italian woman carrying out a caesarean on herself created a great deal of surprise in 1886. A twenty-three-year-old single woman, seven months pregnant, was talked about and faced a great deal of questioning from her family as to the reasons or her increase in weight. Fearing the shame, she cut open her

---

100 Baudelocque, 1801
101 Young, 1944
102 Young, 1944
103 Young, 1944

abdomen with a sharp carving knife and brought out the baby in pieces. In the evening she took a cloth soaked in blood a few miles to her sister's house to prove that she had menstruated. Her subsequent illness led to medical attention and the operation being noted in the medical records. *The Lancet* wrote to the doctors involved in the case and received confirmation and further details.[104]

Interestingly it appears that women 'doing it for themselves' at this time were actually safer than those undergoing so-called professional procedures. An American medical historian, R. P. Harris, recorded a 66 per cent survival and recovery rate for women performing the operation on themselves compared to a rate of 37.5 per cent for American physicians up to 1888, and 14 per cent for their British counterparts.[105] This is possible considering that the woman was more likely than the hospital surgeon to be using clean implements and was less likely to be using equipment that had just been used to carry out a post-mortem or to perform surgery on a patient with a fatal infection. However, also important was that the women who carried out the operation on themselves were on average in better physical shape than the women being given a caesarean after all else had failed. Furthermore, the unusual case of a successful caesarean was more likely to be reported to the medical journals than an unsuccessful one.

This phenomenon was not entirely unheard of in the twentieth or, indeed, the twenty-first centuries. In 1901 a woman at full term in her fifteenth pregnancy is said to have self-performed the operation believing herself to be about to die from tuberculosis. Her wound was sewn by her thirteen-year-old daughter and both mother and child recovered. Another woman is reputed to have admitted herself to hospital in 1913 with an abdominal wound which was found to contain remnants of placenta. The child had apparently been allowed to drop into a bucket of water in which it drowned. The woman recovered.[106]

More recently (2003) doctors in a hospital in Mexico reported a case of a woman who, fearing a repeat of a previous stillbirth following an obstructed labour, cut open her abdomen with a kitchen knife using 'her skills at slaughtering animals'. The baby was delivered alive and breathed immediately. The mother then told one of her eight other children to fetch a local nurse before she lost consciousness. The nurse came and stitched the wounds with ordinary needle and thread and the woman was transferred to hospital, an eight hour drive away. The incisions were repaired at the hospital where the mother remained for ten days. The authors suggest that such extreme actions are occasionally taken by women to preserve their offspring even when it means endangering their own lives and point to lack of health care facilities as well as social and educational measures.[107]

---

104 Baliva & Serpierri, 1886
105 Young, 1944
106 Young, 1944
107 Molina-Sosa et al., 2004, p.288

3 Caesarean birth in Britain in the twenty-first century

'We feel that the current delivery of maternity services, which is generally led by acute general hospitals, over-medicalises birth. ...Primary Care Trusts should be given a lead role in ensuring there is choice and community-led services for women, wherever they live.' [1]

AT THE TURN OF THE CENTURY BRITAIN'S CSR was just below 22 per cent. Latest data (2004) puts it at almost 23 per cent.[2] Assuming an optimal rate of around 12 per cent, this means that around 55,000 women a year are having unnecessary operations. Caesarean sections are more expensive than vaginal deliveries. Based on the estimate that a caesarean costs about £1,500 more than a vaginal birth,[3] the NHS could save over £80 million annually if it halved the caesarean rate.

Since the Winterton Report was published in 1992, followed by the *Changing Childbirth* report in 1993, the number of women giving birth spontaneously without induction, use of instruments or CS has fallen from 63 per cent to 53 per cent in England in 2003.[4] Public attention and debate now focus on how the decision to perform caesareans are being made (mother's choice/doctor's influence), the relative benefits or disadvantages in terms of maternal and perinatal mortality and morbidity, as well as the high cost of CS as opposed to vaginal birth. Concern about rising CSRs prompted the National Childbirth Trust (NCT), Royal College of Midwives (RCM) and the Royal College of Obstetricians and Gynaecologists (RCOG) to host a conference entitled 'Caesarean Section: a public health issue' in 1999. In October 2001 the RCOG Clinical Effectiveness Support Unit published their 'National Sentinel Caesarean Section Audit Report', a Department of Health commissioned audit of births, the aims of which were:

---

1   HoC, 2003b, 'Choice of who should provide care', p.4
2   BirthChoiceUK, 2005
3   NICE, 2004
4   HoC, 2003b, section 4, p.1

- To determine the frequency of caesarean section in all maternity units in England, Wales and Northern Ireland
- To evaluate demographic, clinical and organisational factors associated with variations in the caesarean section rate
- To assess the quality of clinical care against agreed standards, derived from published literature
- To survey maternal views and attitudes to caesarean section and the sources of information that women use and value when they are forming their views about how they wish to have their babies
- To explore clinicians' attitudes towards, and threshold for, caesarean section.[5]

The RCOG audit was comprehensive, collecting data on 99 per cent of births that took place in England, Wales and Northern Ireland over a three-month period in 2000. The objective was to provide essential and relevant data to inform the development of guidelines for CS and provide a baseline for continuing audit of the CSR. The Government recognised a need for national standards and clinical guidelines in this area and in 2004 the National Institute for Clinical Excellence (NICE) published detailed guidelines for CS. Later that year, the Department of Health issued a standard on maternity services which formed part of their National Framework for Children, Young People and Maternity Services. This framework stressed that pregnancy and labour should not be viewed as pathological or potentially so, but rather viewed as normal physiological processes, urging a commitment to a reduction in unnecessary interventions, including CS. It went on to state that in cases of clinical need maternity services should comply with the NICE guidelines for CS. It is clear that caesarean birth has been established as a current health issue. Only time will tell what effect this ultimately will have on our CSRs.

At the beginning of the twentieth century, the main reasons for women having their first caesareans were:

- Presumed fetal compromise (28 per cent)
- Dystocia: failure to progress (25 per cent), and
- Breech presentation (14 per cent).

For women having subsequent caesareans, the main reasons were:

- Previous caesarean (44 per cent)
- Maternal request [as reported by doctors] (12 per cent)
- Dystocia: failure to progress (10 per cent)
- Presumed fetal compromise (9 per cent), and breech presentation.[6]

Overall, over 85 per cent of caesareans were carried out for one of four main reasons:

---

5   Thomas & Paranjothy 2001, p.xix
6   Thomas & Paranjothy, 2001

- Repeat caesareans (29 per cent)
- Fetal distress (22 per cent)
- Failure to progress [dystocia] (20 per cent) and
- Breech presentation (16 per cent).[7]

Repeat caesareans

Repeat caesareans account for a considerable proportion of all caesareans. As primary CSRs rise, an inevitable increase in the number of repeat caesareans follows, despite a wealth of evidence showing VBAC to be a viable and preferable alternative to repeat caesareans.[8]

The practice of repeat caesareans began in the early 1900s when the rationale behind it had a logical medical basis. At that time the vertical incision in the body of the uterus (classical) predominated and such incisions were prone to rupture, particularly during the rigours of labour. However, the low segment transverse uterine incision in general use today is much less vulnerable to coming apart and is associated with lower incidence of maternal and fetal morbidity and mortality. One report put the risk of uterine rupture at 1 per cent of attempted labours.[9] A US review of VBAC literature between 1985 and 1990 found a rupture rate of less than 1 per cent (0.18 per cent) in developed countries[10] and the average estimate is about 0.5 per cent.[11] Latest UK data put the rate at 0.35 per cent.[12] Thus the risk of uterine rupture is relatively low although there is a small risk of scar dehiscence (when the scar comes apart slightly). The old dictum of 'once a caesarean, always a caesarean' appears to be changing and in our latest survey of obstetricians very few agreed with this tradition. Twenty years ago the World Health Organisation (WHO) stated:

> There is no evidence that caesarean section is required after a previous transverse low segment caesarean section birth.[13]

In 2000, 67 per cent of women with previous sections had repeat caesareans.[14] One way to stem the increasing tide of repeat caesareans is first, to reduce the number of primary caesareans being performed and secondly, to increase the proportion of women encouraged to attempt VBAC: vaginal birth after caesarean (see chapter 9). As the rate of unnecessary operations rises the success

---

7   Thomas & Paranjothy, 2001
8   McGarry, 1969; Paul et al., 1985; Molloy et al., 1987; Nielson & Hökegård, 1989;
    Paterson & Saunders, 1991; Savage & Francome, 1993
9   Bucklin, 2003
10 Childbirth.org, 1995-1998
11 Gaskin, 2003
12 NICE, 2004
13 WHO, 1985
14 Thomas & Paranjothy, 2001

rate of VBAC after two caesareans rises and this practice should be encouraged in suitable women.

Fetal distress

In 2000, presumed fetal distress accounted for 22 per cent of the overall CSR. In general, fetal distress means that the baby is showing evidence of suffering from lack of oxygen (asphyxia). The commonest signs are that the baby becomes tired and moves less, it passes the contents of its bowels into the amniotic fluid, or that its heartbeat becomes abnormal. The increased use of this diagnostic category over the past thirty years can be associated with increased use of EFM (electronic fetal monitoring). EFM has been associated with increased CSRs generally despite a paucity of evidence to suggest improved fetal outcomes.

Fetal blood sampling used in conjunction with EFM has been shown to reduce the caesarean rate to that of labours monitored by intermittent auscultation (listening to the baby's heartbeat).[15] This practice was recommended by the Scottish Health Department in 2001[16] and reiterated by the NICE guidelines in 2004.[17] The aim of the guidelines is to ensure the appropriate use of EFM and reduce the numbers of unnecessary interventions in birth, including CS.

Failure to progress (dystocia)

This term is used to describe a variety of different classifications of abnormal labour. Most commonly the term relates to complications regarding the length of labour but can be extended to include other problems occurring during the process of labour itself. During the 1990s dystocia was recognised as one of the major indications for CS and its role in the worldwide increasing caesarean rate firmly established.[18] In 2000 this condition contributed 20 per cent to the CSR in the UK.[19] In some cases failure to progress can be treated by the administration of drugs such as oxytocin to increase the strength of contractions and may prevent the need for CS. However, the rate at which oxytocin is used for this condition varies from 47 to 100 per cent in UK hospitals.

Breech presentation

Breech presentation means that the baby is positioned feet or bottom down for the time leading to birth instead of the usual position of head first (vertex

15 MacDonald et al., 1985
16 SPCERH, 2001
17 NICE, 2004
18 How et al., 1995
19 Thomas & Paranjothy, 2001

presentation). The proportion of babies who present in breech has remained static at around 3-4 per cent. Statistics for the 1980s in Britain show that about 40 per cent of breech presentations were delivered by caesarean, by the 1990s this number reached a staggering 72 per cent of breech presentations in one health authority region in this country.[20] One study found that planned caesareans for breech singletons reduced the risk of mortality or morbidity for the mother or child, compared to vaginal birth. However, when the results were included in a Cochrane review with other studies, it showed the risk of short-term morbidity to be significantly higher in women who had been given caesareans for their breech deliveries.[21]

At the beginning of the twenty-first century breech presentations contributed 16 per cent to the overall CSR. One reason for the reduction may be the re-introduction of external cephalic version (ECV), a process of turning the baby in the uterus prior to birth. The RCOG recommended this in the mid 1990s, however by 2000 it was found to be offered in only 33 per cent of cases.[22]

Other factors that appear to influence the caesarean rate are: maternal age, multiple births and maternal choice.

Maternal age

Obstetric complications and interventions are more common in older women[23] due to diseases such as diabetes mellitus and pre-eclamptic toxaemia.[24] It is usually assumed that the higher rates of interventions experienced by these women are a consequence of the increased risks of childbirth as the woman ages. Indeed, increased maternal age does appear to be associated with higher CSRs and it has been suggested that the fact that many women are delaying childbirth until they are in their thirties or forties is a reason for increasing caesarean rates. However, the actual number of older mothers in the population has not increased in real terms. Women under thirty years of age are choosing to both delay childbirth and have fewer children.[25] What this means is that older mothers constitute a larger proportion of all maternities. Only 6 per cent of mothers were over thirty-five years of age in 1975, by 1995 11 per cent were over thirty-five[26] and in 2000 16 per cent of mothers were thirty-five or over.[27] In the UK the caesarean rate for mothers aged forty to fifty years was 33 per cent compared to 20 per cent for mothers under the age of twenty.[28]

20 Thorpe-Beeston et al., 1992
21 Hannah, 2004
22 Thomas & Paranjothy, 2001
23 Berkowitz, 1990
24 Al-Turki et al., 2003
25 ONS, 2000
26 DoH, 1997
27 POST, 2002
28 Thomas & Paranjothy, 2001

There is a debate about whether older mothers require CS more often but no conclusive evidence to suggest increased obstetric complications in older mothers necessitating the increased caesarean rates.[29] One study found that the correlation between higher maternal age and CSRs persisted even when obstetric complications were controlled for.[30] What is more, countries in Scandinavia have experienced similar demographic changes but have not encountered corresponding increases in CSRs.[31] The Scottish Health Department report suggests that clinicians may adopt different selection criteria for CS in older mothers and it is this that pushes up the caesarean rate for these women.[32]

Multiple births

Twins account for about one in eighty births in the UK and the incidence of triplets is normally about one in 6,000. In 2001 only 1.49 per cent of deliveries were multiple births; 1.45 per cent of births being twins, 0.04 per cent triplets or more.[33]

Many twins and most triplets are now born by caesarean and there is debate over the efficacy of this practice. It is usually safe for twins and triplets to be born vaginally except where the first or second twin is in transverse lie.[34] Some researchers have suggested that it is safer for twins to be born by caesarean.[35]

Quadruplets and higher order births are usually born by caesarean, but the evidence of this practice is scant. The number of pregnancies resulting from IVF treatment is affecting the number of multiple births. The Human Fertilisation and Embryology Authority has recently advised that the number of embryos implanted during IVF should be reduced from three to two. This would reduce the number of multiple births from IVF treatment but the number of twins may not be affected. However, caesarean rates for multiple births present a minor contribution to overall CSRs.

Maternal choice – are more women choosing to deliver by caesarean?

The *Changing Childbirth* report (1993) promoted the right of women to be involved in decisions about birth and be given a choice in childbirth.[36]

---

29 Martel et al., 1987; Bell et al., 2001
30 Bell et al., 2001
31 Thomas & Paranjothy, 2001
32 SPCERH, 2001
33 Social Trends 33, 2001
34 PatientPlus, 2004
35 Smith et al., 2002
36 DoH, 1993

Anecdotal evidence suggests that one of the reasons for rising CSRs is because of women choosing to deliver surgically and requesting this instead of a vaginal birth. CS without medical indication is cited as a factor in the increasing rate of caesarean birth in modern obstetric practice.[37] Thus is it user demand that underlies high CSRs. Such beliefs are fuelled by the media where the 'too posh to push' cliché has been promoted with stories of celebrities choosing caesarean above vaginal birth. To what extent this assertion of choice has filtered down to the rest of the population is debatable. However, if more women *are* asking for the operation then two important questions need to be posed: first, on what information are women basing their requests? And second, what is the role of health care professionals in this 'choice'?

Results from our studies of women's experiences of caesarean birth over two decades have shown that women are relatively unprepared for caesarean birth unless they have experienced it previously. Thus if women are requesting caesareans for their first babies they may be doing so on the basis of little or no clinical information. One study showed some women did prefer caesarean birth because they had fears about labour 'going wrong'. However, they appeared to base their decisions on their own fears about vaginal birth rather than clinical evidence about the risks of caesarean birth for themselves or their babies.[38] In Thailand, women who choose caesarean without medical indication were found to be older, more educated and have accessed prenatal care. The researchers suggest that women are basing their decisions on inappropriate information rather than rational scientific evidence when selecting their mode of birth.[39] Due consideration is rarely given to the influence of obstetric risk for women who may request CS or the information they use to make their decisions.[40] Further, there is no scientific evidence of the benefit in paediatrics or psychosocial medicine of planned caesareans on request and the disadvantages outweigh any perceived advantages.[41]

Myths and stereotypes about caesarean birth abound. For example, that caesarean birth is a 'soft option' as women do not go through the pain and uncertainties of labour or that caesarean birth is quick, easy and convenient. Anyone who has experienced caesarean birth is likely to disagree with this. Caesarean birth is not just another way to deliver a baby. It involves major abdominal surgery which carries not only increased risk of maternal mortality and morbidity, but also considerable pain and discomfort as well as a lengthy recovery period during which the mother will find it difficult to stand, walk, reach for or lift her baby. This is neither a soft option nor a convenience.

---

37 Penna & Arulkumaran, 2003
38 Weaver, 2000
39 Yusamram et al., 2004
40 Gamble & Creedy, 2000
41 Schucking et al., 2001

Other reasons why women might opt for a planned caesarean is the belief that it will prevent health problems in the future, in particular urinary and/or anal incontinence, and belief that a caesarean birth would be safer for themselves or their babies. Whether or not CS provides protection from bladder or bowel incontinence has yet to be proven.[42]

However, despite the media creating a moral panic on this issue, there is no reliable evidence to suggest caesarean rates are rising because more women are asking for them. In our most recent survey of almost 200 women having caesareans, only thirty-nine women said they had asked for the operation, the vast majority of those women (almost 70 per cent) had had previous caesareans and requested another because of pre-existing conditions or in an attempt to pre-empt the situation leading to an emergency operation. Only six women asked for the operation.

These results are supported by the findings of other studies on whether women's choice of CS is causing rates to rise. Studies have found that the majority of women would choose a vaginal birth rather than a caesarean and relatively few women actually wish to have a caesarean.[43] In 2000 in the UK only 5 per cent of mothers reported that they would prefer to deliver by caesarean. Women who had had a previous caesarean were more likely to express this preference.[44]

In an often misquoted study of the birth choices of eighty-five female obstetricians in London, 31 per cent said that they would prefer a planned caesarean rather than a vaginal birth for an uncomplicated singleton pregnancy at term.[45] The study (which had some methodological flaws) is frequently misquoted as evidence that over 30 per cent of female obstetricians would choose a caesarean.[46] But if anything, it only showed that twenty-six women out of eighty-five expressed this preference in *certain circumstances* and that 69 per cent *would not* prefer to have a caesarean. Similarly, a survey of Midwives' preferences for birth revealed that over 95 per cent would prefer a vaginal birth.[47]

In a review of the literature on maternal request for CS, Gamble and Creedy found that few women request a caesarean in the absence of current or previous obstetric complications.[48] The NSCSA (National Sentinel Caesarean Section Audit, 2001) conducted a review of the literature finding maternal request to range from 1.5 to 28 per cent. A significant proportion of respondents in the

---

42 MacLennan et al., 2000
43 Donati, 2003; Hildingsson et al., 2002; Lee et al., 2004
44 Thomas & Paranjothy, 2001
45 Al-Mufti et al., 1997
46 For example: Amu et al., 1998; Dickson & Willet, 1999
47 Dickson & Willett, 1999
48 Gamble & Creedy, 2000

studies reported that they would like more information about the risks and benefits of caesarean birth. The priority for the majority of women was the safest option for the baby, followed by concerns about their own safety, a quick recovery and ability to breastfeed. The potential impact of birth on future sexual function did not feature highly in women's concerns in the UK[49] as has been suggested in other cultures.[50]

The evidence appears to suggest that our attention should focus on the doctors' role in influencing women's choice. It has been suggested that the focus on women's request for CS may divert attention away from physician-led influences on continuing high CSRs.[51] Studies in the UK and Brazil have concluded that doctors underestimate their influence on women's decision making.[52] In Brazil, a country with one of the highest CSRs in the world, doctors promote the view that the caesarean rates are so high (36 per cent) because women are choosing surgical birth. However, it could be that doctors actively encourage women to 'choose' caesarean birth as there is little evidence that women, particularly first-time mothers, demand CS. It has been suggested that it is doctors who benefit from high CSRs in terms of being able to schedule their working days, see more patients (particularly important in private practice) and experience fewer disruptions to their private lives. Thus the benefit of high CSRs goes to the doctors in terms of their time management and being able to attend more patients which, in a private health care or pay-for-treatment system, means more money.[53]

Interestingly, studies carried out in countries with relatively low CSRs as in Scandinavia have also questioned doctors' willingness to perform caesareans where there is no medical indication. A Danish study found that obstetricians in Denmark would prefer women to deliver vaginally in uncomplicated pregnancies, but nearly 40 per cent agreed with a woman's right to request a caesarean.[54] A study in The Netherlands found that doctors' willingness to perform planned caesareans on request ranged from 17 to 81 per cent depending on the case presented to them. The main reasons why they would perform the operation were: autonomy, an unfavourable course of birth in the absence of motivation for a natural birth and litigation. The reasons the doctors gave for refusing planned caesareans were higher rates of maternal morbidity and mortality and the absence of medical indications for the operation. The authors concluded that a woman could always find a doctor willing to perform a CS for non-medical reasons. They further found that this willingness increased with

49 Thomas & Paranjothy, 2001
50 Nuttall, 2000
51 Gamble & Creedy, 2000
52 Thomas & Paranjothy, 2001
53 Hopkins, 2000
54 Bergholt et al., 2004

personal characteristics of the doctor such as increased age and experience, and that doctors were more willing to accept the request if it was based on unfounded, but understandable fear.[55] In Britain, some commentators have argued for women's right to choose planned caesarean birth so long as women are fully informed.[56] However, this position has subsequently been criticised.[57] Our study of 100 consultant obstetricians found that forty-four mentioned maternal request as a reason for the rising CSR (see chapter 8).

The International Federation of Gynecology and Obstetrics (FIGO) in 2003 issued ethical guidelines on caesarean birth for non-medical reasons. It stated that as vaginal birth is safer for both mother and child and that there is a 'natural concern in introducing an artificial method of birth in place of the natural process without medical justification'. It concluded 'caesarean section for non-medical reasons is ethically not justified.'[58]

In the US the ACOG (American College of Obstetricians and Gynecologists) released a statement saying that it was not unethical for physicians to perform caesareans on request where the physician believed it to be in the best interest of the mother and child.[59] However, this directive was widely criticised by a number of women's health organisations who stressed the increased morbidity and mortality associated with the operation.

In the UK 90 per cent of consultants discuss CS in antenatal clinics only when medically indicated. The number of women with no medical indication who are reported to request planned CS ranged from 0-20 per cent. Fifty per cent of consultants said that they had received at least three requests per 100 women seen antenatally and agreed to such requests 50 per cent of the time. Most consultants reported that they would advise vaginal birth in the absence of medical indication if a woman requested CS, but accepted maternal choice for operative birth. Whether or not consultants agreed to CS on request varied according to maternal age and parity. They were more likely to agree to CS in older nulliparous women, and less likely to agree to caesareans on request for younger or parous women.[60]

The Commons Health Select Committee in 2003 urged the NHS to limit caesareans to medical or psychological need not 'lifestyle' choice. They stated:

> The NHS does not generally provide other major operations for patients when there is no clinical need, nor does the NHS tend to offer choices of treatment to

55   Kwee et al., 2004
56   Paterson-Brown et al., 1998; Amu et al., 1998
57   de Zulueta et al., 1999
58   FIGO, 2003, pp.41-2
59   ACOG, 2003
60   Thomas & Paranjothy, 2001, p.107

patients when one costs, on average, £760 more per patient than the alternative... We would like to see a distinct shift in emphasis to ensure that elective caesareans as a 'lifestyle choice' are not supported by the NHS and that caesarean section should be a procedure undertaken only when medically or psychologically necessary and after appropriate support and counselling.[61]

In 2004 the NICE clinical guideline for CS stated:

• When considering a caesarean section (CS), there should be discussion on the benefits and risk of CS compared with vaginal birth specific to the woman and her pregnancy.

• Maternal request is not on its own an indication for CS and specific reasons for the request should be explored, discussed and recorded. When a woman requests a CS in the absence of an identifiable reason, the overall benefits and risks of CS compared with vaginal birth should be discussed and recorded.[62]

Caesarean section on request without medical indication is not an acceptable routine procedure[63] and beneficence-based clinical judgement still favours vaginal birth.[64] However, in England the ratio of planned to emergency caesareans has remained constant over the past twenty years,[65] which seriously calls into question any argument suggesting that caesarean rates are rising because of maternal choice.

Ethnicity

White women in England and Wales have lower CSRs (21 per cent) than black African (31 per cent) or black Caribbean women (24 per cent).[66] This may be due to the fact that some complications of pregnancy are more prevalent in black mothers, diabetes and hypertensive disorders for example. Maternal medical disease was found to be the most influential factor in more caesareans amongst black women than their white counterparts.[67]

Regional variations

Latest data for the UK (2004) showed slight differences in rates between the different countries. England had the lowest rates at 22.7 per cent, 1 per cent below Wales at 23.8 per cent, almost 2 per cent below Scotland at 24.4 per cent, and 3 per cent below Northern Ireland which had a rate of 25.8 in 2002.

---

61   HoC, 2003a, Conclusions & Recommendations, p.3
62   NICE, 2004
63   Schucking et al., 2001
64   Minkoff et al., 2004
65   BirthChoiceUK, 2004
66   Thomas & Paranjothy, 2001
67   Thomas & Paranjothy, 2001

Caesarean section rates also vary according to region.

Region	CSR %
England	22.7
Anglia	24.2
Essex	26.8
Hertfordshire	24.3
London	25.5
Kent & E. Sussex	23.8
Mersey	22.8
Northern	20.1
North Western	21.3
Oxford	23.8
South Western	22.3
Surrey & W. Sussex	24.5
Trent	20.0
Wessex	23.8
West Midlands	23.6
Yorkshire	21.0

Table 3.1
Caesarean section rates by
region (England) 2004

BirthChoiceUK, 2004

In 2004 the caesarean section rates across England ranged from 20.0 per cent in the Trent Region to a high of 26.8 per cent in Essex. It is interesting to note that the areas where health is generally poor, where mortality and morbidity rates are high, that is, in the North of the country, CSRs are at their lowest. It is the healthier, more affluent women in the southern regions who are experiencing the higher CSRs.

As well as there being regional variations in CSRs, there are also variations according to different hospitals.[68] The Royal Shrewsbury Hospital in the West Midlands had the lowest caesarean rate in England in 2004 at 14.4 per cent of births. Hospitals with a high rate in 2004 include the West Suffolk Hospital (31.0 per cent), University Hospital Lewisham (31.3 per cent) and the Queen Mother's Hospital Glasgow (31.1 per cent).[69]

There will be some differences in the populations of women served in these areas which may affect CSRs to a certain extent. Further, some hospitals with specialist units will receive pregnancies which are at greater risk. However, such extensive regional and hospital variations cannot be wholly accounted for in

68 Thomas & Paranjothy, 2001
69 BirthChoiceUK, 2005

terms of differences in the populations of women served by these regions or hospitals, but rather, point to differences in obstetrical practice and policy.

Anxiety and fear of litigation

Anxiety among the medical profession is an underlying factor in the rise in intervention rates in childbirth generally. A recent factor which has increased anxiety among health care professionals in Britain is fear of litigation. If there are problems associated with the birth then the doctor can be sued. Whereas if a caesarean is carried out, any resulting problems (including the death of the mother) are considered to be a normal risk of the operation. In our previous study (1992) almost half (46.8 per cent) of doctors surveyed said that the caesarean rates were rising in Britain because of fear of litigation. By 2005 fifty-four of the 100 consultants questioned cited litigation and defensive medicine as reasons for the rise in caesarean rates. Claims following problems at birth doubled during the 1980s.[70] Between 1995 and 2001 80-90 per cent of claims in obstetrics and gynaecology were related to damage caused to the baby during birth.[71] Thus the fear of litigation has pushed up the CSR.

In 2003 the Chief Medical Officer's paper 'Making Amends' recommended the development of an NHS Redress Scheme to provide no-fault compensation for patients who suffer adverse outcomes as a result of sub-standard care, including damage to babies during birth.[72] However, there is no evidence to show that the introduction of no-fault compensation has any effect on the practice of defensive medicine. The paper also recommended the introduction of a 'Duty of Candour' on health care professionals, that is, an obligation to admit when things might have gone wrong. The idea being that professionals would then be personally exempt from disciplinary action unless they had committed a criminal act, were clinically negligent or where it would be unsafe for them to continue to practice.

The situation in the Netherlands may be instructive here as there is no tradition of medical litigation there and this is one reason why they have maintained consistently lower CSRs than other countries. Doctors who have been negligent are dealt with accordingly but there is no 'compensation' to pay for care of a child injured at birth. The social support system provides fully for this so parents have no need to sue health care professionals.[73]

Private versus public health facilities

As in other countries of the world, CSRs in Britain vary according whether women attend NHS hospitals or opt for private health care. Internationally

---

70 Macnair, 1992
71 POST, 2002
72 DoH, 2003c
73 Smulders, 1999

caesarean rates are higher in private facilities than they are in publicly provided health care. For example, the Portland Hospital in London (private) has a section rate of 44 per cent whereas the highest rates in NHS hospitals are around 30 per cent. Most health insurance companies state that they only cover caesareans carried out for medical indications. In Britain only 0.5 per cent of births take place in private hospitals so this is unlikely to affect overall caesarean statistics.

Staff and skill shortages

Lack of midwives and the inexperience of junior doctors may be pushing up CSRs as there is a link between high rates of CS and low levels of staffing. The ideal is for one midwife to give one-to-one attention to a woman in labour. However, in some units there are not enough midwives and so they have to care for several women at once. In England in 2002, 59 per cent of all midwifery post vacancies remained unfilled for over three months and in London, recruitment and retention of midwives constitutes a major problem in maternity services.[74] Fewer than 33,000 of the 92,000 registered midwives in the UK were practicing in 2002.[75] In response, the Department of Health is making an investment to increase the number of midwives working in the NHS by an extra 2000 by 2006. The Royal College of Midwives (RCM) attribute the increasing problem of staff shortages to the ways that midwives are expected to work. Because of the way that maternity care is organised, midwives are unable to give the quality of care they feel necessary, or continuity of care to their patients.[76] The Department of Health has suggested that increasing choice in maternity services for women might increase job satisfaction amongst midwives and improve retention.[77]

The vacancy rate in obstetrics is also increasing and there is some evidence to suggest that the number of junior doctors choosing to specialise in obstetrics is in decline.[78]

In 2003 the 'Commons Health Select Committee on Health Fourth Report' stated:

> Evidence we heard throughout our inquiry has led us to conclude that it will be difficult to invest sufficient time to allow midwifery and medical staff to gain experience of normal birth but it is crucially important to the range of skills they practise and the quality of care they provide.[79]

The Committee went on to stress:

---

74 HoC, 2003a, section 4, p.5
75 Macfarlane et al., 2002
76 Boseley, 2000
77 HoC, 2003b, section 6, p.1
78 HoC, 2003a, section 4, p.19
79 HoC, 2003a, section 4, p.8

We are concerned that some women undergo unnecessary sections on the recommendations of doctors who lack experience owing to the time limitations imposed by the New Deal and the European Working Time Directive on their training.[80]

In our survey of 100 consultant obstetricians lack of supervision of juniors was mentioned by three consultants and another said 'The training of junior doctors is a major factor in the rising CSR'. Two consultants mentioned the inexperience of senior doctors and another said the CSR was rising because of 'new consultants' lack of confidence'. Demands are also placed on consultants' time by clinical governance and other organisational factors.[81]

The increasing rate of technological management of labour over the past thirty or more years means that medical students, doctors and midwives in training do not see as many normal deliveries as they need to in order to understand the individual pattern and differences between women. Interventionist protocols in the labour wards have led to a deskilling of midwives and doctors leaving them unable to deal with anything other than the most straightforward of deliveries.

REDUCING THE CAESAREAN SECTION RATE

In 2004 the NHS clinical guideline for CS recommended the following strategies to reduce the CSR:

- External cephalic version for women with uncomplicated breech pregnancy
- Continuous support during labour from women with or without prior training
- Offer induction of labour beyond forty-one weeks
- Use of a partogram with a four-hour action line to monitor progress of spontaneous labour with an uncomplicated singleton pregnancy at term
- Involvement of a consultant obstetrician in the decision making
- Fetal blood sampling in cases of suspected fetal acidosis where there are no contraindications rather than relying on electronic fetal monitoring alone
- Support for women choosing VBAC.[82]

Other strategies that have been proved to be successful in reversing the trend of rising CSRs are discussed below.

Ensuring 'choice' in childbirth is informed

As we have seen, there is no reliable evidence to suggest that more women are choosing to deliver by caesarean. This is particularly true for first-time mothers.

---

80   HoC, 2003a, Conclusions & Recommendations, p.4
81   Thomas & Paranjothy, 2001
82   NICE, 2004

If women with previous caesareans are asking for the operation then any attempt to reduce the CSR must include adequately detailed information to enable women to make informed decisions and a commitment to encouraging women to attempt labour after previous caesareans (see discussion on VBAC, chapter 9).

Reducing use of Electronic Fetal Monitoring (EFM)

EFM is widely used in most industrial countries despite debates about its efficacy and effectiveness and is associated with higher rates of CS. There is no evidence to suggest that EFM reduces perinatal mortality or the incidence of cerebral palsy.[83] Thus there appears to be no value to the continued use of EFM to women at low risk. Better definition of the deliveries in which fetal monitoring will be useful in the diagnosis of fetal distress and thus a more conservative application of this equipment may help to reduce CSRs generally.

Giving support during labour and continuity of carer

The provision of one-to-one trained support during labour has been shown to reduce the CSR.[84] Women in labour appear to value the special relationship of trust that 'being with women' entails and continuing support in labour may influence CSRs.[85]

Management of breech presentation

Evidence on whether caesarean birth for breech presentation leads to better outcomes for mothers and babies is contradictory. There is some evidence to suggest that planned caesarean birth for breech presentation improves outcomes[86] (see discussion on p.91). Other research suggests it is not associated with better perinatal outcomes or neurological development,[87] and external cephalic version has been shown to reduce the CSR.[88] There is evidence to suggest that such obstetric skills have been lost over time due to increasing reliance on the technological management of birth. However, encouragement, education, practice and re-skilling can reverse this trend and help reduce the CSR.

The active management of labour (AML)

The aim of AML is to achieve birth within twelve hours of the onset of labour.[89] However, the onset of labour is difficult to assess and different practitioners take

---

83 Walsh, 1998
84 Walker et al., 2004
85 Thomas & Paranjothy, 2001
86 Hannah, 2004
87 Whyte et al., 2004
88 Walker et al., 2004; Hindawi, 2004
89 O'Driscoll et al., 1984

different indications. In addition, the assumption that individual women's labours will fit into a strictly defined timescale has been questioned.[90] With AML, if the labour does not progress within the specified timescale the procedure is accelerated by the use of drugs (oxytocin intravenously). If the cervix fails to dilate at the rate of one centimetre per hour, artificial rupture of the membranes is performed.

AML has been shown to reduce the CSR[91] without detriment to mother or child.[92] After examination of the indications for performing caesareans, practitioners in one Glasgow hospital concluded that AML could be the most useful approach to reducing the CSR.[93]

Audit and target-setting

It appears that placing a close audit or monitoring programme on obstetric practice leading to CS can affect caesarean birth rates.[94] Accurate data collection is particularly important with regards to CSRs as the identification of trends and the use of evidence can inform policy and practice, improving care for women.[95] A French study found that providing maternity units with expected CSRs provides a reference point for comparing actual rates and is likely to have an impact on birth practices.[96] Moreover, the reduced caesarean birth rates have been shown to have no detrimental effect on perinatal or maternal mortality or morbidity.[97]

In 2003 a Department of Health report on maternity services concluded that rigorous audit, along with experienced staff in the labour wards would benefit care of women and reduce CSRs. It stated that there should be an:

> ...implementation of evidence-based protocols and policies and an investment in staff establishments so that doctors and midwives can spend time giving information, advice and reassurance to women before labour; so that they can support women during labour; and so that experienced doctors can make decisions to undertake a caesarean section. [98]

Repeat caesareans are a significant factor in high rates and therefore a reduction in the overall rate cannot be achieved without serious consideration of the use of caesareans for first-time mothers. Rigorous auditing of caesarean rates may help.

---

90 Savage, 1986b; Axten, 1995
91 Hindawi, 2004
92 Boylan et al., 1991
93 Macara & Murphy, 1994
94 Dillon et al., 1992; Tay et al., 1992
95 Thomas & Paranjothy, 2001
96 David et al., 2001
97 Maher et al., 1994
98 HoC, 2003a, section 6, p.2

Thus in the first few years of the twenty-first century we are experiencing the highest CSRs ever in the UK. Many commentators blame the mothers themselves for the increasing rates, suggesting that more women are requesting CS as a lifestyle choice. Evidence does not support this and rising rates are more likely to be based on outdated practices (for example, repeat caesareans) the use of EFM and personnel issues such as staff shortages and lack of experienced practitioners in the labour wards. The results of our survey of 100 obstetricians further suggest that attitudes and a demoralisation of some obstetricians may be as important.

The removal of the majority of antenatal care and birth from hospitals into the care of small autonomous teams of midwives working in the community will help to lower caesarean rates. Dissemination of accurate and appropriate information, empowerment of parents and collaboration between policy makers, the NHS, health care professionals, the media and childbearing women is also required to reduce CSRs.

4 International information

What is clear from an analysis of worldwide caesarean data is that the important issue is finding a balance, finding the right level of CS for the population of women served.

INCREASES IN CS RATES OVER THE LAST THIRTY-FIVE YEARS are, with a few notable exceptions, international phenomena, although there are marked differences between countries.

In looking at the international data for CS rates, caution is advisable as data collection and audit practices differ between, and are often inconsistent within countries. The data referred to in this chapter represents information collated from numerous studies and is presented as an example only. The most striking factor when considering this information is that rates of CS have been rising in the vast majority of countries where data are available, and the trend is no longer confined to industrialised countries. In 1985 the WHO recommended a CSR of 10-15 per cent stating that above this there were no additional health benefits:

> Countries with some of the lowest perinatal mortality rates in the world have CSRs of less than 10 per cent. There is no justification for any region to have a rate higher than 10-15 per cent.[1]

As this chapter shows, caesarean rates in many countries have been above the recommended limit for a decade or more.

The highest recorded CSR is in Chile, which was at 40 per cent in 1999. South Korea was also approaching that rate in 2000. Some South and Central American countries have produced consistently high CSRs. Brazil has long been seen as the caesarean capital of the world, consistently recording amongst the highest rates, latest data (2000) showing that over one in three (36 per cent) births were by this method.[2]

---

1   WHO, 1985, p.437
2   Hopkins, 2000

The United States had one of the highest rates in the world reaching nearly one birth in four by the late 1980s. The number of caesareans being performed there levelled out in the mid 1990s, but has been on the increase again (see discussion below, p.65). Further, it used to be the case that some of the lowest rates of CS were identified in European countries. This pattern has changed. Data for the year 2000 put Italy in fourth place after South Korea, Chile and Brazil, with a caesarean rate of 33.3 per cent,[3] Taiwan was next with a rate of 32.3 per cent[4] followed by Greece[5] and Turkey[6] with rates around 30 per cent. Australia[7] and the US[8] were showing section rates of 23 per cent, and Canada 20.5 per cent. In the same year in Britain, Wales had the highest rate at 22.9 per cent, followed by Scotland (20.8 per cent) and England with the lowest at 20.6 per cent. The latest data (2004) show that rates for all countries in the UK have risen by an average of 2 per cent despite the recommendations of the National Caesarean Section Audit report published in 2001.[9]

The Nordic countries (Denmark, Finland, Norway and Sweden) did not witness the rapid increases in CSRs experienced in other parts of Europe and the world, with national rates reaching around 14 per cent by the year 2000.[10]

We have collected data from different countries and Table 4.1 shows some of the information we have gathered. A striking feature is the great variation between societies of similar social organisation and ethnic types. Higher CSRs do not correlate to better outcomes for mother or child. The Netherlands has consistently had much lower perinatal mortality rates than the United States, despite its low caesarean rate. In India, maternal and perinatal mortality rates are high despite high CSRs. What is more, Sweden halved its perinatal mortality rates at the same time as reducing the number of caesareans performed, suggesting that it is possible to lower the CSR on a nationwide basis without increasing risks to infants.[11]

Caesarean section rates in a given country depend on many variables including population and cultural characteristics. However, the overwhelming predictor of high CSRs relates to how health care is organised. Studies have shown that caesarean rates differ drastically according to payment status and that private health care provision encourages higher rates of surgical intervention.[12] This was

3   Saporito et al., 2003
4   Lin & Xirasagat, 2004
5   Tampakoudis et al., 2004
6   Koc, 2003
7   Walker et al., 2004
8   MMWR, 2002
9   Thomas & Paranjothy, 2001
10 nationmaster.com, 2000
11 Nielsen et al., 1994
12 Chile: Murray & Pradenas, 1997; China: Cai et al., 1998; Brazil: Hopkins, 2000; South
    Africa: Lawrie et al., 2001; Italy: Saporito et al., 2003; Egypt: Khawaja et al., 2004; Taiwan:
    Lin & Xirasager, 2004

Table 4.1 Caesarean rate by year in selected countries 1970 – 2004

Country	1970	1973	1975	1980	1981	1982	1983	1985	1986	1987	1988	1989	1990	1992	1994	1995	1996	1997	1998	1999	2000	2001	2002	2003	2004
Australia	4.2		8.2	13.2					16.9		15.9		17.0					21.0		21.9	23.0				
Austria						7.0	7.5										13.1	14.0	14.5		17.2				
Belgium						8.0	8.1			9.8											15.9				
Brazil														32.0						27.1	36.0				
Canada	5.7		9.6	16.1						18.3	19.9					18.0[1]			19.0		20.5	22.1[2]			
Chile									27.7						37.2					40.0					
China										16.6[3]								22.5[4]		27.4[5]					
Denmark	5.7		7.5	10.7		11.7	12.8				13.9									13.7	14.5				
Egypt																					22.0				
England	4.9					8.2	10.0	10.5				12.0	11.3	12.8	15.0	15.5	16.3	17.0	18.2	19.1	20.6	21.5	21.9[6]	22.0	22.7
Finland	6.0		8.2								14.4								15.5	15.1	15.7				
France		6.1[7]			10.9											15.3				17.5	17.1				
Greece							13.8[8]					16.7									29.9[9]				
Holland	2.1		2.7	4.7		5.3		6.3		6.8	7.2			7.4[10]	8.5[11]			10.4	11.2[12]		12.9				
Hungary	6.2		6.5			9.2					10.2													22.0	
India						6.2									21.8[13]					25.4[14]			32.6[15]		
Ireland																			17.8	20.4	21.3				
Israel						10.0[16]				17.5	10.2									22.5					
Italy							14.5									22.0	27.9				33.3				
Jordan														8.0[17]								10.9[18]			
N.Z.						9.8												18.2	19.2	20.4	20.8	22.1	22.7		
N.Ireland																					20.2	23.9[19]	25.8		
Norway	2.2		4.1	7.2		9.0	9.4												13.6	12.6	13.7				
Portugal								11.1		14.1	15.5	16.5						27.0							
Scotland	5.0		8.1	11.3	11.6	12.0	12.7	13.0		13.2	13.5	14.0	14.2	14.6	15.5	15.9	16.0	17.5	18.5	19.7	20.8	22.1	23.5	24.2	24.4
S.Korea																					40.0[20]				
Spain							9.9		11.7	12.5	12.3	14.9													
Sweden	3.9	5.0	7.8	12.0			12.3						10.8			11.7		12.9	13.4	14.2	14.4				
Turkey											5.7								26.1			30.0			
USA	5.5		10.4	16.5		18.5	20.3	22.7		24.4	24.7	23.8	23.5			21.0				22.0	22.9	24.4	26.1		
Wales						10.6				12.3	12.4	13.4			16.6	17.1	18.2	18.9	20.9	22.5	22.9	23.8	23.9	24.1	23.8

1 1994-5
2 2000-1
3 Hong Kong
4 Shanghai

5 Hong Kong
6 2001-2002
7 1972
8 1977-83

9 1994-2000
10 1991
11 1993
12 1997-8

13 1993-4
14 1998-9
15 Madras City (Chennai)
16 Estimate

17 1990-1992
18 1999-2001
19 2000-2001
20 Approx.

the basis of the high rates in the United States for many years and remains the case in Brazil where up to 90 per cent of private patients have caesareans.[13] Here it is clear that medical indications are not the only cause of high section rates, particularly in the private hospitals[14] and have been attributed to doctor-induced demand.[15] It is the wealthier women who suffer the highest caesarean rates despite these women being at lower risk during childbirth than their poorer counterparts.[16] In Chile the private health insurance sector has consistently higher caesarean rates, 59 per cent compared to 28.8 per cent in national health fund facilities.[17] In Italy the private hospitals have a higher rate of caesareans than the public ones, 54 per cent as opposed to 46 per cent.[18]

In this chapter we consider birth practices in a few selected countries beginning with those countries with the highest CSRs.

Chile (CSR 40 per cent in 1999)

Until the 1980s all salaried workers in Chile contributed to a national health fund. Private health schemes were not launched until 1981 but by 1994 a quarter of the population were covered by them. Maternity care in the private health care system is provided by obstetricians whereas midwives are the senior professionals present in the majority of deliveries taking place in local health centres and hospitals. Chile's high CSR correlates with the increase in privately insured patients over the same period and may be explained by the doubling of the number of women being attended in birth by a 'personal' obstetrician rather than a 'duty' practitioner.[19] The reasons for the higher rates of caesareans in the private sectors are not straightforward and are more likely to do with convenience and time-management factors than the cost of care alone.[20]

Brazil (CSR 36 per cent in 2000)

Brazil has maintained exceptionally high CSRs on a worldwide scale. Here, as in other countries, the CSR varies according to not only the private/public health care dichotomy, but also to economic and socio-cultural factors such as education and place of residence. It might be expected that poorer women would have inferior diets and so be more likely to suffer from labour problems. However, private patients were three times as likely to be so classified. The more educated a woman is, the more likely she is to give birth by caesarean;

---

13 Hopkins, 2000
14 Fabri & Murta, 2002
15 Hopkins, 2000
16 Barros et al., 1991; Taffel et al., 1992
17 Murray & Pradenas, 1997
18 Saporito et al., 2003
19 Murray & Pradenas, 1997
20 Murray, 2001

correspondingly, less educated women are less likely to be delivered by caesarean. Similarly there are regional variations in CSRs. One striking feature is the urban/rural divide with women living in urban areas having twice the CSR of rural women. Variations appear to reflect affluence with the most economically developed region of São Paulo having double the caesarean rate of the least developed region.[21] However, it is unlikely that women's education or place of residence will affect CSRs per se, and is more likely to do with their ability to pay for private practitioners to attend them at birth, a factor that, as we have seen, increases rates of caesarean delivery.

Doctors in Brazil often blame excessive rates of caesarean birth on patient demand. That is, they argue that women are asking for the operation. It has been suggested that as doctors have more power in the clinical setting, they can use their expertise and authority to convince a woman to 'choose' a caesarean. As such, Brazilian obstetricians are very active in the culture of caesarean birth in Brazil.[22]

In 1980, the Brazilian government, concerned about the financial incentives underlying excessive rates, attempted to reverse the upward trend for caesarean births by equalising reimbursement payments for vaginal and caesarean deliveries.[23] However, this did not stem the rising caesarean rate because hospitals then claimed higher rates for caesarean patient care and accommodation.[24]

There may be other cultural and organisational factors at work which contribute to high CSRs in Brazil. All births are attended by obstetricians, which will increase CS rates as births supervised by midwives have lower rates of intervention. As the caesarean rate has been so high for so long, doctors have lost the skill in delivering all but the least complicated births. Delivery by caesarean carries a certain amount of status in Brazil, and there have been suggestions that caesareans are preferred to maintain female genitalia for sexual reasons.[25]

One contributory factor to the high CSR in Brazil is that it affords the opportunity for sterilisation. Despite female sterilisation being illegal as a form of contraception, it is the most widely used form of family planning in the country.[26] Tying of the ovarian tubes can be performed during a caesarean delivery. The government pays for the caesarean but doctors are being paid privately for this 'extra service'.[27] The Brazilian Code of Medical Ethics permits

---

21 Hopkins, 2000
22 Hopkins, 2000
23 Carson & Francome, 1983
24 Hopkins, 2000
25 Nutall, 2000
26 Eggleston, 1995
27 Lopez, 1998

sterilisation in 'exceptional cases' and it appears that having had at least three caesarean deliveries constitutes an exceptional case as no doctors have been prosecuted for illegal sterilisations.[28] Medically unnecessary CSs are performed in order that the mother may be sterilised and are pushing up overall caesarean rates in Brazil.[29]

Italy (CSR 33.3 per cent in 2000)

Italy has amongst the highest CSRs in the world, 33 per cent in 2000[30] and in the Campania region they were as high as 52 per cent in 2000. One study of childbirth practices in this region highlighted certain aspects of physician convenience and the limited role of fetal risk factors in influencing the caesarean rates. Sixty-three per cent of caesareans were recorded as being performed in the morning and 93 per cent on working days.[31]

Turkey (CSR 30 per cent in 2001)

In Turkey, one study found that the CSR was associated with socio-cultural as well as health care service factors. For example, maternal age and education, household welfare, access to prenatal care and place of delivery all related to high caesarean levels. The author of this study suggested that women with higher socioeconomic status are more likely to accept CS than women with lower socioeconomic status,[32] but as with other countries, it may be that private hospital care is having an impact on rates.

United States (CSR 26.1 per cent in 2002)

In the US, maternity services for those who cannot afford private care are funded by 'Medicaid', a partnership between state authorities and the federal government. Midwifery was illegal in many states until the 1990s and because of variations in legislation from state to state, not all states have certified midwives. Nurse midwives predominate and in some states, lay midwives practise. Obstetricians lead deliveries in the majority of cases, particularly in the private sector.

Intervention rates in the US are high. By the late 1980s the caesarean rate had risen until one in four births was delivered this way. The rise was a subject of public concern, and numerous publications on the topic were produced.[33] A US Government Task Force reported in 1981 that breech presentation, repeat CS,

---

28 Eggleston, 1995
29 Eggleson, 1995
30 Donati et al., 2003
31 Saporito et al., 2003
32 Koc, 2003
33 See for example Cohen, N & Estner, LJ (1983) *Silent Knife* (Greenwood Press)

dystocia and fetal distress were the diagnoses which had contributed most to the tripling of the rate between 1968 and 1977 when it was 13.7 per cent. The Task Force tried to halt the rise but despite this the caesarean rate in the United States rose until one in four births were by this method by 1988.

One of the Task Force's recommendations, pushed for by the user representatives, was that doctors should end the dictum 'once a caesarean, always a caesarean' and allow a vaginal birth after a previous caesarean. A second recommendation was for an end to the increasing trend in the United States of routinely performing a caesarean for a breech presentation.

Another factor in the US's previous high rates was what was labelled 'defensive medicine'. In the 1980s we carried out a study of British and US doctors asking them for the reasons that the caesarean rate had risen so high. From the results we reported that 90 per cent of the US obstetricians mentioned fear of litigation or made a comment such as 'too many lawyers'.[34]

Another variable affecting the US section rate was their system of health care provision. We have seen that the effect of private practice is to increase intervention rates compared with non-paying patients,[35] and yet the women who can afford to pay for care or insurance are usually taller, less likely to smoke, less likely to be young teenagers, and more affluent. So by all criteria they should be more likely to deliver normally. It has been suggested that in the United States many insurers reimburse doctors by the amount of treatment given.[36] Consequently more tests and procedures per woman mean greater profit.

Other factors that appear to affect whether women in the US will be delivered by caesarean are race and ethnicity. A 1999 study showed that African Americans have a higher rate (21.8 per cent) than either whites (20.7 per cent) or Hispanics (20.2 per cent).[37]

Strategies aimed at reducing the CSR in the US were successful for a while. The success was in reducing the number of operations being performed during the first five years of the 1990s. Following a rise in caesarean rates to a high of almost 25 per cent in 1988, the US Department of Health and Human Services' Healthy People (HP) 2000 Working Group set targets for a primary CSR of 15 per cent and a VBAC rate of 35 per cent by the year 2000.[38] This was followed by the American College of Obstetricians and Gynecologists (ACOG) in 1991 setting targets to increase VBAC rates to 40 per cent by 2000.[39] Such target

---

34 Francome et al., 1993
35 Murray & Pradenas, 1997; Cai et al., 1998; Hopkins, 2000; Lawrie et al., 2001; Khawaja et al., 2004
36 Stephenson, 1992
37 Ventura et al., 1999
38 PP&BS, 2000
39 Thomas & Paranjothy, 2001

setting placed a renewed emphasis on trial of labour and had a significant effect on CSRs. By 1995 the US section rate had dropped to about 21 per cent. The VBAC rate rose 33 per cent between 1991 and 1996 but fell 17 per cent between 1996 and 1999.[40] Following a paper in the influential *New England Journal of Medicine* documenting the risks of poorly carried out trial of labour in women with scarred uterus[41] some obstetricians considered that the original policy of 'once a caesarean, always a caesarean' was safer. So in 1998 and again in 1999 the ACOG issued new guidelines on the use of VBAC in which they reversed their earlier recommendations stating that VBAC should be approached with more caution and that facilities and personnel for emergency caesarean should always be available. As few US hospitals have the capability to provide twenty-four hour emergency cover, the effect has been to reduce the number of VBACs offered. In some areas of the country VBAC is not offered at all. It has been suggested that rather than being based on empirical and clinical evidence regarding the safety of VBAC and negative effects of caesareans, following some highly publicised cases, the ACOG's decision was based on the recurring fear of litigation.[42] Thus we can see the CSRs in the US rising steadily again from the low of 21 per cent in 1995 to an all time high of 26 per cent in 2002.[43] We may yet witness further increases in caesarean rates in the US.

Canada (CSR 22.1 per cent in 2001)

Like the rest of North America, the CSR in Canada did appear to stabilise during the 1990s, although the rate does appear to be rising again. This rise was attributed to increases in primary caesareans for dystocia and planned repeat CSs.[44]

Maternity services in Canada are funded by the Canadian Public Health System. Because the population of Canada is concentrated in the large urban centres near the US border, it is often necessary for women from the rest of the country to travel long distances to give birth. This is especially problematical because Canada was for some time the only country in the world without a legalised system of midwifery care.

In 1986 the Canadians published a statement, following a national consensus conference on aspects of caesarean birth, which was circulated widely in an attempt to reduce the national caesarean rate. They set criteria for vaginal breech delivery, for VBAC and the diagnosis of difficult labour, as well as defining areas which required further research. A year later little change had occurred and more direct action was being piloted in an attempt to influence doctors to change

---

40 Menacker & Curtin, 2001
41 McMahon et al., 1997
42 Gaskin, 2003
43 England & Horowitz, 2003
44 Liu et al., 2004

their practice.[45] This educational exercise also failed but a later initiative, using a peer group leader, was successful in reducing the rate of caesareans.[46] One of the reasons for the rise in the caesarean rates in Canada during the 1970s and 1980s may well have been the decline in the number of deliveries carried out by family physicians.

By 1990 they were performing less than a third of deliveries and the trend was towards specialist obstetrician/gynaecologists. Family doctors gave a number of reasons for stopping obstetric practice. One was the conflict with family life of having to carry out deliveries in unsocial hours and a second was the high malpractice insurance that had to be paid by family doctors who practise obstetrics.[47] This led to a serious shortage of medical providers of obstetric care.

The shortage of doctors and the changes in attitudes towards delivery have led to a strong demand for midwifery care. Midwifery existed in the early days in Canada but had almost disappeared by the end of the nineteenth century because of medical opposition and legislation. One suggestion was that doctors began incorporating midwifery within their practices after seeing how lucrative it could be. They succeeded in convincing pregnant women that childbirth needed medical assistance and midwives began to be regarded as unsafe practitioners. As women were denied access to medical schools, only men were trained as doctors and so childbirth was taken over by men in a way which also happened in the United States. The revival of midwifery owes its roots to the counter-culture movement of the 1960s as women began to seek a more natural state in life and began to question the high level of technical intervention in childbirth. Midwifery has become increasingly well organised since the mid-1970s.[48] In 1986 the Ontario government announced its intention of licensing midwifery as an autonomous, self-governing profession.

There are now registered midwives in some states, but only to a limited extent. In 2001 only 3 per cent of deliveries were overseen by a midwife in Ontario. Intervention rates are still relatively high but the movement towards midwifery is likely to influence CSRs in Canada.

Australia (CSR 21.7 per cent in 2000)

Australia has a national health service funded by taxation (Medicare), more extensive than in the UK, alongside a private health care system. The majority of publicly funded births are attended by a midwife but in the private sector obstetricians carry out most deliveries.

---

45 Lomas, 1988
46 Lomas, 1991
47 Enkin, 1991
48 Enkin,1991

The pattern of caesarean birth in Australia has followed a similar trend to that in Britain. In Australia the section rate rose by 35 per cent during the 1990s to 22 per cent of births in 2000.[49] Regional variations are apparent. For example South Australia had a CSR of almost 25 per cent in 1999 when the rate in the Australian Capital Territory was 19.6 per cent.[50]

Ireland (CSR 21.3 per cent in 2000)

By the year 2000 the CSR in Ireland was up to 21.3 per cent, an increase of over 81 per cent since 1991.[51] This figure put the Irish caesarean rate close to the UK average rate of 22 per cent in the year 2000.

In Ireland free maternity care is provided for all women by the health boards. The majority of births (99 per cent) take place in hospital and the tradition of midwifery stemming from the eighteenth century, when obstetricians wrote textbooks of midwifery, is still strong. However, midwives do not have to register their intention to practise annually as they do in the UK, thus making it difficult to collect reliable data on the number of midwives practising currently.

Over 40 per cent of babies are born in one of the three maternity units in Dublin. In the Dublin Maternity there is a commitment to low levels of intervention from all the staff members. The midwives are in charge of the day-to-day running of the hospital and junior doctors are there to learn from them.

In the National Maternity Hospital in Dublin they had a record of *relatively* low CSRs due to their pioneering 'Active Management of Labour' (AML). The active approach to labour promised a woman having her first baby that she would not labour for more than twelve hours. It was important to establish whether she was in labour and if not she was sent home. Once labour was established, if her progress was not 1 cm dilation of the cervix per hour, contractions would be strengthened with synthetic oxytocin. The regime included induction or breaking the waters to assess their amount and colour. If clear, they assumed that fetal distress is unlikely, but if stained with the baby's faeces (meconium) then the woman was regarded as being in a different category and in need of greater supervision and monitoring.

The Dublin evidence on caesareans is instructive. O'Driscoll and Foley reported that, during the years 1965-80, when caesarean rates increased dramatically in centres across the United States from less than 5 per cent to more than 15 per cent,[52] the Dublin caesarean rate rose only from 4.2 to 4.8 per cent and perinatal mortality rate (PMR) fell from 42.1 to 16.8 per 1,000 for infants born weighing

---

49   Walker et al., 2004
50   EGAMS, 2002
51   Condon, 2004
52   O'Driscoll & Foley, 1983

500g or more, which is a greater fall than occurred in the United States. They concluded that these results did not support the contention that the increase in caesarean births had contributed significantly to the decline in perinatal mortality.

When the Dublin approach to labour was introduced in Houston, Texas, the duration of labour was reduced from an average of nearly thirteen hours to nearly eight and the caesarean rate fell from over one birth in five (23 per cent) to one birth in ten (10 per cent). However, since then CSRs have increased in Ireland and the USA.

New Zealand (CSR 22.7 per cent in 2002)

The caesarean section rate in New Zealand has followed the global trend but the rise started later than in the US. The rate remained below 10 per cent until the late 80s. National data on caesarean rates has only been collected since the late 1990s but latest figures show a rise from 18.2 per cent in 1997 to 22.7 in 2002.[53]

Over the last thirty years there has been a shift in the pattern of services. In the early 1970s general practitioners did the bulk of antenatal care outside the main centres. They were assisted by midwives, who could not practise autonomously but only under the supervision of a doctor, and delivered the majority of women in hospital using forceps and later vacuum extraction. They only referred pregnancies with complications to obstetricians and often continued to share care.

In 1990, after a major battle, an amendment to the 1977 Nurses Act gave midwives autonomy and since then midwives have taken over much of the primary maternity care. This amendment also gave midwives parity with GPs as far as funding was concerned and led to bitter and divisive arguments between these two branches of the professions caring for pregnant women. In 1992-95 a number of reviews of the maternity services were undertaken because of the increase in costs, anxiety about quality of care and duplication of work as women saw GPs and midwives separately. In April 1994 after a report by Coopers Lybrand Cabinet, funding for a Lead Maternity Carer (LMC) in primary care was agreed and the money for this was separated from the funding for secondary facilities. This was implemented in 1996 as a Section 51 Maternity Notice but doctors were unhappy. Consultations with users took place. In 1997 recommendations about referral were made[54] and in 1998 Section 51 was amended to separate the fee for a doctor LMC who used midwives employed by hospitals. These changes were evaluated in 1999 and a report published.[55]

---

53 MoH, 2003
54 RHA, 1997
55 HFA, 1999a & HFA, 1999b

In November 2000 the Health Funding Authority published a review of the historical changes and made recommendations for a strategy for maternity service provision for the next two years. They commented: 'Views on maternity services remain polarised'. They reiterated the government 1990 vision. 'Each woman and her whanau [family] has a safe and fulfilling outcome to her pregnancy and childbirth, through provision of programmes and services that are based on partnership, information and choice. Pregnancy and childbirth are a normal life stage for most women, with appropriate care available for those women who require it'.[56]

Sadly, during that decade the rates of induction and CS continued to increase although episiotomy rates fell and assisted vaginal delivery remained much the same. The latest available figures are from 2002 and show that the CSR is now over 22 per cent.[57]

The variation between tertiary hospitals (average 27.4) was striking, with Waikato having a rate of 33.7, and Middlemore in South Auckland a rate of 15.9 per cent. A study published in 1995 suggested that their low CSR was in part due to obstetric policies.[58] The proportion of all CS carried out in tertiary hospitals was over half of all operations (53.2 per cent). Secondary level hospitals (without a neonatal intensive care unit or all specialties) performed 41 per cent of the CS and had an average rate of 23.1 with a range from 16.7 per cent in Rotorua to 33.8 per cent in Southland. 5.8 per cent were delivered in primary care facilities with an average rate of 5.8 per cent raised by the inclusion of a private hospital with a 58 per cent rate.[59]

By 2002 midwives were named as the LMC for 73.1 per cent of women registering for antenatal care whilst GPs accounted for 9.6 per cent and obstetricians for 11.2 per cent and the remainder were unknown. At birth there was little change with 72.3 per cent still having a midwife as the LMC although the number of women having a normal birth was only 67.7 per cent.[60] So despite the increased involvement of midwives in maternity care the rates of intervention have continued to rise.

The CSR does rise with age for reasons not fully understood although it has been argued that this is physiological[61] and in the 1999 report rose from 8 per cent in women seventeen and under to 18 per cent at age thirty and almost 30 per cent at age forty.[62] But whether this is due to clinical need is questioned. Elective

---

56 New Zealand Information Service, 2004, p.40, table 3.9
57 New Zealand Information Service, 2004, p.40, table 3.9
58 Johnson & Ansell, 1995
59 New Zealand Information Service, 2004
60 New Zealand Information Service, 2004, p.37, table 3.5
61 Rosenthal & Paterson-Brown, 1998
62 MoH, 1999, p.7, figure 2.4

operations rose from 13 per cent in younger women to 45 per cent at age thirty-five and half of these were not repeat sections. The rates of CS were lower in Maori and Pacific island women who are more likely to be socio-economically deprived and would have been expected to have higher rates if based on clinical need, as has been witnessed in other parts of the world. In 2001 a survey of all obstetricians and heads of midwifery in NZ collected data which gave a CSR of 20 per cent based on 61.5 per cent of births (later government published figures were 22.1 per cent.[63]) The response rate was poor, 34 per cent of midwives, only half of whom gave opinions, and although 69 per cent of 221 obstetricians replied only twenty-two expressed opinion about the rising rate. Asked about the optimal CSR for NZ, midwives gave a rate of 11 per cent (independent) and 12 per cent (heads of departments). Clinical directors suggested 16 per cent and O&G specialists 18 per cent. Half the midwives thought the rate was 'about right' in their unit as did fourteen obstetricians but seven thought it was too high. Some obstetricians suggested that NZ women were unfit: 'NZ women tend to sit around during their pregnancy, becoming obese and unfit. They just do not have the ability to bear down effectively. There is also virtually no antenatal preparation for labour.' One midwife said 'Less children, more parental time, liberalism, guilt, professional/solo so more pampering of children, less tolerance of pain. Around here still immense pride in being tough'. Here was a predominantly Maori area and CSR for booked patients (after transfer from midwifery unit was 7.6 per cent). Another retired obstetrician said:

> Prior to my retirement (1971-1994) CS were done by general surgeons and the rates were high.... CSR was reduced to 5-6 per cent over a period of time. 1) I gave total personal care and attention to the mothers-to-be. 2) Educating local GPs-guidelines for referral. 3) Worked in a team with midwives.[64]

This seems an ideal way to look after pregnant women and achieve the kind of CSR which a healthy well-fed population like New Zealand should have.

Obstetricians considered that litigation and maternal request were the major non-clinical reasons for the rise and breech, reduction in forceps induction of labour and improved neonatal survival were the main clinical reasons. Midwives put litigation, maternal request and epidural anaesthesia as the main reasons although six of the fourteen thought midwifery inexperience an important factor.

In November 2000 the Health Funding Authority published 'Maternity Services: A Reference Document' which was a blueprint for ensuring that women got good care. Specific attention was to be given to formulating guidelines for CS and they refer to the 1994 WHO recommendation for a range

---

63   MoH, 2003
64   Savage, 2001 (from the author)

of 5-15 per cent for the CSR globally.[65] New Zealand, as a wealthy developed country, should be at the lower end of this range and let us hope that with public health doctors monitoring the situation the rate will start to fall.

Scandinavia and the Netherlands

Scandinavian countries and the Netherlands have experienced consistently low CSRs, currently within WHO recommendations at around 14.5 per cent. Sweden has a national health service providing all elements of maternity care. The majority of births are attended by a midwife who refers to an obstetrician only when necessary. Most births take place in hospital (99 per cent) so home births are rare. The Swedish CSR fluctuated between 11 and 13.4 per cent since 1980 but remained quite stable in the 1980s when most other countries experienced dramatic rises in section rates.[66] This was due to the fact that obstetricians in Sweden took action, agreeing a common policy to try and stem the rise seen elsewhere. The infant mortality rate in Sweden is one of the lowest in the world relating to the high standard of living and consequent low rate of pre-term birth which is a major contributor to PNM.

In Norway free maternity care is provided by the state health scheme and is used by 99 per cent of women. Midwives take care of the majority of low-risk women and most births take place in hospital with a corresponding low home-birth rate of less than 0.5 per cent. The caesarean rate in Norway was 13.7 in 2000. However, as expected, the pattern of caesarean births varies greatly according to ethnicity. For example, in Norway the CSR ranges from 10 per cent among mothers from Vietnam to almost 26 per cent in women of Filipino origin.[67] In Sweden too, Asian women have an increased frequency of caesarean delivery.[68]

There is a long tradition of home birth in the Netherlands. In the early 1970s, 70 per cent of births were delivered at home with a corresponding low CSR of 2 per cent. By the late 1970s home births had halved to 35 per cent due to changes in training needs of health care professionals which meant midwives brought more of their clients in to the hospital setting. Following action and campaigning from midwives this situation changed and the rate of home births began to rise again, to 35-38 per cent in the 1980s. The situation in the late 1990s was that 46 per cent of births were attended by a midwife, 8 per cent by GPs and 46 per cent by obstetricians.[69] However the CSR does appear to be rising. Whilst within WHO guidelines of 10-15 per cent, latest estimates put the CSR in Holland at almost 13 per cent in 2000.

---

65 WHO, 1994
66 Devries et al., 2001
67 Vangen et al., 2000
68 Devries et al., 2001
69 Smulders, 1999

Less Economically Developed Countries (LEDCs)

There are few countries in the world where data on CSRs are systematically collected and reliably collated. This is more so in LEDCs where there are weak health information and registration systems. Estimates on all types of births tend to rely more on household surveys.

The debate on the efficacy of caesarean birth takes on a different meaning when considering the position of women in the developing world. High rates of maternal mortality and morbidity are due to a number of factors, the most important of these being women's lack of access to adequate emergency obstetric services that would enable prompt management of obstetric complications.[70] Rather than concern being raised about rising section rates and unnecessary operations, concentration is switched to focus on issues of lack of access to health care services and the corresponding absence of facilities, equipment and personnel to perform caesareans which may save the lives of women and babies.

Obstetric complications are the leading cause of death and disability amongst women of reproductive age in developing countries. It has been estimated that 529,000 maternal deaths each year are due to problems of pregnancy or childbirth and a lack of sufficient obstetric care.[71] West African countries have some of the highest maternal mortality rates in the world. Here, an estimated one woman dies from problems associated with pregnancy or labour compared with one in 4,000 in northern Europe.[72] For every maternal death in sub-Saharan Africa, a further thirty women suffer injury, infection or disability from maternal causes. This means that fifteen million women per year are affected by this type of death, illness or disability, leading to a cumulative total of 300 million or, put another way, more than a quarter of the female adult population in the developing world. Women in sub-Saharan Africa face a one in thirteen chance of dying from complications of pregnancy or childbirth compared to the one in 4,085 chance experienced by women in more economically developed countries. This susceptibility to obstetric risk for women in LEDCs starts early in life. For example, women whose growth has been restricted by malnutrition are more at risk of obstructed labour. Furthermore, female genital mutilation increases risks during childbirth and this affects an estimated two million girls every year.[73]

In 1987 the Nairobi Safe Motherhood Conference drew attention to the problem of maternal mortality in the developing world and in 1990 the WHO set a target

---

70 Okonofua, 2001
71 UNICEF, 2005
72 Murray & Lopez, 1997
73 UNICEF, 2003

of halving maternal mortality by the year 2000. Two major international conferences in the 1990s echoed the concerns of the Nairobi conference – the International Conference on Population and Development in Cairo in 1994 and the Fourth World Conference on Women held in Beijing in 1995 pressed for safe motherhood as an essential right of all women and urged immediate action.[74] In 1998 the WHO reiterated 'Safe Motherhood' as its slogan for the World Health Day. However, despite the efforts of the safe motherhood campaign the target of halving maternal mortality by the year 2000 was not achieved. In fact, work on ascertaining the rates of maternal mortality increased the number of deaths recorded.

The many-faceted factors that cause maternal mortality and morbidity in LEDCs also affect the chances of survival for the infants. The estimate of infant deaths occurring just before birth, during delivery or in the first week of life is eight million.[75] There have been limited pockets of success with programmes such as the WHO Mother-Baby package consisting of eighteen basic interventions that have proven to reduce infant and maternal mortality in areas where resources are scarce.[76]

As most obstetric problems cannot be predicted or prevented, access to emergency obstetrical care and skilled personnel are essential in the reduction of maternal mortality and morbidity. Women are in most need of skilled care during delivery and in the immediate post-partum period when around three-quarters of all maternal deaths occur. Further, access to trained personnel is low and maternal mortality high in countries where women have low status and poor access to basic and routine health services.[77] The number of women attended in birth by skilled personnel is woefully inadequate in many parts of the world (see Table 4.2). Around 99 per cent of the estimated 500,000 maternal deaths each year take place in LEDCs[78] (see Table 4.3). Insufficient maternal care is responsible for 529,000 maternal deaths and an estimated four million neonatal deaths.[79] In 1998 the World Health Day was dedicated to safe motherhood, one of the recommendations being that governments work with private health providers and insurance companies to ensure that safe motherhood initiatives are included in their plans. Thus the priority is not about reducing CSRs, but rather in improving access to medical services for women in those countries.

One study which concentrated on eight sub-Saharan countries[80] found the CSR to be less than 2 per cent in four countries and less than 5 per cent in the other

---

74 Ghada, 1998
75 UNICEF, 2003
76 Ghada, 1998
77 UNICEF, 2005
78 UNICEF, 2003
79 UNICEF, 2005
80 Burkina Faso, Cameroon, Ghana, Kenya, Madagascar, Niger, Tanzania and Zambia

Table 4.2 Percentage of births attended by skilled personnel 1995-2003

Region	Per cent
Sub-Saharan Africa	41
Middle East/North Africa	72
South Asia	35
East Asia/Pacific	87
Latin America/Caribbean	82
CIS/CEE*	92
Industrialised countries	99
Developing countries	59
Least Developed countries	32
The World	62

Source: UNICEF, 2005
*Commonwealth of Independent States/Central
& Eastern Europe

Table 4.3
Maternal mortality 1995

Region	Per cent
Sub-Saharan Africa	49
South Asia	30
East Asia/Pacific	10
Middle East/North Africa	6
Latin America/Caribbean	4
Industrialised countries	<1
The World	n= 515,000

Source: UNICEF, 2003

countries except Kenya. In fact the number of caesareans performed in these countries was found to have declined in five countries during the 1990s.[81] Thus it appears that access to health care facilities and CS is not improving in sub-Saharan Africa and may in fact be getting worse. This is a cause for concern as maternal mortality in these areas is extremely high and indicates a lack of effect of 'safe motherhood' programmes in these areas. It has been suggested that better access to CS is required in sub-Saharan Africa and that a CSR of between 3.6 and 6.5 per cent is necessary to address the obstetric problems in these countries.[82] However, there is little data on the extent to which timely CS can reduce maternal mortality and morbidity rates in developing countries.[83]

In the Rivers State of Nigeria, caesarean delivery has been made free of charge thereby removing financial barriers to women seeking operative birth. Yet the effect of this policy is unclear as, whilst it removes the expense of surgery, it does not tackle cultural norms and beliefs, nor does it ensure that women will be able to access prompt and professional assistance when required. In some cultures women who cannot deliver vaginally are stigmatised. For example, in

81 Buekens et al., 2003
82 Buekens et al., 2003
83 Okonofua, 2001

rural Eastern Nigeria women fear CS as they might be considered abnormal for not being able to deliver vaginally. CS is also threatening to them because they fear blood transfusion or involuntary sterilisation (practised in some hospitals after repeat caesareans). To those women CS may mean more than the delivery of a healthy baby or the saving of their lives. The abdominal scar will act as a constant reminder of their incapacity to deliver vaginally. Women may be considered to have been 'mutilated' by those who represent western customs and ignore traditional norms.[84]

What is clear from an analysis of worldwide caesarean data is that the important issue is finding a balance, finding the right level of CS for the population of women served. Despite some of the more economically developed countries showing signs of levelling out in terms of CSRs (or at least a reduction in the rate of growth of caesarean rates) for many of us the level is still too high. In the less economically developed countries the problem is reversed: women who need surgery are unable to obtain a CS. The WHO set an optimal level at between 10 and 15 per cent in 1985; we have stressed that there is no benefit in terms of outcome of a CSR over 12 per cent at the most. In Britain, the current rate of caesarean birth is almost 23 per cent, more than 11 per cent above necessary levels, and showing no signs of slowing down. It is hoped that a combination of the NICE Guidelines, the genuine anxiety expressed by some obstetricians and midwives, and increased understanding by women will halt the rise and, in time, lead to a decline in the CSR.

---

84 Engelkes & van Roosmalen, 1992

5 Is a caesarean really necessary?

'Caesarean [birth] rates in the US have increased each year since 1965. Yet there is no evidence that maternal and child health has improved as a result of this increase.'[1]

'In general maternity units, no benefit is apparent from a CSR above 10 to 12 per cent on the singleton population as a whole. The case against a CSR below 10 per cent rests on a single variable, onset of respiration at one minute.'[2]

MUCH OF THIS CHAPTER IS BASED UPON THE EXPERIENCE and views of one of our authors, Wendy Savage, and it is from her perspective that it is written. Wendy has thirty-five years experience in Obstetrics and Gynaecology, twenty-five of which were at the London (then Royal London) Hospital where she was appointed as Senior Lecturer at the London Hospital Medical College in 1977, with an honorary contract with Tower Hamlets Health Authority.

The quotations at the head of this chapter come from public health physicians. They were the first in the US to raise the alarm about the rising rate of CS thirty years ago.[3] In *Healthy People 2000* they set targets for the primary CSR of 15 per cent and 35 per cent for vaginal birth after caesarean section (VBAC) and for a while the US CSR rise was reversed.[4] Joffe et al. looked at a large data set from the North West Thames Region to reach their conclusion. We have seen that the caesarean rate varies a great deal between different countries, hospitals and individual obstetricians. Some women will have the operation before labour begins (planned caesarean) while other women presenting with identical or similar problems in another setting will be encouraged to deliver vaginally and often do so. We can divide the reasons for performing a caesarean into two separate categories – the absolute reasons for which women will always need a

---

1   DHHS, 1991, p.378
2   Joffe et al., 1994, p.406
3   US Task Force, 1978
4   PP&BS, 2000

77

caesarean and the relative indications where practice will vary. There are situations where the only safe option for either the mother or the baby, or for both, is to have a caesarean.

We have drawn heavily in this chapter on the National Sentinel Caesarean Section Audit (National Audit) which found a 21.5 per cent CSR. Phase 1 was carried out in three months in 2000 and covered 99 per cent of births in England and Wales in 213 NHS, ten midwifery-led and three private units. Phase 2 was carried out in January 2001 on a random sample of units. Women's views were sought but the response rate was only 37 per cent whereas of 224 obstetricians surveyed it was 77 per cent.[5] This is the most up-to-date information nationally. The guidelines for CS commissioned by the National Institute for Clinical Excellence (NICE) were written after an extensive review of the literature[6] and provide the basis for current practice in Obstetrics. For an explanation of some of the terms used see the Glossary.

Why a caesarean may be necessary

There are some reasons ('indications' is the word used in medical practice) for which a caesarean section is always needed – the *absolute* indications. In the majority of operations there is an element of judgement or discretion and this is why individual obstetricians may have very different CSRs despite having similar populations of women or working in the same hospital. Table 5.1 gives an estimate of the likelihood of the generally agreed indications which have remained much the same over the last thirty-five years, during which time the overall CSR has risen five-fold in England and Wales from 4.9 per cent to just over 23 per cent in 2004.[7]

These figures were originally calculated from data from the London Hospital obstetric database, and from the 1958 Perinatal Mortality Survey[8] (when few interventions were possible), and published in the paper 'The rise in caesarean section – anxiety or science?'[9] The estimates for feto-pelvic disproportion and fetal distress reflect the way reasons were coded. It is interesting that in the National Sentinel Caesarean Section Audit, which looked at all CS in the UK in 2000, very similar figures were obtained for some of these reasons.[10]

When these data were compiled, intervention was done only when really necessary. Abnormal lie or presentation were given as reasons for 0.7 per cent of CS, placenta praevia for 0.5 per cent, abruptio placentae for 0.2-0.4 per cent

---

5   Thomas & Paranjothy, 2001
6   NICE, 2004
7   Chamberlain & Chamberlain, 1972; BirthChoiceUK, 2005
8   Butler & Bonham, 1958
9   Savage, 1992
10   Thomas & Paranjothy, 2001

Table 5.1 Reasons for Caesarean Section

Maternal reasons	%	Fetal reasons	%
Transverse lie with ruptured membranes*	0.2	Severe fetal distress	1-2
Face (chin-posterior) and brow presentation	0.5	Primary maternal herpes at term	0.01
Breech with extended neck (stargazing)	0.1	Mother HIV positive	0.01
Type 3&4 placenta praevia	0.5		
Severe abruption with baby alive	0.2-0.4	Cord prolapse before full dilatation of cervix	0.1
Absolute feto-pelvic disproportion	?1-2		
Eclampsia/severe PET before term	0.5-1	Total fetal reasons	1.0-2.1
Total maternal reasons	3.0-4.7	**Total reasons**	**5.0-6.9**

* Very unusual in a first pregnancy; relatively new indications not used in 1958
\# The incidence of placenta praevia, though uncommon, rises with each CS operation

and cord prolapse for 0.1 per cent. From Table 5.1 one can see that between 5.0 and 6.9 per cent of women are likely to need a CS either to preserve their own life or health or that of the baby. Some CS are planned before labour starts and are called 'elective' or 'planned'. When the need for a CS does not become apparent until labour starts, it is called an emergency CS. You can see from Table 5.1 above that most conditions will not occur until labour is in progress, so that the planned CSR should not be more than 2 per cent in primigravidae. Some cases of placenta praevia, herpes and HIV can be planned as can repeat CS in women having a subsequent child. According to the National Audit, two-thirds of CS operations were emergencies, so about 37 per cent were planned.

The majority (two-thirds) of healthy women will have a normal vaginal birth without any complications in the present system of care, although we consider this figure too low: at least 80 per cent of healthy women should be able to deliver normally as shown by results of mainly midwifery practice.[11] Even women with pre-existing diseases like diabetes or cardiac problems can usually deliver their baby safely vaginally.

The most common reasons given for CS in England, Wales and Northern Ireland as found in the National Audit are given in Table 5.2.[12]

11   Van Alten et al., 1989; Rockenschaub, 1990; Durand, 1992; Rockenschaub, 1990; Independent Midwives, 2004; Smulders, 2005 (personal communication)
12   Adapted from Table 4.6 on p.23 of Thomas & Paranjothy, 2001

Table 5.2 Leading Reasons for Primary CS, National Audit 2000, England and Wales

Reason for CS	% of women	% of CS	Regional range % of CS
Presumed fetal compromise	4.7	22	14.3 NI – 23.4 L
Failure to progress	4.4	20.4	17.9 NW – 23.8 W
Repeat CS	3.0	13.8	12.5 NE – 23.9 NI
Breech presentation	2.3	10.8	7.9 L – 12.4 NE,SW
Maternal request*	1.6	7.3	5.7 WM – 8.4 SE
Malpresentations/unstable lie	0.73	3.4	2.8 SE – 3.9 NE
Placenta praevia	0.67	3.1	2.4 NE – 3.7 WM
Eclampsia, PET, HELLP**	0.5	2.3	1.7 EM – 2.7 L
Other fetal	0.5	2.3	1.8 SW – 2.8 WM
Maternal medical disease	0.41	1.9	1.5 SE – 2.0 WM,W
Abruptio placentae/APH/IPH	0.39	1.8	1.5 SW – 2.6 NW
Previous traumatic birth	0.37	1.7	1.3 NE – 2.3 SW
Multiple pregnancy	0.26	1.2	0.8 NI – 1.4 L,NE,SE

* Maternal request as reported by clinicians so may include cases where there was a medical indication.
** A syndrome where platelets fall and liver function tests are abnormal.
Region where the consultants practise:
L=London, SE=South East, SW=South West, NE=North East, NW=North West, EM=East Midlands, WM=West Midlands, NI=Northern Ireland, W=Wales

Presumed fetal compromise: 22 per cent of CS, 4.7 per cent of women

This is now the leading cause of CS and was diagnosed and acted upon in almost one woman in twenty. Babies who grow poorly in the womb use their stores of starch (glycogen) which are laid down to enable the fetus to withstand the reduction in blood supply during the height of a contraction if they are getting insufficient nourishment through the afterbirth or placenta. When the woman goes into labour the fetus may show signs of distress. One of these is the passage of meconium, the contents of the fetal bowel which can be emptied into the amniotic fluid surrounding the fetus. This is what is called a 'soft' sign and does not require immediate action especially if old and not very thick, but warrants watchfulness for other signs of fetal distress. These may be changes in the fetal heart rate as recorded by an external transducer fixed over the woman's abdomen or a clip attached to the baby's head. This information about the fetal heart rate is fed into a machine is called a cardio-tocograph or CTG for short. These changes in the heart rate are often misleading and early studies showed that if fetal monitoring was done without checking by doing fetal blood sampling then the CSR rose yet the outcome for the babies was no better than if a CS had not been done. More recent reviews have confirmed this.[13] The consensus is that for healthy women with a normal pregnancy routine EFM is not indicated and neither is an admission trace.[14]

These are usually unplanned operations and if fetal distress is diagnosed after the cervix is sufficiently dilated (4 cm is usually taken as the point at which fetal blood sampling is possible although at 3 cm one can usually get a sample of blood from the baby's head) a fetal blood sample should be taken to confirm whether the baby is truly distressed or whether this is a 'false positive' change on the CTG trace. If the baby's heart beat instead of showing decelerations which recover rapidly, falls and stays low then this usually means that the baby needs to be delivered immediately by CS. However, one situation where the baby is not in danger is if the head has been high and as it enters to pelvic brim and is suddenly compressed the heart rate falls and may remain low for some minutes. It then returns to the normal rate (at term) of 120-160 beats per minute.

Rarely, the baby's growth may be so poor that this is detected in the antenatal clinic, as the height of the uterus (fundal height) does not increase as it should and the bulk of the uterus also falls as the liquor volume falls. Ultrasound scans comparing the circumference of the baby's head and abdomen can help to distinguish between a small normal baby that does not need to be delivered early and one whose abdominal stores of glycogen are being used up. If the baby is active and liquor volume is normal and, in some units, doppler tests show good blood flow to the uterus, labour can be induced early in the hope that the baby will be able to go through labour without becoming distressed. If the tests suggest that there are no reserves then a planned CS may be performed. However it was shown some years ago that over-cautious management could increase the CSR without improvements in the survival of the babies.[15] There have been no randomised controlled trials (RCTs) to compare planned CS with planned vaginal birth for infants that are small for their gestational age, and the NICE guidelines recommend that planned CS should not be offered outside a research context.[16] CS before labour was carried out in the National Audit in 1.2 per cent of women having their first pregnancy and 1.4 per cent of those having subsequent pregnancies but the reasons for these operations are not given. Some would have been for suspected fetal compromise and some for maternal disease as well as previous CS in the subsequent pregnancies.

It seems unlikely that true fetal distress or compromise requiring CS has increased so markedly in the last thirty years. Zuspan et al. put the incidence of true serious fetal distress at 1.0 per cent in US hospital practice.[17] It is probable

---

13 Thacker & Stroup, 2001
14 RCOG, 2001d
15 Kiwanuka & Moore, 1987
16 NICE, 2004, p.32
17 Zuspan et al., 1997

that at least half of these babies did not need to be delivered surgically. Although there may be differences in the way that consultants in the National Audit coded the indications for surgery, the discrepancy between Northern Ireland (where 14.3 per cent of CS were done for this reason) with London (where almost a quarter were similarly coded) suggests that there is over-diagnosis of this condition. In the Scottish Audit, 69 per cent of CS for fetal distress did not have fetal blood sampling.[18] In the National Audit, 16.2 per cent of CS were said to be done because of an 'immediate threat to the life of the woman or fetus' but only 51 per cent fulfilled the criteria, which did include severe fetal ECG changes or a FBS below 7.2. Of the half that did not fulfil the criteria, 59 per cent were said to have presumed fetal compromise. The CTG was said to be normal in 8 per cent and abnormal but not severely so in 89 per cent. Nineteen per cent of these had an FBS done and in none was the level below the danger line of 7.2. This suggests that at least 1 to 2 per cent of women had a CS for presumed fetal compromise before it was really necessary.[19] In the next category 'Maternal or fetal compromise not immediately life threatening', just under a third of operations showed marked variations between units from 7 per cent to 36 per cent of CS but the proportion who had FBS is not given.

Comment

When EFM was introduced in the late 1970s it was thought obvious that checking the fetal heart continuously, instead of listening with a Pinard stethoscope using the midwife or doctor's ear every fifteen minutes, was an advance.[20] However, it was not for another fifteen years that the first RCT to check this assumption was carried out in Dublin.[21] This showed that it was not in the long term better for the baby and increased intervention in the mother. It took another fifteen years before a guideline for the use of EFM was produced by the RCOG and, despite this, some units still routinely subject women to continuous EFM and some midwives feel uneasy without recording the fetal heart in this way. Does the anxiety produced by this technique of monitoring affect the woman's own response so that both she and the baby become distressed, resulting in a raised heart rate? Are younger doctors unable to deal with their own anxiety in the way that older doctors who practised before EFM and the relative safety of CS had to learn how to do, with watchful waiting and careful observation of the woman? Are doctors intervening too early with a much lower threshold and thus creating an unnecessarily high CSR in the first pregnancy which naturally then affects the second pregnancy (see p.88). Does the whole way that antenatal care is conducted these days – with constant

18 McIlwaine et al., 1998
19 Thomas & Paranjothy, 2001, p.51
20 Sibanda & Beard, 1975
21 MacDonald et al., 1985

monitoring by different people and routine ultrasound scans (also, like EFM, introduced without an RCT to demonstrate the pros and cons of this procedure on a large scale) – induce anxiety in the woman? Does this undermine her own feelings about the pregnancy and her capacity to nurture the developing fetus adequately?

Failure to progress (FTP) or dystocia ('difficult labour'): 20.4 per cent of CS, 4.4 per cent of women

This was the second most likely diagnosis given by consultants for doing a CS in the National Audit and a fifth of CS were for this reason. This is almost one woman in twenty-three, yet in the 1958 Perinatal Mortality Survey (which looked at all births in one week in England and Wales)[22] the PMR did not rise in first births until the woman had been in labour for more than forty-eight hours and, in women having a subsequent baby, twenty-four hours. Whilst one would not advocate labours lasting this long today, only 4 per cent of women having their first baby and 2.7 per cent of those having a subsequent child fell into these categories. At this time when synthetic oxytocin[23] was not widely available and induction of labour was only embarked upon with caution, this survey gives an indication of how natural labour progressed. The number of babies dying before birth and in the first week of life per 1,000 total births is known as the perinatal mortality rate (PMR) and the biggest factor contributing to this is premature birth. Although only 0.6 per cent of women had their labours accelerated by the use of oxytocin in the 1970 survey,[24] only 5.1 per cent had labours lasting over twenty-four hours; but unlike the 1958 survey, eighteen hours was taken as a long labour. Is eighteen hours now considered too long?

In 1970 O'Driscoll and his colleagues in Dublin reported a trial in which they took twelve hours as the limit for a first labour and actively managed women whose labours were going slowly by artificially rupturing the membranes and using oxytocin.[25] They showed that the CSR reduced without detriment to the babies and this approach was enthusiastically taken up in both the UK and the USA. Subsequent work found variable success rates[26] and the NICE guidelines state that 'active management of labour and early amniotomy have not been shown to influence the likelihood of CS for FTP and should not be offered for this reason.'[27]

---

22 Butler & Bonham, 1963
23 I will use the shorthand 'oxytocin' for 'synthetic oxytocin' after this: oxytocin is a naturally occurring hormone and cannot be collected and stored.
24 Chamberlain & Chamberlain, 1972
25 O'Driscoll et al., 1970
26 Thornton & Lilford, 1994
27 NICE, 2004, p.49

One aspect of the policy was that the woman had continuous attention from the same midwife, something not always possible in other centres. That continuous support from a trained laywoman, a 'doula', reduced the CSR was shown in 1991 by RCTs carried out by Klaus and Kennell.[28] This was confirmed in the latest systematic review of fifteen RCTs encompassing 12,791 women in both developing and developed countries with trained and untrained women, including family members, supporting the labouring women. The relative risk of having a CS was 0.9 in the supported women and where the support was not provided by a member of staff the chance was even lower at 0.74.[29] Thus the midwifery support may explain the success of the Dublin policy when selectively applied. When up to 40 per cent of women were having their labours speeded up with oxytocin (as I saw when I visited Dublin in the late 1980s) one can surmise that the policy was being almost routinely applied.

Occipito-posterior position as a cause of failure to progress

My own view is that the original good results may have been due to success in dealing with the dysfunctional labour that may be the reason for, or may follow, the abnormal position of the fetus known as occipito-posterior (OP). In about 6 per cent of women the fetus is lying with its back against its mother's back instead of her tummy wall so that the back of the head is next to her spine and the face looks towards the pubic bone in the front of the pelvis. In the normal position with a head first (or vertex) presentation, the baby's occiput is towards the pubic bone and the baby faces the sacrum at the base of the mother's spine. With the OP position the baby's head has to rotate more as it descends in the pelvis and this takes longer. In a woman having her first baby, the cervix usually dilates at 1 cm per hour once she is in active labour which fits with the mean length of labour of twelve hours – although the range can be between six and twenty-four hours in the majority of women. With an OP baby the dilatation may be only 1 cm in two hours but as long as progress is steady, the baby in good condition, the head descending and rotation occurring, there is no need to speed up the labour. Backache is very prominent in these presentations and here an epidural may transform the experience for the woman. The neck may be more extended than usual so that there is a bigger diameter of the baby's head coming down through the pelvis and sometimes at full dilatation the head becomes stuck in the transverse position and requires help with the vacuum extractor, fingers or forceps to flex the head and complete the rotation, so that the baby can be delivered in the usual way. It is this skill to assist vaginal birth that obstetricians in our survey said that younger doctors lacked.

28 Kennell et al., 1991
29 Hodnett et al., 2003

In my experience the diagnosis of OP is often missed these days; yet it is not difficult to make and, when this is done, one can help the woman to adjust to the idea of a longer labour. The options for pain relief and the use of oxytocin if progress is slow can be discussed. If the membranes rupture before the onset of strong contractions, the midwife feels the tummy and thinks the head is engaged and then on vaginal examination finds the head is 2 cm or more above the ischial spines s/he should immediately think that the baby is lying in the OP position. Usually when s/he listens to the fetal heart, it is on the opposite side from where s/he thinks the back of the baby is lying and this may even alert her/him before s/he does the vaginal examination. Sometimes, in the case of a direct OP, all s/he feels is limbs. It is possible, with the increase in obesity, that palpation of the abdomen (feeling the baby through the tummy wall) is more difficult; or it may be that, because a woman is strapped to a fetal monitor and abdominal palpation is done less often, skills in this technique in both midwives and doctors have declined.

It may also be that the incidence of OP is increasing with our sedentary lifestyle and more frequent use of cars, as postulated by a midwife who advocates exercises to prevent or help reposition the baby.[30] No RCT has been done but she has had good results in her own practice.

When progress is slow, I think that speeding up the labour and using an epidural earlier rather than later can increase the rate of vaginal birth and decrease the rate of CS, but I do not have figures to prove this. Doing an RCT is difficult because of the late diagnosis of this condition. With about a fifth of women who start labour with an OP, the baby does not rotate but (providing the mother has a good-sized pelvis) is born in this way, face to pubis. Because there is usually a bigger diameter of the baby's head an episiotomy is recommended earlier rather than later.

Cephalo-pelvic disproportion (CPD) or feto-pelvic disproportion (FPD) as a cause of FTP

CPD and FPD both involve there being insufficient room for the baby to pass through the mother's pelvis. Although absolute or severe disproportion was common in this country in the nineteenth century – because of poor nutrition, which leads to rickets thus affecting the growth of the pelvis – and is still common in developing countries like Africa, these are uncommon in the UK today.

It can rarely be diagnosed before labour begins and almost never in a woman having her first baby. Today fractured pelvises from road accidents are the most

---

30 Sutton & Scott, 1996

common cause, though still uncommon. Most babies present head first so CPD is much more common than breech pelvic disproportion; therefore this term will be used for the rest of this section. Shorter women are more likely to have a CS than taller women and five feet two inches was taken as warning signal when I trained. However, within this broad range some really short women are able to deliver large babies and so factors such as height, shoe size and clinical assessment of the pelvis are hardly considered today.

Where CPD is suspected clinically, because the head is high at term and does not easily enter the pelvis, it was common practice to assess the relative sizes of the outlet of the pelvis and the baby using clinical palpation, X-rays and/or ultrasound to assess fetal size.

Recent studies have shown that such attempts to assess whether or not the baby can pass through the pelvis are unreliable predictors. Some women whose pelvises have been shown to be 'radiologically inadequate' have succeeded in giving birth vaginally, and some women whose pelvises have been shown to be 'radiologically adequate' have required emergency caesareans so the Royal College of Obstetricians and Gynaecologists (RCOG) does not recommend this.[31]

In the National Audit only 6 per cent (Regional range 2-12 per cent) of women who had had a previous CS had pelvimetry and this had influenced the decision to perform a repeat CS in 40 per cent.[32] One RCT showed that women who had X-ray pelvimetry were more likely to have caesareans than those who did not.[33] This may be because obstetricians interpret the findings wrongly. The inlet of the pelvis should be between 10 and 12 cm (with a mean of 11 for British women) and the average baby's head at term has a biparietal diameter of 10 cm. I vividly recall a woman from a District General Hospital referred by her cardiologist. She had a heart condition and had been booked for a planned CS of her first baby on the basis of an X-ray pelvimetry done locally. The pelvis had a good shape and the inlet was 10 cm so it was within normal limits. The baby clinically was not large and she had a successful trial of labour and delivered a healthy 2.9kg baby after six hours. Both she and her cardiologist were delighted with the outcome.

It was my practice to do an X-ray pelvimetry after a woman had had a CS. I think that talking though the tangible evidence of the X-ray picture of the bones of the pelvis often helped women to labour more confidently in the next pregnancy. Occasionally, one did come across a pelvis with an unfavourable shape and could discuss the likely effect of this on labour; but the X-rays were used as an aid to the management of a vaginal birth after a CS, not to predict that

31   Pattinson, 2001
32   Thomas & Paranjothy, 2001, p.46
33   RCOG, 2001a

planned CS was necessary. This is because it is rare in British women to have an abnormal pelvis these days. Again, I have no RCT evidence that this approach reduced the CSR but women booked under my care had a higher rate of successful VBAC than those booked under my colleagues (who did not routinely use X-ray pelvimetry even before the RCOG guideline). (See Figure 3, Appendix D).

In the National Audit, 81 per cent of women who had a CS for FTP had received oxytocin strengthening during their labour. This ranged from 74-84 per cent between regions and 47-100 per cent between units.[34] Those who had not had oxytocin contributed 2.6 per cent to the overall CSR of 21.5 per cent.

Of those CS classified as urgent which were done for FTP, 12 per cent did not meet the criteria laid down by the researchers and in 57 per cent of these the CTG was said to be normal.[35] This may mean that the woman was tired and the obstetricians acting compassionately or it may mean that action was taken earlier than necessary and given more time the woman might have delivered vaginally.

Comment

The increase in CS due to failure to progress does not seem likely to have been due to an increase in small or abnormal pelvises as women today are taller and had better nutrition in childhood than their mothers. The proportion of large babies has not increased compared with the 1958 survey when the CSR was 2.8 per cent. Attitudes about the length of labour and how rapidly it should progress may have changed as stated by some of the consultants we surveyed and it is possible that women are less fit than they used to be. However, it again seems intrinsically unlikely that so many women really need a CS for this reason – unless our modern system for delivering women in large units, with a variety of often unknown people looking after them, really affects the way that women labour. The NICE guidelines state that healthy women with an anticipated normal pregnancy should be informed that delivering at home halves their chance of having a CS.[36] The Home Birth study does suggest that something about hospital births affects the chances of a woman delivering normally[37] and I suspect that the labour ward with its bright lights, ringing telephones, bleeps going off and frequent interruptions does militate against successful labour. Women need peace and quiet, as few professionals as possible involved and privacy, as was recognised by the Winterton Committee.[38] Intuitively one feels that the sound of other women labouring is not conducive to relaxation and the state of inner concentration that women need to deliver normally.

---

34 Thomas & Paranjothy, 2001, p.46
35 Thomas & Paranjothy, 2001, p.51
36 NICE, 2004, p.39
37 Chamberlain et al., 2003
38 HoC, 1992

Repeat CS: 13.8 per cent of CS, 3 per cent of women

This was the third-commonest reason for CS in the National Audit and of course only applies to women who have had at least one baby before. Three per cent of pregnant women had a CS and 13.8 per cent of CS were for this reason. The contribution of women with a uterine scar towards the overall CSR was 29 per cent. The VBAC rate for England and Wales was 33 per cent, the regional range was 27-38 per cent and between units 6-64 per cent. Of those women who had a CS, 44 per cent said they had been offered a trial of labour and this ranged from 39-49 per cent between regions and 8-90 per cent between units.[39]

Within units consultants may also vary as shown in figure 1 in Appendix D taken from the Royal London Hospital database in 1990.

The usual practice in the UK is to offer a trial of labour or trial of scar to women whose first operation was done for a reason which is unlikely to recur in this pregnancy such as breech presentation or antepartum haemorrhage (see later in this chapter). If the operation was done for FTP thought to be due to CPD, most consultants would advise a CS but as the late Professor Ian Donald said in relation to pelvimetry: 'the best pelvimeter is the fetal head'. Even when the first CS was done for CPD, McGarry showed that 20 per cent of women were able to deliver vaginally – and this was at a time when the CSR was under 5 per cent.[40]

The position of the baby, its weight and the likelihood that a second labour will be more efficient than a first, all point towards the best option for the woman being to try and deliver vaginally. Clearly if she has had a difficult labour, often because of poor management, she may feel that she does not want to try, but given a supportive consultant who is available, she may be able to see the benefit of this. It is good for the baby to have some squeezing from contractions and some labour may make the operation easier as the lower part of the uterus becomes thinner so even if the woman ends up with a CS there are these advantages. My policy with women who had had a previous CS was to write in the notes that I should be informed by the registrar when she is admitted in labour, after s/he had done the vaginal examination. Thus the woman knew that I would pass on to the registrar the points that were important to her about her previous labour. I also thought it important that the same registrar did all the vaginal examinations (although with the current shift system this may be more difficult to arrange). Apart from the subtle changes that may take place in the flexion and moulding of the head and the consistency of the cervix, which may not be appreciated if different people do the examinations (an important part of learning how to monitor a labour), women appreciated the continuity. I would always see the woman when I was free to do so and I would warn women when

---

39 Thomas & Paranjothy, 2001
40 McGarry, 1969

I was going on holiday so they were not disappointed, reassuring them that the colleague I worked closely with knew my views and shared most of them.

RCTs have not been done comparing planned CS with trial of labour and so the NICE guidelines group consider that the risks and benefits are uncertain. However, observational studies have given us information about the risks and benefits although few have looked at how the woman copes when she goes home. My second daughter, who had a CS for grade 4 placenta praevia with her first baby, was very pleased that she delivered vaginally the second time. She felt she could not have coped with an active toddler as well as the newborn baby and the after effects of a CS.

The NICE guidelines refer to uterine rupture after a CS but this is a misnomer. A scar rupture is rarely a rupture in the way that occurs in obstructed labour – as I have seen in Africa, for example. What usually happens is that the scar gives way – 'dehiscence' is the medical term – or comes 'unzipped'. There is only a little bleeding and there is enough time to take the woman to theatre and do a CS. With a uterine rupture, the muscle of the upper part of the uterus tears apart possibly down to the uterine arteries and there is massive bleeding and a desperate emergency for the mother. The baby is usually expelled into the abdominal cavity and the placenta separates so the baby dies. In the scar dehiscence there is time before the baby is affected as the contractions tend to stop and the head may be going down into the pelvis and is unlikely to be pushed out of the uterus initially.

The risk of scar dehiscence given in the NICE guidelines[41] is 3.5 per 1,000 for women having a trial of labour compared with 1.2 per 1,000 in women having a planned CS. In the study from Dublin in 1987 of over 2,000 consecutive cases of trial of scar eight women had scar dehiscence and 90.8 per cent achieved a vaginal birth. No babies died.[42]

NICE reviewed thirty-nine studies and found that the range of scar dehiscence was from 0 per 1,000 to 28 per 1,000 and twenty-eight studies found no difference in the relative risk of scar dehiscence. Flamm et al. in California did a prospective multicentre study and found a risk of less than 1 per cent in over 7,229 women with a previous uterine scar.[43] The NICE guidelines do not come out strongly in favour of VBAC which one would have expected in a publication which followed public, professional and governmental concern about the rising rate of CS. They say that, in childbirth following CS:

> ...the decision about mode of birth should consider maternal preferences and priorities, general discussion of the overall risks and benefits of CS (specific risks

---

41 NICE, 2004, p.95
42 Molloy et al., 1987
43 Flamm et al., 1994

and benefits uncertain), risk of *uterine* rupture [my emphasis, discussed above] and perinatal morbidity and mortality... Women who want VBAC *should be supported* [my emphasis].... [44]

They then go on to list the risks taken from the systematic reviews. The majority of these studies are not from this country. Practice in the US is different in some ways and their experience of trial of scar is much less than in this country because it is only relatively recently that the policy 'Once a CS always a CS' has been questioned. However, since the NICE review Smith et al. in Cambridge have analysed the Scottish database for births between 1991 and 1999 and confirmed a higher rate of perinatal death in the women having a trial of scar which was related to scar dehiscence.[45]

Comment

In my view VBAC should be the preferred option offered to women with a uterine scar. In well-conducted units the risk to the baby is not as high as the loss of one baby in 1,000 calculated from the systematic reviews compared with one in 10,000 for those women having a planned CS.

If you give women the results from these pooled studies and say without any further explanation that there is a ten-times greater risk of the baby dying and twice the risk of the scar rupturing most women will agree to or even ask to have a repeat CS. I think doctors need to use the correct language in an objective way so that the risks are not overemphasised. They should analyse the results in their own hospitals so they can give the local risks which are more relevant to the woman than studies where the skills of personnel and organisation of services may differ significantly from their own unit.

As the risk of the woman dying, whilst low, after CS is still higher than that of vaginal birth[46] and the mother has the problems following any surgical operation, higher rates of haemorrhage, infection and thrombosis this tips the balance in favour of trial of labour to our minds. In addition, the longer recovery time and difficulties in coping with the baby have not been measured in any RCT and so do not appear in these reviews; but they are important factors for women and their doctors to take into consideration.

Smith et al. in Cambridge have attempted to produce a model which predicts the chance that a woman will deliver vaginally based on maternal height, weight and age. Using women who were induced with prostaglandin in the Scottish database they correctly predicted that women with a low risk of CS would have

---

44 NICE, 2004, p.16
45 Smith et al., 2004
46 McMahon et al., 1996

a CS, with 8.6 per cent having one as against the 7.9 per cent expected.[47] Further work on this idea may help women to decide whether it is worthwhile trying to deliver normally.

Breech presentation: 10.8 per cent of CS, 2.3 per cent of women

The proportion of women having a CS for breech in the National Audit was 2.3 per cent and breech was the reason for 10.8 per cent of the total CS operations. Women whose first pregnancy was breech had a 91.9 per cent CSR and those who had had a baby before had a 98.2 per cent CSR so even before the Term Breech Trial, nine women out of ten at term were having a CS. There has been debate for many years about the best way to deliver a baby presenting bottom first instead of head first. Because the baby is more likely to be breech earlier in the pregnancy and premature babies are more likely to die, this complicated crude comparisons of the PMR. Also, some babies with congenital anomalies are more likely to present by the breech and more likely to die.

Small scale RCTs did not show convincing evidence that CS was preferable for the baby and, of course, the mother has the problems that follow any surgical operation, as discussed above.[48] The Term Breech Trial was a large RCT with participants from many countries.[49] It appeared to be well designed and had a steering group that decided to end the trial before recruitment had finished, after it had analysed the interim results. Many obstetricians think that this is the definitive answer that the profession and women have been looking for; this is certainly the view of the NICE guideline group, which recommended that planned CS should be offered to women with a term singleton breech presentation.

However there are a minority of obstetricians, of which I am one, and many midwives who are not convinced by this study. Roosmalen and Roosmalen pointed out that several of the thirteen perinatal deaths in the planned vaginal group were not related to breech birth. One was cephalic and one was a stillborn twin and therefore should not have been in the trial at all![50] Glazerman has concluded that the original term breech recommendations should be withdrawn[51] and that outcomes in the babies were similar.[52]

I have a problem: one cannot enter a patient into an RCT unless one is unsure about the treatment being assessed (being unsure which treatment is better is known as 'equipoise'). As I believe that it is safe to deliver babies by the breech

---

47 Smith et al., 2004
48 Collea et al., 1980
49 Hannah et al., 2000
50 Roosmalen & Roosmalen, 2002
51 Glazerman, 2006
52 Whyte et al., 2004

and have been doing so successfully for some years, I could not enter the trial. If this is true of other experienced obstetricians then maybe those who took part were not very experienced. Certainly, I find three of the four babies who were said to have had a 'difficult' vaginal birth to have been of surprisingly low weight to have got into difficulties (the four weights being 2,400, 2,550, 3,000 and 3,500gm). The other problem is that half of the centres provided less than ten cases which makes one wonder whether they were experienced in breech birth.

Kotaska, a Canadian obstetrician, recently pointed out that most of the 131 centres were in North America where the overall rate of vaginal breech birth was 13 per cent. In the trial this rose to 57 per cent suggesting to him that doctors were pushing vaginal birth to the limit and learning on the job.[53] He also noted that the study protocol allowed a rate of progress of half a cm per hour whereas most people expect a rate of 1 cm per hour and consider slow progress a warning sign. Up to 3.5 hours were allowed in the second stage. Again, most obstetricians would not expect more than 2 hours in the second stage even with an epidural.

However, supporting the conclusions of the Hannah trial, another Dutch study has just been published looking at the mode of birth and perinatal outcome from routinely collected data before and after the publication of this study.[54] They found that before the trial the CSR for term breech was 50 per cent with a PMR of 3.5 per 1,000. Within two months of its publication the CSR rose to 80 per cent and has remained there. The PMR fell to 1.8 per 1,000. Fifty per cent of women now have a planned CS and the remainder are allowed a trial of vaginal birth. Thirty per cent of the group end up with an emergency CS and 20 per cent still deliver vaginally. So 40 per cent of those who had a trial of labour delivered vaginally.

A recent report from Shrewsbury of 1,400 term breech babies over a ten-year period showed that 38 per cent were delivered by planned CS, just over 32 per cent had a CS in labour and 29 per cent had a vaginal breech birth. The overall PMR was 2.8 per 1,000. One baby delivered by CS died from lethal congenital anomalies. Three were born vaginally, one followed an abruptio placentae (see later) which could have happened whether breech or cephalic, one died from a traumatic breech birth and one death followed sub-optimal care. Babies presenting head first can also die from sub-optimal care so there was one death directly attributable to breech birth.[55]

Women faced with a breech presentation at term may be offered External Cephalic Version (ECV) where the doctor attempts to turn the baby round to a head-first position using manual pressure. Like everything in life this procedure

53 Kotaska, 2004
54 Reitberg et al., 2005
55 Pradhan et al., 2005

is not completely without risk and for some years in the 1970s and 1980s its use fell out of fashion. There may be transient fetal heart changes in up to 16 per cent of women and 3 per cent will be admitted for induction of labour. One per cent will have painless vaginal bleeding and in a similar number there will be some separation of the placenta according to a systematic review by Hofmeyer.[56] Despite the anxiety that this will produce in women, the RCOG issued a guideline in 2001 recommending that all women should be offered this procedure.[57]

In the National Audit, a third of women who had a CS had been offered this but there is no data about how many women had a successful version. A recent systematic review concluded that there was significant reduction in breech births and CS in women who had had an ECV compared with those who had not.[58]

Women's views may differ from those of obstetricians. After publication of results from an analysis of routinely collected data in the North West Thames Region showing a higher PMR with vaginal breech birth than CS, the authors were surprised that women declined the offer of a CS.[59] Benna Waites, when faced with a breech presentation was shocked by how little information was available to women. After researching the area, she published a very useful and readable book reviewing the literature and dealing with her emotional reactions which I am sure women will find helpful.[60] AIMs has produced a breech edition of its newsletter with an article by Mary Cronk, a midwife with immense experience in breech birth, which gives some useful advice.[61]

Comment

The difficulty for women is that younger obstetricians have often little or no experience in breech birth and so in effect it is safer to have a planned CS than a badly managed vaginal breech birth. However, it is not difficult to learn the skills needed and the Advanced Life Support Obstetrics (ALSO) course has trained over one thousand midwives, GPs and obstetricians since its inception (see www.also.org.uk). It was imported from the US where family doctors became worried when obstetricians deserted rural communities and they were left to cope with birth.

The important thing with a breech birth is to let the baby descend on its own through the birth canal and not to pull the body down. Patience is the answer and

---

56 Hofmeyer, 2001
57 RCOG, 2001b
58 Hofmeyer, 2001
59 Thorpe-Beeston et al., 1992
60 Waites, 2003
61 Cronk, 2005

we were taught to 'sit on our hands'. Once the head enters the pelvis, the blood supply to the baby is cut off and it is essential to look at the clock because the minutes seem like hours, the baby often making attempts to breathe whilst the body is hanging down. Latterly, before my retirement, I encouraged women to adopt the upright or kneeling position. This seems to help the natural process of birth and is certainly preferable to the 'stranded beetle' or lithotomy position (where the woman lies on her back with her legs supported by stirrups) favoured by conventional obstetrics. It is important that the art of breech birth is not lost as there will always be women who labour rapidly and come in with the breech on the perineum. Staff need to know what to do as a CS at this late stage is not good for mother or baby.

Maternal request: 7.3 per cent of CS, 1.6 per cent of women

This was the fifth most common reason given in the National Audit by consultants and 7.3 per cent of CS were said to be done for maternal request, accounting for 1.6 per cent of women. Whether there were medical reasons for the woman's request is not known. In the phase 2 research, 5.3 per cent of women said they would like a CS (3.3 per cent of women having their first and 7 per cent of those having a subsequent baby), so it appears that about a third of women had their wishes granted.[62] Obstetricians estimated that from one to twenty women per hundred seen in the antenatal clinic requested CS in the absence of any medical or fetal reason for this. They agreed to about a half of these requests but they exercised discretion depending on the clinical circumstances. Only 3.7 per cent would agree to book a planned CS in the absence of any medical indication if the woman was a healthy twenty-five-year-old having her first pregnancy, whereas 30.9 per cent would agree if she was forty-two. Only a quarter would decline to do this and refer her to another colleague in the first case, and 6.8 per cent in the second. The remainder would not advise CS but accept it if the woman has said she wants a CS. Seventy-eight per cent of consultants agreed that planned CS was not the safest option for the mother and views on the baby were almost equally divided with 51 per cent believing that planned CS was safer for the baby.[63]

There is considerable literature about maternal request which is well reviewed by Susan Bewley and Jayne Cockburn[64] and in the NICE guidelines (p.37), and which is also covered in chapter three of this book.

Having dealt with the major reasons for CS which are in the main relative indications I will now deal with the absolute reasons. These are much less frequently cited as the reason for a CS.

62 Thomas & Paranjothy, 2001, p.101
63 Thomas & Paranjothy, 2001, p.107
64 Bewley & Cockburn, 2003

Malpresentations and unstable lie: 3.4 per cent of CS, 0.7 per cent of women

The normal way for the fetus to lie in the womb is with the head flexed so that the vertex (a point on the skull between the two soft areas, the fontanelles) is the lowest point of the head. This means that the smallest diameter of the head will be traversing the bony pelvis and the head is well flexed. If the head is extended, either the face or the brow present. The diameter when the brow or forehead is the leading part of the head of a term baby is too large to go through the average pelvis and a CS is inevitable. With a face presentation, if the chin is at the front (mento-anterior) the head can be born if flexion occurs but if the position is with the chin at the back of the pelvis the head gets stuck and CS is needed.

Normally the fetus lies with its axis parallel to that of the mothers body and womb, but if the fetus lies across the womb (transverse lie) or is oblique or swinging around from one position to another there is a risk of cord prolapse when the woman goes into labour. Once the waters have broken with a transverse lie and the liquor has drained away, the uterus clamps round the fetal body and a CS is needed. Waiting for labour to start with an oblique lie may allow the woman to deliver naturally as the contractions often straighten up the lie. Unstable lie is more likely in a woman who has had several children, so waiting in hospital until labour starts is an (unattractive) option for her. However, if she understands what to do when she feels contractions or the waters break, I think it is safe to allow her to go home. If the waters break before she is in labour the cervix is likely to be closed and as the head is not in the pelvis, in the unlikely event of a cord prolapse, she can adopt the knee chest position to prevent pressure on the cord until she gets to hospital. With a transverse lie, a scan will show whether there is a low-lying placenta, fibroid or ovarian cyst preventing the head from entering the pelvis, which would indicate the need for a planned CS.

Problems with the placenta

Bleeding from the vagina during pregnancy should always be taken seriously and reported to a midwife or doctor. However, in the majority of cases the bleeding stops and may be due to 'incidental causes' such as a polyp or a cervical infection or to a cause that is never ascertained. However, there are two serious causes: placenta praevia and placental abruption.

Placenta praevia: 3.1 per cent of CS, 0.7 per cent of women

Placenta praevia is the name given to an abnormally situated placenta which is in the lower part of the uterus rather than the upper part. If the placenta completely covers the cervix or encroaches on it (grade 3 or 4) the woman must be delivered by CS as otherwise the bleeding during labour will kill her. If the

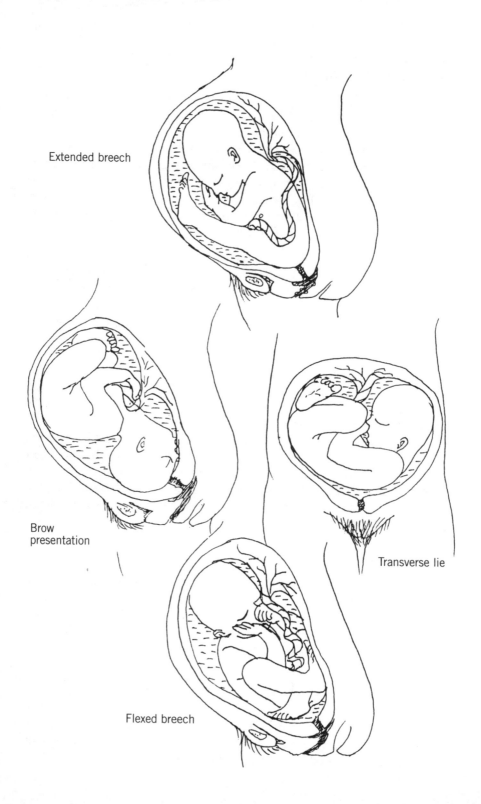

Extended breech

Brow presentation

Transverse lie

Flexed breech

placenta is less far down (grade 1 or 2) a vaginal birth is possible. With the practice of routine ultrasound scanning many women are told they have a low-lying placenta at 18-20 weeks but the majority of these (90-95 per cent) will be drawn away from the lower part of the uterus as this grows during the pregnancy. It is usual to repeat the scan at 32 weeks to see if that has happened, but I used to wait until 36 weeks if there had been no bleeding. This was because another scan is needed at 36 weeks if the placenta is still low at 32 weeks, and often there is no problem by then. In the majority of cases when there is a major degree of placenta praevia there will be bleeding and, unless the baby is mature, it is reasonable to transfuse the woman. At 38 or 39 weeks a planned CS is carried out,

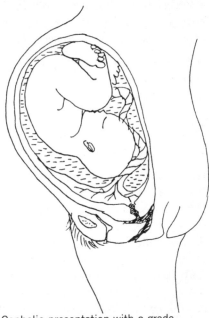

Cephalic presentation with a grade 3–4 placenta praevia

although if there has been no bleeding it is reasonable to check in theatre that the ultrasound pictures are accurate. This is done by performing an 'examination without anaesthaesia', with everything prepared to do a CS if necessary. A sterile vaginal examination is done, the head pushed into the pelvis with one hand and one feels through the tissues lateral to the cervix (the fornices) to see if the head can be felt. If it can, then one cautiously introduces a finger through the cervix and feels round until one does or does not feel the edge of the placenta. If it is not felt and there is no heavy bleeding, the membranes can be ruptured and an oxytocin drip put up to induce labour and ensure that the fetal head presses on to the placenta and compresses it against the bony pelvis. The fetus is not particularly at risk with a placenta praevia and so maternal considerations come first. A description of this procedure using a general anaesthetic is given in chapter six.

Abruptio placentae or placental abruption: 1.8 per cent of CS, 0.4 per cent of women

In this condition the placenta separates from the wall of the uterus. If the separation is massive the baby dies instantly and the woman becomes shocked by the pain and the blood loss. If she is in labour, rupturing the membranes may allow her to deliver vaginally. However, if the cervix is closed, a CS to relieve the pressure in the uterus will make it possible to treat the blood-clotting disorders which frequently follow. Fortunately this is rare and if the fetus is alive, swift action to perform a CS will save the baby and treat the mother. This condition is more likely to occur in a woman who has high blood pressure.

If there is only a small amount of bleeding, the pregnancy can be allowed to continue with careful checking to ensure that the placenta is transferring enough oxygen to the baby.

Eclampsia, pre-eclampsia (PET) and HELLP syndrome: 2.3 per cent of CS, 0.5 per cent of women

High blood pressure can exist before a woman becomes pregnant but it more frequently develops during pregnancy. The cause of this is still unknown – although poor formation of the placenta in early pregnancy may cause raised blood pressure in order to compensate for its poor functioning.[65] It usually develops after 24 weeks and it seems to me that there are two types: an early onset, often rapidly progressing type between 28 and 34 weeks; and a late onset, fairly benign condition later on in the pregnancy. Birth cures the condition so the objective is to allow the baby to grow and mature as long as possible whilst controlling the blood pressure so that the woman does not suffer ill effects. The triad of oedema (swelling), high blood pressure and protein in the urine is known as PET (and also as pregnancy related hypertension, PRH or pregnancy induced hypertension) and is more common in first pregnancies and in African or Afro-Caribbean women. If the disease is progressing fast and induction of labour seems unlikely to succeed then a planned CS is performed. In the uncommon but life-threatening condition of eclampsia, when the woman has fits, a CS may be life saving for her and the baby. In the HELLP syndrome (which seems to be increasing in incidence), platelet numbers decline and there are changes in the liver function tests so there may be problems with blood clotting. Early birth is advisable.

Other fetal reasons: 2.3 per cent of CS, 0.5 per cent of women

Cord prolapse is a life-threatening condition for the baby and requires immediate CS in a cephalic presentation as the blood supply to the baby can be cut off as the head enters the pelvis. This occurred in about one in a thousand pregnancies in the past but the National Audit does not give exact figures for this. Sometimes a CS is done if the baby is small for gestational age but I presume this was classified under 'presumed fetal compromise' so am unsure what all these other operations were done for. Some babies with congenital

---

65 Redman & Walker, 1992

abnormalities may need to be delivered by CS but this is rare. HIV may be included in this category as surgery is of questionable benefit for the mother. Primary herpes simplex in the last trimester of pregnancy is an indication for birth by CS to reduce the risk of transmission of the virus to the baby but both of these indications are rare.

Maternal medical disease: 1.9 per cent of CS, 0.4 per cent of women

Diabetes is probably the most important of these although far fewer women today have a planned CS for this cause now that diabetic control is much better. However, the baby may be large and it may be considered that a planned CS is preferable to a long difficult labour. Certain neurological conditions do not allow the woman to push so a CS should be done. Many women with cardiac disease are safer having a vaginal birth than a CS with the added problems in the recovery period, but some obstetricians still advise a CS as being less stressful than labour. Women who have had a vaginal repair for prolapse are advised to have a planned CS so that the repair holds.

Previous traumatic birth: 1.7 per cent of CS, 0.4 per cent of women

This could be for emotional or physical trauma. Some women do develop faecal incontinence following vaginal birth or have a bad tear of the cervix and vagina which makes repeat vaginal birth inadvisable. The audit does not break this down any further but it is a sad commentary on the state of obstetric and midwifery services if the previous birth was so emotionally traumatic that the woman required a CS in the next pregnancy.

Multiple pregnancy: 1.2 per cent of CS, 0.3 per cent of women

The incidence of multiple pregnancy has increased with the advent of in-vitro fertilisation to fifteen per thousand. Fifty-nine per cent of twin pregnancies were delivered by CS, half before thirty-seven weeks and 37 per cent as planned CS, mostly because the first twin was breech. The use of CS for multiple pregnancies has increased without good evidence of benefit.[66] Triplets for example can safely be delivered vaginally[67] yet only three sets achieved this in the National Audit, 92 per cent being delivered by CS. In 3.5 per cent of cases CS was done for the second twin after vaginal birth of the first twin and this is a situation where internal version

---

66 Rhudstrom et al., 1990
67 Wildschut et al., 1995

and breech extraction can be done if the second twin is not presenting as it should. Again, this is a skill that younger obstetricians may not be acquiring. Expecting that labour will progress normally to a vaginal birth even if the first twin is breech would be appreciated by many women. Emma Mahoney spoke movingly about how she had to fight to experience delivering twins normally at a meeting of the Forum of Maternity and the Newborn at the Royal Society of Medicine in 2004 and has written a delightful book about her experience.[68]

The future

The NICE guidelines call for further research to evaluate the place of planned CS in preterm births including preterm breech, twin and triplet pregnancies, small-for-gestational-age infants and complementary therapies. In the meantime, their review of the literature did not find that on the basis of RCTs the following factors had any influence on the risk of having a CS.[69]

- Walking in labour
- The position in the second stage of labour
- Immersion in water
- Epidural analgesia
- Drinking raspberry leaf tea.

Conclusion

As the primary CSR rises, it increases the rate of repeat CS – the biggest contribution to the overall CSR was the 8 per cent of women who had a scarred uterus. Of these, 63.5 per cent had a repeat CS and this contributed almost a quarter (23.1 per cent) to the overall CSR. Robson, in an attempt to compare different hospitals and populations, divided women into groups. Using this tool shows that women having their first baby who had a spontaneous onset of labour had an 11.8 per cent CSR whereas those who were induced had more than double this (27.9 per cent).[70] Whilst some of these women may have had other problems which made a CSR more likely such as PET or SGA babies, reduction in unnecessary inductions might reduce the CSR. Careful evaluation of the woman is needed and I do not believe this is a task for midwives who are the experts in normal birth. These induced labours, along with CS before labour in primigravidae, contributed the second largest number of CS to the total (17.8 per cent). So, better management of this group could reduce the primary CSR and increased use of VBAC could reduce the number of repeat CS. This could make an immediate impact on the CSR which has risen inexorably since the last edition of this book in 1993 from 13 per cent to 22.9 per cent in 2004.

---

68 Mahoney, 2005
69 NICE, 2004, p.46
70 Robson et al., 1996

Whilst 50 per cent of women felt that they had the right to have a CS and 73 per cent a vaginal birth under any circumstances, only 63 per cent agreed with the statement that 'giving birth was a natural process that should not be interfered with unless absolutely necessary'.[71] In contrast 80 per cent of consultants agreed with this statement.[72] As only two-thirds will give birth normally, are women being realistic whilst consultants delude themselves? Have women lost their confidence in their own ability to give birth naturally? Only 3 per cent of women having their first baby wanted a CS and Ryding has shown how psychological help can reduce these requests which are often due to fear of labour.[73] About a fifth of women who had had a previous CS wanted another and they were the majority of those (7 per cent) who had had a baby and wanted a CS. All but two of the 162 consultants who responded also agreed that the threshold for doing a CS was lower. The median CSR accepted was 20 per cent – a considerable rise since our survey in 1990.

If the consensus is that the CSR is too high and detrimental to the health of women then we must change the culture amongst obstetricians, midwives and women so that CS is not accepted as an easy way for women to give birth.

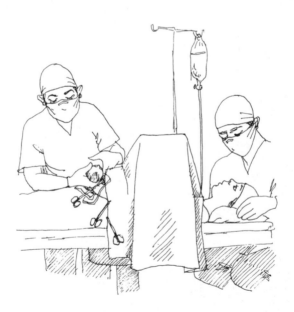

71 Thomas & Paranjothy, 2001, p.101
72 Ibid., p.105
73 Ryding, 1993

6 The modern caesarean operation: coping with a caesarean – for parents, midwives and teachers

If a woman is awake for the operation, every effort is usually made to explain to her and her partner or friend what is going on and to make the experience as positive as possible.

IN THIS CHAPTER WE DISCUSS HOW TO PREPARE FOR A CAESAREAN; we describe what to expect during the procedure and after; we give advice to midwives caring for women after a caesarean; and throughout we present the sort of information that antenatal teachers might pass on to expectant parents.

Preparation for a caesarean

The extent to which a woman can prepare for a caesarean depends in large part on whether it is a planned or an emergency operation. A planned caesarean is one which is planned in advance before the woman goes into labour. An emergency caesarean is usually performed during labour when the mother's or the baby's life may be considered to be at risk or when labour is not progressing. Many women having a caesarean may never have had an operation, or regional (epidural or spinal) or general anaesthetic before, so they may have to come to terms with this as well as the fact that they will be giving birth by caesarean rather than vaginally. The NICE guidelines suggest that women should be given evidence-based information about caesareans during the antenatal period as one in five of them will have a CS.[1] This recommendation is not based on hard evidence but is the informed opinion of the group preparing the guidelines and we have some reservations about this. If a leaflet is given without any discussion, will this influence the way the woman approaches labour? It seems possible that fear and anxiety might well increase the number of women asking for a planned CS unless there is time for adequate unbiased discussion and where will this time come from? As our survey of obstetricians' attitudes

---

1   NICE, 2004

(chapter 8) confirmed, there is still a wide spectrum of views and it gives an opportunity for those obstetricians who believe that the best way to deliver is surgically to put that view across. Lastly, whilst overall the rate is one in five, for a woman going into spontaneous labour at term the risk of having a CS is more like one in twenty for a first pregnancy and one in 100 for a subsequent birth.[2] The NSCA was published in 2001[3] but there is no agreed leaflet available for hospitals to give women – perhaps this is something that could be taken up by the All Party Maternity Care Working Party.

Women having a planned caesarean can ask their doctor and midwife about the operation. They should be able to discuss the kind of anaesthetic to be used, whether their partner or friend can be present and any questions they may have about the procedure and their postnatal care. It is especially important to discuss what support will be available in hospital if a woman intends to breastfeed her baby. If a woman does not speak or understand English, it is essential that her midwife ensures that she has access to an interpreter or link-worker so that she can prepare for the operation.

Some women having a planned caesarean may feel uncomfortable about continuing to attend NHS or NCT antenatal classes. However, many women still find these valuable in order to enable themselves and their partners/friends to prepare for the birth and for life with a new baby. Breathing techniques for labour can help women remain calm if they are frightened at the prospect of the operation or if they are alarmed at the physical sensations often experienced during a caesarean. They also help with coughing and clearing the chest of secretions after a caesarean, particularly one under general anaesthetic. The relaxation techniques, as well as being skills useful for life in general, can help a woman cope with the caesarean itself, with post-operative pain and with breastfeeding.

Women and couples attending a well-run group often find the support from other members of their class invaluable. If they do not have a friend or relative who has had the same experience, the midwife or antenatal teacher may be able to put them in touch with another woman or couple who have recently had a caesarean. Raising the subject at a class can also help prepare those women who may have an emergency caesarean, particularly if the chances of having a caesarean are presented in a realistic yet non-alarming way.

One of the respondents in our first survey of women commented: 'I think much more should be taught about caesareans at antenatal classes to prepare women for the after-effects as it seems commonplace nowadays.'

---

2   Savage, 2005, unpublished data from four hospitals, from the author
3   Thomas & Paranjothy, 2001

Another woman who participated in a NCT survey said:

> At thirty-six weeks caesareans began to be mentioned and/or trial of labour. This was the hardest part, to decide what to do. I made contact with the local NCT and found a lady who had had the same problem. The hospital held a 'Caesar Evening' which was very helpful. I feel more information about caesareans should be given antenatally. For me it was not such a shock as I was able to find out so much beforehand.[4]

Women expecting a planned caesarean have the opportunity to gear themselves up mentally for the operation. They can make arrangements in advance for practical support when they come home with the new baby, particularly if they have other children, and for the time when their partner, if they have one, may have gone back to work. It is also possible for women who use a homeopath or herbalist to take advice about which remedies will aid their recovery after the operation (although little or no evidence is available about the efficacy of these remedies). If a woman intends to breastfeed, it is important for her to let her midwives know and to have this written into her notes, particularly if she is having a general anaesthetic, as regrettably it is not always assumed that a woman will breastfeed. The NICE guidelines should improve this position as they state that women should be informed that they are not at higher risk of difficulties with breastfeeding. The evidence is that the delay in putting the baby to the breast is the major factor: if women are encouraged to put the baby to the breast within two hours they are as successful at breastfeeding as women who have had a vaginal delivery.[5] She can also learn about the most comfortable positions for breastfeeding after the operation (see 'Further Information for Parents', p.269).

The preparations for an emergency caesarean are similar to those for a planned one, but everything happens faster. This can be bewildering for the woman, particularly if she does not understand English or is deaf, and so it is even more important that staff help by explaining to her and to her partner or friend what is happening and the reasons for it. If the baby has become distressed, the woman will probably be asked to lie on her left side. This shifts the weight of the uterus away from the big blood vessels in her back. She may also be given oxygen to breathe through a mask. These are both ways of helping to give the baby more oxygen. The woman can use the breathing techniques learned for labour to keep calm.

A respondent in our survey of women's experiences said that more information before the caesarean may have helped her post-operatively:

> When they finished stitching, I started to be sick and then felt like I could not get air into my lungs, as though someone was sitting on my chest. This lasted for

---

4   NCT, 1992
5   NICE, 2004

three hours. When talking to the doctor a couple of days later she assured me that this was entirely clinical, to do with my blood pressure and temperature, and that this was quite common. Talking to other caesarean women on the wards later, we had all experienced this to some degree and felt that if we had been told this may happen beforehand then we would not have panicked as much at the time.

Both before and during an emergency operation the woman's partner or friend will have an important part to play in supporting the woman and helping her understand and come to terms with what is happening. This is particularly so if she is exhausted after a long labour or drowsy from the use of pain-killing drugs. The partner or friend can take a photograph of the baby when it is first born and, if present during the operation, can describe the birth to the woman so she knows about the first few precious moments of her baby's life. 'Precious moments lost forever' was how one of the women in our survey described her caesarean under general anaesthetic.

If the partner or friend is not present (often the case if a general anaesthetic is used), it is important that the woman's midwife or other member of staff present sees the woman after the operation to describe the birth and to answer any questions she may have. Sometimes it is possible for a member of staff or a student to take photographs. Doctors may not invite the partner or friend into theatre, thinking that he or she may be shocked by the tubes going into the unconscious woman. If you want to be present, ask whether you can come in once the anaesthetist has done his or her job.

> I had nothing but praise for the sensitive way my emergency caesarean was handled – I was consulted then at every stage.[6]

Going into hospital

Women having a planned caesarean may be admitted to hospital during the afternoon or evening before the operation. They can spend the time finding out about the postnatal ward to which they will go after the operation. They can begin to meet some of the midwives and feel a little more at home. Women who would rather spend the night at home may ask to come in on the day of the operation. This is often possible and a time is given after which the woman must not eat or drink anything if a general anaesthetic is planned or in case it should prove necessary. A visit to the ward can be arranged a week or so beforehand.

It is important for the woman to be told what is happening at every stage, including who is responsible for her care (particularly after any change in shift), and to feel that she can ask about anything she needs to know.

---

6   NCT, 1992

Choice of anaesthetic

My first section was done under a general anaesthetic and the second under spinal. I felt so much better and brighter in myself after the spinal. I could still feel involved in the birth, have my partner present and see my baby as soon as she was born.

The 1991 study of women's experiences revealed that 60 per cent of women were asleep for their caesarean and 40 per cent were awake for the operation. Of the latter group, most women had an epidural block, while a few had a spinal block. Because women have said that they missed the first precious moments of their baby's life, and because of the increased risk of general anaesthetics, most doctors advise women whenever possible to have a caesarean under epidural or spinal. The recent study found that the consultants estimated that 80 per cent of women were awake for emergency operations and 90 per cent for planned surgery. Of the 100 consultants asked this question, the majority gave a figure of over 90 per cent for all surgery and the increased use of spinal block rather than an epidural was notable. In our most recent study of women's experiences (chapter 7), 18 per cent reported having a general anaesthetic.

The other disadvantages of a general anaesthetic are:

- A woman may feel quite drowsy and disorientated for the first two or three days after delivery
- The drugs may make the baby sleep and cause difficulties with breastfeeding
- The woman's partner or friend is not usually present during the operation, and may have to press to be allowed into the theatre
- Small but real medical risks of aspiration/failed intubation and, rarely, death.

However, some women prefer to be asleep for a caesarean and, if that is the case, they should feel able to ask for a general anaesthetic because the risks for an individual woman are small.

The main advantages of an epidural or spinal anaesthetic for a caesarean are that:

- The woman can be conscious for the operation
- Her partner or friend is normally invited to be present
- An epidural can be used for more effective pain relief postnatally
- The woman is easier to care for afterwards
- The baby can be put to the breast earlier.

The main disadvantage of an epidural for caesarean is the small risk (1 per cent) of a dural tap (see below).

When an emergency caesarean is necessary, there may or may not be time for an epidural to be administered but a spinal anaesthetic can usually be given. If a woman already has an epidural in place for routine pain relief, it can be 'topped up' with a larger dose of local anaesthetic to give the total pain relief necessary for abdominal surgery.

Spinal block

> With chronic back stiffness, I have been frightened for years of the idea of an epidural or spinal. I initially wanted a general anaesthetic. The anaesthetist persuaded me spinal was better for the baby. I was very pleased with the result – it worked very well.

A woman may be unable to have an epidural because there is insufficient time, or a general anaesthetic may be inadvisable for medical reasons – or may be unacceptable to the woman. In these circumstances, the anaesthetist may be able to offer her a spinal block. A spinal block is a single injection of local anaesthetic given between two vertebrae in the lower spine, below the site of an epidural (see illustration below). A spinal block is quicker to perform and takes effect faster than an epidural, but lasts less time.

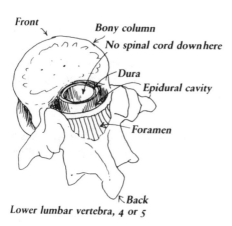

Spinal anatomy showing the bony vertebra and spinal cord with its coverings

Front

Bony column

No spinal cord down here

Dura

Epidural cavity

Foramen

Back

Lower lumbar vertebra, 4 or 5

In the past, spinal block for caesarean was quite rare, possibly because of the risk of a severe headache afterwards from loss of spinal fluid following dural puncture. Now that doctors use finer needles and the technique carries less risk of leakage, it has become more widely available. Because a spinal block can be performed only once, some anaesthetists also insert an epidural before the operation proceeds. This combined spinal/ epidural procedure is used in case anaesthesia is needed for longer than anticipated, and also allows pain relief to be administered after the operation. It means anaesthesia is obtained more quickly than in an epidural on its own but it cannot be used if there is a serious emergency as general anaesthetic is still quicker to induce.

In some hospitals, a spinal block alone is offered routinely instead of an epidural for both planned and emergency caesareans in order to save anaesthetists' time. Some women find that although they may experience more post-operative pain (because of the absence of the epidural tube for optimal pain relief), the quicker anaesthetic procedure makes the operation more acceptable.

Procedure for administering an epidural block

An intravenous drip is always inserted into the woman's arm before the procedure in order that a serious fall in blood pressure (which can adversely affect the baby) may be corrected quickly. The woman must then remain still for this skilled procedure, usually lying on her side or sitting on the side of the bed with her head bent forwards. After an injection of local anaesthetic has been given to numb the skin of the lower back, the anaesthetist inserts a needle closed with a stilette (removable centre) between two vertebrae in the lower back into the epidural space around the spinal cord (see illustration below). Once the epidural space is identified, the stilette is withdrawn and a fine plastic tube is threaded through. The tube is taped securely to the woman's back and a small filter attached at the level of her shoulder. Some women find they have more sensation than others during the procedure: most do not feel anything, while a few feel quite uncomfortable. A test dose of local anaesthetic is given and, if all is well, the needle is withdrawn leaving the fine plastic tube in place. Experienced anaesthetists may withdraw the needle before injecting the test dose. While the epidural is taking effect, the baby's heart rate is monitored continuously and a careful check kept on the woman's blood pressure in case it drops suddenly.

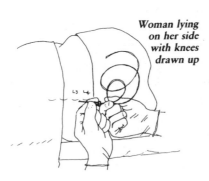

Woman lying on her side with knees drawn up

Introducing a catheter through a needle into the epidural space

There is a small risk of a dural tap when an epidural is inserted (1 per cent). This is when the needle goes in too far, punctures the protective sheath around the spinal cord and causes cerebrospinal fluid (the liquid that bathes the spinal cord and brain) to leak out. This can cause a woman to have a severe headache for several days. If a dural tap occurs, the woman is immediately asked to lie down. The headache is more severe when she sits up, so she is advised to lie down for as long as is necessary after the birth. This obviously makes life with a new baby much more difficult. Another more common problem is that the epidural does not work evenly or provide effective pain relief, so a general anaesthetic may be needed.

Some anaesthetists correct a dural tap by performing a 'blood patch'. This is done by drawing up some of the woman's blood into a needle and injecting the blood into the site of the dural tap. In many cases this prevents a headache. The risks of a dural tap are lower when an epidural is administered by an experienced anaesthetist skilled in the procedure.

The operation is not allowed to start until the anaesthetist is satisfied that the anaesthetic is effective. This is tested by using a very cold spray or a sharp needle. Once the sensation of pain and cold are gone, the epidural is giving total pain relief.

Procedure for administering a general anaesthetic

One concern about general anaesthesia is that acid stomach contents may reach the lungs and cause problems. Most maternity units do not allow women to eat or drink once they are in the active phase of labour and some give regular doses of antacids routinely to all labouring women. NICE guidelines suggest that isotonic drinks are safe (i.e. not concentrated glucose drinks) and that although a low residue diet increases the amount of fluid in the stomach the effects on general anaesthetic are uncertain.[7] It is too early to know whether this has made any difference in practice to hospital policies. There are differences of opinion among anaesthetists as to the best regimes. Prior to a general anaesthetic, drugs may be given to neutralise or reduce the stomach contents.

The anaesthetic is introduced by means of a plastic cannula in a vein in the woman's arm or hand. The drug passes into the bloodstream and leads to the woman being asleep in about thirty seconds. During this time the anaesthetist's assistant applies pressure to the woman's neck, pressing on the cricoid area to prevent any acid stomach contents reaching the lungs and causing damage. The anaesthetist next gives another injection which relaxes all the muscles. A tube is then introduced over the back of the throat and into the windpipe, after which the cricoid pressure can be released. The tube is then attached to a ventilator which breathes for the woman during the operation, ensuring she has the right amount of gas to keep her asleep and oxygen both for herself and the baby. Oxygen levels (using a clip on the finger), blood pressure and pulse are recorded throughout and displayed on a screen next to the anaesthetist.

Procedure for caesarean section

The woman will be wearing a hospital gown, will have removed any jewellery and contact lenses and may have had a little of her pubic hair shaved to clear the usual site of the caesarean section, slightly below the 'bikini line'. Shaving is not in fact necessary. The woman's bladder is emptied by a catheter which most maternity units leave in place until the next day. The catheter is always left in for at least twelve hours after the last epidural top up as regional anaesthesia interferes with bladder function. A soft metal plate is strapped around one of the woman's legs. This is the diathermy equipment that allows special forceps to be used to burn ('cauterise') small blood vessels in the wound and so control

---

7   NICE, 2004

bleeding. A vertical screen is also positioned at the level of the woman's waist to protect her from the diathermy. However, if she wishes, a mirror can be positioned to enable her to see what is going on. The operating table is tilted fifteen degrees, usually to the left, so that pressure on the large blood vessels is avoided as this can lead to a fall in blood pressure. This is even more likely to happen with regional anaesthetic but about 6 per cent of women suffer from 'supine hypotension' in the last few weeks of pregnancy and feel dizzy or sick if they lie flat.

The operating theatre, usually within the labour suite, contains the main operating table with large circular theatre lights above it. In addition there is a trolley for resuscitating the baby with a heater above it to keep the baby warm, and an oxygen supply. There is a cot and, should it be needed, an incubator.

There are usually four doctors present: an anaesthetist who will be at the mother's head, an obstetrician, an assistant, and a paediatrician who will check the baby after the birth. There are also several midwives including the 'scrub nurse', in charge of handing the instruments to the obstetrician, and the woman's midwife. In teaching hospitals there may be students and trainee anaesthetists as well. If a woman is awake for the operation, every effort is usually made to explain to her and her partner or friend what is going on and to make the experience as positive as possible. Many women find that a cheerful and positive attitude on the part of the staff in the theatre makes the caesarean a less daunting experience than often anticipated.

> I felt frightened but confident at the same time. The theatre staff made me feel very special, I had lots of attention. I was overwhelmed with gratitude when they delivered our baby.
>
> The staff were very supportive and were always reassuring me throughout the whole birth because it was my first birth and having a hard time as well. If I have to have a caesarean again I would hope that I would be fortunate enough to have similar staff as I had for my first.[8]

All staff wash their hands thoroughly and wear sterile gowns and gloves. The anaesthetist will have ensured that the woman is sufficiently anaesthetised. He or she may use a needle or ice cube on different parts of the woman's abdomen to test for sensation. The woman's abdomen is exposed and cleaned with antiseptic solution, then sterile towels are draped over it, leaving only a small opening through which the operation will be performed. During the procedure some women feel nausea or dizziness (particularly after the baby is born), and some women vomit. Oxygen can be administered through a small mask to alleviate this, or anti-emetic/anti-sickness drugs are given.

---

8   See chapter 7 for women's experiences of CS

To deliver a baby by caesarean, an incision or cut is made first in the wall of the abdomen and is generally about five or six inches long. This is usually horizontal and sometimes called the 'bikini cut'. NICE recommends a slightly higher cut, the Cohen incision rather than the Pfannensteil which has been used for thirty years.[9] Rarely, if the baby is in a transverse position or if there is placenta praevia or some other medical reason, a vertical incision might be used. Even if the woman has a previous vertical scar, a horizontal incision may be used to make post-operative recovery more rapid. Even with good regional anaesthesia, a caesarean can be full of strange sensations for the woman, who may panic if she is not prepared for this and wonders what she might feel next. If she hates the sensations and finds that she cannot cope with being awake for the operation, she should tell the anaesthetist and, if she prefers, ask to have a general anaesthetic. Women have reported feeling 'as if someone were drawing on your skin with a pencil', 'feeling slightly tickly' or 'a sharp pain over the pubic bone' as the obstetrician made the first incision. Pain sensation is more easily abolished than stretching feelings. One anaesthetist described it more vividly: 'You may feel something, like someone rummaging around inside you, but it's weird rather than painful'.

One woman in our survey said that she 'did not anticipate so much tugging and pulling. I did not know how I would be stitched or stapled. The number of people around me was disquieting.'

It normally takes only five to ten minutes to deliver the baby. The uterus is in the middle of the abdomen with the bowels above and behind. The bladder lies over the lower part of the uterus and is pushed down so that the obstetrician can reach the thinner lower segment of the uterus. A second horizontal incision is made in the lower segment of the uterus. Both incisions may be cauterised to minimise blood loss. Women have reported a 'sensation of wet' as the warm amniotic fluid runs down between their legs after the second incision. An electric pump is used to suck out the amniotic fluid and any blood from the uterus; some parents comment on the 'slurping' noises. The doctor's hand then reaches deep into the uterus and delivers the baby through the opening. If the baby is head down, the doctor may be able to cup a hand under the head and lift it through the opening, but if there is difficulty in delivering the baby's head, small forceps are used instead. Once the head is through, the rest of the baby's body usually slips out easily in a similar manner to a vaginal birth. However a small proportion of women end up with J or T incisions if the surgeon is not speedy and the uterus contracts around the neck. In addition there is evidence that the risk of head entrapment in premature babies is the same at vaginal and CS delivery at about 5 per cent[10] because the premature baby has a larger head

---

9   NICE, 2004
10 Bewley, S. (personal communication)

in relation to its body. A woman who is awake for the operation may feel a variety of sensations as the baby is delivered, but should feel no pain. Women have described sensations as if someone were 'rummaging around the bottom of a drawer' or a 'shopping bag'. The baby usually splutters and gasps and may cry. The umbilical cord is clamped and cut immediately. The paediatrician will normally want to check the baby and suck out any fluid from its nose and mouth. The doctor will then deliver the placenta and membranes by gently pulling on the umbilical cord. If the woman has not been in labour (as in a planned caesarean), some doctors stretch the cervix open from inside the uterus to allow drainage (of blood and other fluids) into the vagina. Others consider this unnecessary and think it may increase the risk of infection.

Under general anaesthetic, the level given to the woman during the birth is relatively light so that the baby is not born too drowsy. Because of this, women sometimes have an awareness of voices or things happening but there should be no sensation of pain. After the baby is born, the level of anaesthetic is increased and the much longer process of putting the uterus and abdominal wall back together again begins. This usually takes about thirty to fifty minutes. Dissolving sutures are used to sew the wound in the uterus. The final layer of the skin is nowadays usually closed by a continuous hidden stitch kept in place by beads at either end or by staples which are removed after four or five days, when the outside of the wound has healed. Rarely, it may be beneficial to remove any blood collected in the wound with a small plastic drain coming from the side of the wound and leading into a small glass bottle but the routine use of drains is not recommended by NICE.[11] The wound is covered either by spraying on a plastic protective layer, or with gauze and sticking plaster or similar sticky tape. Antibiotic prophylaxis (one dose by injection) against infection is now recommended routinely for all women.[12] Anti-clot prophylaxis is given to prevent clots on the legs and lungs. Whether a woman just has TED (thromboembolic elastic) stockings or has injections to thin the blood depends upon her risk status. Obese women are more at risk of clots and should ensure they have the full treatment.

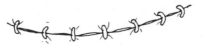

Running stitch under the skin, fixed with beads

Wound clipped together with curved staples

After the birth, the woman is given an injection of syntometrine to minimise the risk of heavy bleeding from the uterus (postpartum haemorrhage) and the baby is given vitamin K. After a caesarean under general anaesthetic, the woman is transferred to the recovery room

---

11 NICE, 2004
12 NICE, 2004

where she is brought round and shown the baby. It is common for women to fall asleep again and to wake up on the postnatal ward wondering what has happened. If the woman's partner or friend can stay with her until she wakes up again, this can be very helpful.

The baby

The baby is more likely to have breathing problems following a planned CS and may have to go to the Special Care Baby Unit (SCBU). The condition, transient tachypnoea of the newborn or TTN, is short lived. However, if the baby is born too early as well as not having the squeezing of the chest that occurs during labour and vaginal delivery, respiratory distress syndrome may occur and this can be severe and, rarely, fatal. Therefore it is recommended that planned CS is arranged for thirty-nine weeks or later for single babies and thirty-eight weeks for twins[13] – although the rationale for having different times for twins is unclear. There is an argument for allowing the woman to go into labour and then performing the planned CS to avoid these problems.

Studies have shown that the risk of cutting the baby's skin is about one in fifty operations.[14] Fortunately the skin of newborn babies heals very well and the cut is very unlikely to leave a scar.

The scar

The modern lower-segment caesarean section gives a stronger scar than a classical vertical one. It heals more quickly and easily, causes less discomfort to the woman during recovery and should withstand any future labour contractions. Occasionally, if there are problems with a lower-segment operation, for example if a large fibroid is obstructing access, then a vertical incision is made in the thicker and more muscular upper segment of the uterus. A vertical or 'classical' incision may also be performed for transverse lie or placenta praevia. What the doctor wants to avoid is a T-shaped incision which is thought to be the weakest scar of all. Sometimes in a very premature delivery a vertical incision in the lower part of the uterus is made.

It is important for subsequent births that women should know the type of

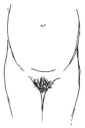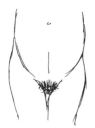

'Bikini' line cut   Vertical cut

---

13 NICE, 2004
14 NICE, 2004

scar they have on their uterus. A vertical scar is more likely to tear in labour than a horizontal one. However, a vertical scar on the abdomen does not necessarily mean a vertical scar on the uterus, which will usually have a horizontal segment scar. If the woman does not know what type of scar she has, an experienced doctor can usually feel a transverse scar during a vaginal examination in early labour.

Care after a caesarean

Some hospitals have single rooms available to which women who have had caesareans are given priority. Other hospitals have 'amenity rooms', private rooms for which NHS patients may pay in order to have this privacy. Many women find the relative peace and quiet of a room to themselves makes a positive difference to the first few days of their recovery.

> I feel very strongly that after such a bad time (my surgeon's own words) I should have been put in an amenity room... and I would have willingly paid but I was in no fit state to ask and it did not occur to my poor husband... it would certainly have aided my recovery.[15]

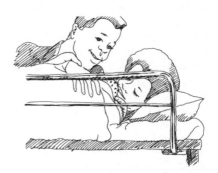

If a baby dies, it may seem even harder that, despite having a caesarean, this has happened. A woman in this situation needs both a great deal of time to talk through the experience and sensitive support on the lines recommended by SANDS (see 'Further Information for Parents', p.270).

Pain relief

It is important for the woman to be made comfortable so that she can become mobile as soon as possible and feel able to feed and get to know her baby. This is particularly the case in the first twenty-four hours after birth when the post-operative pain is at its highest level. If the woman has had an epidural and staffing levels on the postnatal ward are adequate, the tube will be left in for twenty-four hours, because this is the most effective method of administering pain relief. Otherwise, the woman is given injections of pain-relieving drugs into her bottom or thigh. Once the woman is able to drink, she can change from injections to pain-relieving tablets. Some hospitals give a cocktail of soluble pain-killer with peppermint water for wind and an antacid for heartburn. The pain-relieving drugs used are safe for breastfeeding mothers to take as the amounts transferred to the baby are minimal. It is better to have adequate relief from pain and discomfort than to try to manage without. Some women use the TENS machine they have hired for labour for post-operative pain relief. TENS is believed to have no side-effects on mother or baby, but this has not yet been scientifically evaluated. Equally, natural therapies are considered by some people to be helpful at this time, but they too have not been evaluated. Some women cope with the pain of removing sticking plaster from the site of the drip in their arm and the wound by gently loosening it themselves.

Mobility and caring for the baby

The art of recovering after a caesarean is in maintaining a balance between gradually becoming mobile, and being able to care for the baby, with having enough opportunities for rest and not becoming exhausted by doing too much too soon. A respondent in our survey of women's experiences advised other women:

> Don't try and do too much too soon in hospital. You've to be easy on yourself so you can do more later (remember you've had a major operation).

It is vital that sufficient practical support and help in hospital is easily available. Having to ask repeatedly for help increases some women's feelings of inadequacy so that either help should be offered or women should be made to feel free to ask for it.

A respondent in our study said that she felt 'a bit anxious because moving around was so painful and I was completely dependent on the nurses' help.'

Women have the right to this sort of support and should not feel that it reflects adversely on them if they need it. It is important for the woman to have early access to a physiotherapist or a specially trained midwife to show her how to guard her wound and become mobile. Any breathing and relaxation techniques she has learned for labour will be useful at this time.

Women are encouraged to get out of bed and begin caring for their baby as soon as possible because this improves blood circulation and aids recovery. It may seem cruel to make a woman get up on the first day after an operation, but with a lower-segment scar and with good pain relief it is often possible and may be beneficial for a woman's morale as well as her physical well-being.

> Physically, once you're up and walking, keep your back straight![16]

While in bed it is important for the woman to keep her legs moving by circling

---

16   From our study of women's experience (see chapter 7)

her ankles and wriggling her toes. This improves circulation and prevents blood clots. Some women are given injections to help thin the blood until they are fully mobile and most are asked to keep the white TED elasticated stocking on until they are walking properly. If the woman has had a caesarean after a trial of forceps or Ventouse, her perineum may feel stiff and sore and she may need a rubber ring or special inflatable cushion (available for hire from local NCT branches if not available from the NHS) to sit on.

> I can remember sitting crying because I could not do much for him [her baby]. I was stuck in bed with a drip and catheter and he was crying. It was so frustrating.

At first, the woman may need some help to get out of bed and sit on a chair, and later to walk to the lavatory. It helps to keep her bed as low as possible and a monkey bar may also be used so that the woman can pull herself up. Getting out of bed will take time and the woman should try to find the most comfortable way for herself. One way is for her to sit up and gradually shuffle her bottom sideways to the edge of the bed, pushing her hands into the bed to help her lift her bottom. She can then lower one leg at a time on to the floor and swivel her body so that she is sitting on the edge of the bed. When she is ready, she can gently move into a chair or get up and walk (see illustration below).

> Holding and lifting the baby and getting out of bed to the baby were very difficult.

The woman may be surprised at the length of time she needs to get up and walk to the lavatory; she may need someone with her for reassurance and to make sure she is all right. She should allow herself as much time as she needs for getting out of bed, then for standing up. She should not walk until she is standing up straight and should be encouraged to stand as upright as possible, since this aids recovery, as well as her self-respect. Then she can look ahead and think about moving. To walk, she can lean her weight on one foot, then swing the other leg forward, shift her weight to that foot and repeat the movement: by using the momentum of her legs in this way, she puts less strain on the wound.

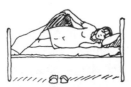

1. Roll onto one side

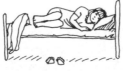

2. Knees up, top hand across onto the bed

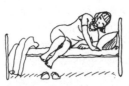

3. Push on top hand, swing feet down gently

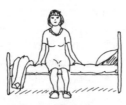

4. Feet apart, push up on both hands

If the woman's baby is in a special care baby unit (SCBU) without beds for mothers, or even in a different hospital, it is vital that staff enable her to see the baby as soon as possible. She can be taken in a wheelchair to see the baby. Even if the woman is unable to feed the baby herself, she can let the baby hear her voice and feel her touch which can be a positive experience for them both. Usually a photograph is taken and given to her to help her cope with the interval before seeing her baby.

Going to the lavatory

As mentioned above, some maternity units leave a catheter in place for the first twenty-four hours to drain the bladder. Otherwise the woman can use a bedpan or ask the midwives to sit her on a commode. If the woman cannot empty her bladder, her midwife may need to insert a catheter to relieve the pressure and prevent the bladder becoming overstretched. After the first night, the woman should be feeling well enough to make her way to the lavatory.

It is very common for women to have a lot of wind after a caesarean, as with any other abdominal operation. This can be uncomfortable, so the woman should be encouraged to pass any wind and to avoid fizzy drinks, including carbonated mineral water. Peppermint water can help with the problem.

The woman is unlikely to open her bowels on the first day but if, as can happen, she becomes constipated, she may wish to take gentle laxatives or suppositories to keep the motions soft and avoid straining. If a woman is breastfeeding, there are certain kinds of laxative she should avoid. Fibre-rich foods can help: some women take dried apricots as a snack in their hospital bag. Occasionally, certain kinds of pain-killing drugs can cause constipation and alternatives should be used.

Food and drink

The intravenous drip is normally kept in place for twelve to twenty-four hours after birth to ensure the woman receives enough liquid. In addition, the woman is given mouthwashes and small amounts of water which are gradually increased. Care should be taken to avoid increasing the liquid intake too rapidly, which may cause the mother to feel sick. Once the woman can drink freely, the drip can be removed. When she is drinking normally and bowel sounds are present, she can start eating solid foods, building up initially from a light diet. NICE (2004) recommend that women who are recovering well can eat and drink as soon as they feel hungry and thirsty but in the last two Confidential Enquiries into maternal death there have been a handful of women who have died from a rare complication of spontaneous bowel ruptures.[17] Those of us who are old

---

17 DoH, 1998; DoH, 2001

enough to have seen problems after surgery when fluids were not restricted still feel that to prevent these rare complications all women should not eat until bowel sounds are present and care should be taken not to give large amounts of fluid, but there is no hard evidence for this view. It may be a consequence of the higher rate of CS, or it may be related to the shortage of midwifery staff and the increasing shiftwork pattern of doctors working fewer hours causing warning signs to be missed.

Coughing

It is important for the woman to cough and clear phlegm from her chest after the operation, especially if she has had a general anaesthetic. If she smokes, the problem can be worse and she could be at risk of a chest infection. A physiotherapist will help her cough and it may be useful to her to have some pain relief before the physiotherapy. The physiotherapist will teach the woman how to support her scar with her hands when she coughs. This is also helpful when she laughs or uses the lavatory.

Sleep

At first the woman will be propped up in bed to sleep and pain-killing injections or tablets will help. It is very important that the woman's sleep is not disturbed by pain. It used to be the practice for the baby to be taken to the nursery in order for the woman to get an undisturbed night's rest. However, many women intending to breastfeed prefer to keep their baby with them all the time and in some maternity units nurseries are no longer used. Where there is a hospital nursery, some women find it helpful for the staff to change and settle the baby for the first two nights after the birth. The baby is brought to the woman just for breastfeeding, so that she gets as much rest as possible. If a woman does have her baby with her, it is essential for her calls for assistance to be answered within a reasonable time should the baby need to be lifted out of the cot for feeding or comforting. The woman should be encouraged to try to sleep whenever the opportunity presents itself, particularly if she has been woken in the night for feeds.

Breastfeeding

It is now accepted that the vast majority of women are physically capable of breastfeeding (97 per cent according to World Health Organisation figures). The superiority of breastmilk has led to the recommendation that all babies should be exclusively breastfed for the first four to six months. Therefore breastfeeding after a caesarean is to be recommended, not only because it is best for the baby, but also because it helps the uterus return to its normal size more quickly. The fact that the woman has had an abdominal operation may make breastfeeding more uncomfortable than after a vaginal delivery, but there are many ways in which she can adapt to the situation. It is important that the people around the mother support her wish to breastfeed and help her remain confident in her ability to do so.

One woman in our survey said that she found breastfeeding difficult because of 'too many attachments [and] inadequate pain relief to enable free movement'. Another said that:

> Debilitation hinders your ability to respond to baby. Pain-killers etc. are unfavourable during breast feeding. It was slow getting the baby skin to skin and feeding after the operation.

Women who have delivered by caesarean need particular help, support and encouragement.

Some women are able to breastfeed immediately after the operation if they are not too drowsy or if they have had an epidural or spinal block. This gives the mother and the baby a chance to be especially close and may give the woman a feeling of normality at being able to feed the baby herself, particularly if she is disappointed at having had a caesarean. There is usually plenty of time while the obstetrician is repairing the wound. Some women ask for the baby to be put to the breast while they are still asleep under the general anaesthetic and the baby can be placed next to the mother so that skin-to-skin contact occurs even before she wakes up. Babies need the smell and comfort of close physical contact. Another way of caring for the baby during this time is for the father or other partner or friend to cuddle the baby next to their skin.

The woman will need help getting into a comfortable position so that the baby can feed without resting on the wound. This can be achieved by the woman either sitting up or lying down. Hospital beds are not ideal places to breastfeed, so she may need to experiment to find comfortable positions, with pillows and lots of help. If the woman needs to be propped upright following a general anaesthetic, she will need help with pillows to be able to feed in a good position without pulling the breast out of the baby's mouth. The back-rest of the bed should be in its upright position with a pillow across her lap and the baby resting on the pillow; or the pillow can be at her side and the baby lying on the pillow with its feet tucked under her arm (also known as the 'football hold' or 'underarm position'). Another way for the baby to feed in hospital is lying on a pillow on the meal table which fits over the bed. Alternatively the woman could sit on a chair with her feet up on a stool to keep her legs higher than her wound. If the woman lies on her side, the baby can lie on his/her side next to her (see illustration opposite).

One woman in our survey said that she found her baby 'slow to latch on and difficult to hold because of painful belly'. Another said she found it 'slightly more difficult to get into a comfortable position for feeding or latching-on'.

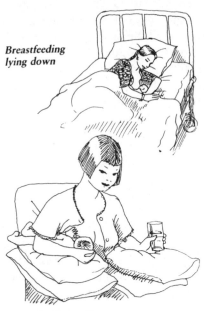

*Breastfeeding
lying down*

*Breastfeeding well
supported in an upright
chair*

Latching the baby correctly onto the breast is very important for all breastfeeding and the mother will be helped at first by the midwives to achieve this. The baby needs to be facing the mother, lying on her/his side, with her/his mouth close to the nipple. The baby's mouth needs to be open really wide, with the bottom lip curled back. When s/he is correctly positioned, her/his chin will be tucked into the breast, with a really good amount of breast tissue in the mouth. Most of the areola, particularly the underside, will be in the mouth, although just how much depends on the individual woman. The mother should not attempt to shape the breast with her hand in order to help the baby fix on. If she feels that the breast needs support, she should support it from below, with the flat of her hand against her rib-cage.

If the baby is latched on well, the top of the ears may wiggle and the muscles at the temples may move as well. The baby will suck quickly at first, and then, as the milk lets down, will change to slower, deeper and more rhythmic sucks, often accompanied by gulping noises. The mother should be encouraged to let the baby finish the first breast by her- or him-self to make sure that s/he gets as much of the higher-fat hind-milk as possible. She can then offer the second side if s/he wants it.

It is vital that the woman receives plenty of support from her midwives in learning how to latch the baby on correctly. Since they will have to lift the baby out of the cot for her, this should not be a problem. The midwives should also help the woman change to the other breast when the baby has finished on the first side, although often the baby will have fallen asleep and come off the breast, having had a satisfying feed from just the one side. If feeding becomes uncomfortable, the woman can remove the baby from the breast gently by putting her little finger into the corner of the baby's mouth to break the suction, before encouraging her/him to latch on correctly before feeding again. In time the woman and baby will learn good positioning together.

Breathing and relaxation techniques learned for labour are good for breastfeeding too, and the woman can be reminded to use them if she forgets. One of the things to be aware of during the early days of breastfeeding after a caesarean is that the pain-killing drugs may cause the pain of a poorly latched-on baby or of sore nipples not to be apparent. It is also possible for a drowsy baby to drift off to sleep during feeds, slide off the nipple a bit, wake up and then start feeding again in a poor position which is likely to cause damage to the nipple. It is therefore important for the woman and her midwives together to try to ensure that the baby always feeds correctly positioned.

Sometimes women who have had a caesarean find that it takes longer for the breastmilk to come in after the colostrum. For example, a woman in our survey said that the 'milk takes longer to come down'. If this is the case, the woman should not be allowed to lose confidence in her ability to feed the baby. Although the anaesthetics used for caesareans have not been shown to be the cause of such a delay, it is thought that there are factors which do not help. These might include the fact that the woman may have been without food and drink for as long as two or three days. Other reasons might be a drowsy baby feeding less often and sucking less strongly than a more alert baby, and a woman reluctant to put the baby to the breast as frequently as a woman who does not have an abdominal scar to contend with.

The woman should be encouraged to feed with colostrum whenever the baby shows signs of being hungry so as to help the milk come in. Sometimes midwives offer to give the baby a bottle to allow the mother an opportunity to rest, particularly during the night. However, this should generally be avoided, as giving bottles of water, dextrose or formula will only serve to delay the milk for longer by depriving the woman's breasts of the stimulation they need from the baby's sucking. It has been shown that supplementary and complementary feeds may ultimately reduce the time a woman breastfeeds her baby.[18] If the milk is delayed for as long as five or six days, as can happen sometimes, it is important for the woman not to lose heart and to remember that colostrum is a valuable food, richer in calories and antibodies than breastmilk. It may be that her system is taking longer to get under way, but the baby will not suffer and her milk will come in eventually.

In order to make breastfeeding as easy as possible, the woman should wear a front-opening nightdress or a loose T-shirt which can be pulled up and a proper nursing bra for good support of the breasts.

If the woman's baby is in a SCBU because of prematurity or sickness, the woman will need even more support for breastfeeding. If the baby is unable to breastfeed at all or for long enough to get sufficient nourishment, the woman will need to

18   Royal College of Midwives, 1991

be shown how to use an electric breastpump to help establish and maintain her milk supply. The expressed milk can then be fed to the baby by tube. This can help the woman feel that she is doing something positive for the baby which no-one else can do. Skin-to-skin contact helps stimulate the milk-producing hormones as well as enabling the woman to be especially close to her baby. Support from a NCT breastfeeding counsellor can be valuable in this situation. Specialist leaflets are available for mothers who have had caesareans and for those whose babies are in special care, giving practical information on expressing and storing breastmilk (see 'Further Information for Parents', p.269).

Washing

It is probably best for the woman to wait a day for the first wash and then to ask for help for a shower. Attempts should be made to keep water away from the area of the wound unless this has the protective plastic covering which is waterproof. After this, the woman will probably be able to wash herself and a shower may be easiest if she finds bending over very painful. It is important for the woman to keep the wound as clean and dry as possible to promote healing and prevent infection. If she has a bath in hospital or uses a bidet, it is essential that these are cleaned before use, with a disinfectant or cream cleanser and her own cleaning cloth. The seat of the lavatory and bidet can be cleaned using antiseptic wipes. If the woman is unfortunate enough to have had stitches in her perineum as well (from an episiotomy for trial of forceps or Ventouse), these will also have to be kept clean and dry. A hairdryer is not recommended for drying stitches.

The wound

As mentioned above, sometimes a small plastic drain will be used to take away into a small plastic bottle any blood that might have collected under the skin. It is usually removed the day after the operation by gently pulling it out. The elastic top of normal briefs may chafe the wound, a situation which may last for many months, so it is usually better for the woman to wear 'Bridget Jones knickers', ones that come up to her waist, and to avoid any sanitary protection which may rub. The soft, stretchy briefs sold by the NCT (Maternity Sales) are ideal as they are elastic enough to hold a sanitary pad in place and to stop any chafing of stitches in the perineum (see 'Further Information for Parents', p.269). Loose, comfortable clothes which do not press on the wound are essential.

There are several ways of closing the caesarean wound in the abdomen. Some stitches are hidden and dissolve so that there is nothing to remove later. Others are hidden but do not dissolve. These are fixed at either end of the wound with a small bead and are easily (and fairly painlessly) removed by cutting one bead free and pulling the other with the thread out of the wound. Alternatively there may be individual stitches, clips and/or staples to remove. In the case of a horizontal cut the stitches will be removed after four or five days, but with a vertical cut they will be left in for seven to ten days.

Some women suffer because the wound becomes infected; it looks red and inflamed and may be painful. This can be helped by making a small hole in the wound with a probe and taking out the pus. A poultice or heat pad placed over the wound may also help to draw out the pus. It is vital to keep the wound as clean and dry as possible. The wound will remain quite sensitive for a while. As it heals, its colour changes back to normal by which time it will probably be covered by the pubic hair which will have grown back again. It may become itchy and this can be eased with a light vegetable oil. It is not uncommon for women to feel numbness around the scar. This sensation may last for several months and in fact a small area may remain permanently numb.

Bleeding from the vagina ('lochia')

This is the same as after a vaginal delivery. The lochia is red at first, but after about five days will change to a brown colour and resemble the discharge at the end of a period. It will finally change to a watery yellow-brown or pink discharge. Many women who breastfeed find that after a feed they experience 'after-pains' when the oxytocin released by the baby's suckling causes the uterus to contract down and a little fresh blood may be found on the sanitary pad shortly after. This is quite normal and the woman will usually be able to deal with the discharge by using sanitary pads. However, she should be advised to tell her midwife if the bleeding becomes heavier, begins to smell offensive or if she passes blood clots. This could indicate an infection in the uterus or that a piece of the placenta or membranes is still inside the uterus and, if necessary, the woman will be taken to theatre and, under anaesthetic, the uterus is gently scraped until it is empty.

Infections

It is possible that the woman may get an infection in her urine, chest, breasts, wound or uterus. If the woman has a persistently high temperature, her doctor will check her for any site of infection and she may need to take antibiotics. These may make the woman feel rather tired and may lead to diarrhoea. If the woman is breastfeeding, the baby's stools may become even looser than is usual with breastfeeding, but this does not usually cause a problem provided that the woman is warned that it may happen. In most hospitals, women are given one dose of antibiotics at delivery as a preventative measure against infection.

Visitors

On the first day after the caesarean, it is probably best if the woman sees as few people as possible so that she can rest. She will probably want to see her partner and other children and will find their support with becoming mobile and caring for the baby helpful. But the woman may want to keep other visitors to a minimum so that she can use her time in hospital to rest and recover as much as she can before going home. It is important for the woman's partner to be aware of her need for support and, when telling family and friends about the new baby, to ask them not to visit until the woman is ready to appreciate their company.

When the woman goes home, it may be necessary to ration visitors then too, particularly if they make her feel she has to rush around tidying up and cleaning and making cups of tea. On the other hand, visitors who come with food and to help with chores may be very welcome!

Coping at home

Nowadays, as the result of the quicker healing of the horizontal caesarean scar, most women stay in hospital for only three to five days rather than the ten-day period which was usual in the past. In some areas women go home even earlier if all is well and they feel ready, and the community midwife removes any stitches on the fifth day.

All women who have had a caesarean need practical support until they have recovered fully from what is, after all, major abdominal surgery. Therefore all genuine offers of help should be accepted, particularly if there are other children and the woman's partner has to go back to work a few days after her return home. Some women have a relative or friend to stay and help or have their friends and neighbours look after the children, do the shopping and drop in with food they have cooked. Other women stay with their mother or other relative so that they can be looked after. Women who are alone or who have difficulties with coping at home may need the practical help and support of a home help or family aide. Either the community midwife or health visitor can make suitable arrangements; if things are very difficult, they can arrange for the support of a social worker. When the community midwife transfers care of the woman to a health visitor, good communication about the caesarean and any other relevant factors is of paramount importance. Some health professionals arrange for this handover of care to take place with the woman present, so that she can be involved too.

It is important in the first couple of weeks at home that the woman is free to concentrate solely on her own rest and recovery and on feeding and caring for the baby. During the first two weeks after birth, babies often sleep a lot as they too recover from the birth and start getting used to the world outside the uterus.

This is a good time for the woman to rest as much as she can so that when, after two weeks, the baby is awake for longer each day (and therefore needs to feed more often) she will be able to cope more easily. Some women find the support of a breastfeeding counsellor from the NCT helpful if they need extra help with breastfeeding.

Gradually, the woman will be able to take on her normal duties at home. Heavy lifting must be avoided for at least six weeks. Women are also advised not to drive for six weeks in case an emergency stop puts a sudden strain on the scar. Once the lochia has ceased, a woman can start having penetrative sex again whenever she feels ready. However, a woman cannot have a coil or other uterine contraceptive device fitted until three months after the birth instead of the usual six weeks.

Emotions

> By the second day I was up, and doing nearly everything by the third day, which caused me stress because I couldn't quite manage because of the pain I was in. It left me feeling inadequate as a mother, and I wanted to do more.

Some women find the emotional aftermath of a caesarean to be of more significance to them than its physical aspects. The resulting emotions and thoughts are likely to carry on for longer than the physical recovery and, in some cases, may not even begin until the woman starts to get back to normal. Immediately after any birth the woman's feelings towards her baby are likely to be volatile.

> When they took me back to the ward after the operation, they brought the baby in and I just said 'get him out of here'. I feel really guilty about my feeling towards him on that first day now, especially after seeing other women on the wards caring for their babies straight away. It was only when I realised that my baby was covered in a bad rash and needed nursing without a nappy on that I got protective towards him and then I knew I could care for him more than anyone else.

Emotions may swing from immense maternal love at one extreme to indifference and feelings of unreality. Studies have shown that about 40 per cent of mothers find that the elation and love for the baby they expected to feel immediately after the birth in fact took several days or even weeks to develop.

If the caesarean came after a long and difficult labour, the woman may be glad that it is all over and be delighted with her baby.

> As soon as they said you will have to have a section, I became very upset and cried a lot, even though I thoroughly understood the circumstances and knew it was for the very best for my baby and me. But as soon as I came round and saw my husband with our beautiful son I was glad it was all over and glad I had a section. I don't regret it one bit.

However, the mother's tiredness and feelings of relief may be so strong that there is no room for other emotions. In order to help the woman relate to her baby, she can be encouraged to hold and examine the baby as soon as possible after the birth. If the baby is dried, it will not lose heat so quickly if the woman wants to take her time. The first feed at the breast is a good way of establishing contact, whenever the woman and baby are ready. Even if the baby does not want to feed at first, being held close will enable the baby to smell, taste and feel its mother as well as recognise her voice. Skin-to-skin contact will also help to stimulate the woman's milk supply. As with any birth, the baby will be getting used to life outside the uterus with its bright lights, loud sounds and intriguing sights.

It is common for nearly all women to experience short-lived 'baby blues' on the third or fourth day after birth. The woman may find herself crying for no reason and she may also be irritable, anxious, forgetful, confused and disorientated. She may fear rejection by her partner. All new parents have concerns about the well-being of their baby and worry that it may not be all right. However, some women may become excessively anxious for no reason and be suspicious that there are things about the baby that they have not been told. Birth may revive unconscious memories and feelings about siblings or herself which may contribute to the woman's distress.

There are other ways in which the baby blues become evident. They may last for only a day but in other cases for a couple of weeks. Ten per cent of women experience postnatal depression, a clinical problem which may need professional help, as well as understanding and support from their family and friends. Postnatal depression is more common after a caesarean than a vaginal delivery. This is due, at least in part, to the fact that in addition to recovering from dramatic changes in hormone levels, the woman is recovering from a major operation with physical discomfort, tiredness and possible infection to compound the usual problems of getting used to feeding and caring for a new baby. It can be depressing for the woman to keep asking for help, to see other women get back to 'normal' more quickly after vaginal deliveries and to find that not everyone is sympathetic. In addition there may be feelings of inadequacy and disappointment at not having had the kind of birth that was planned.

Some women in our survey described their post-operative feelings as 'disappointed because I wanted a natural birth', 'a bit unsuccessful', and 'disappointed, debilitated.'

Some women feel that they were at fault and that they are not a 'real woman'. This may be compounded in some ethnic groups by negative attitudes towards caesarean section by the partner or community.[19] For most women, these feelings will pass fairly quickly, but other women will need extra help and understanding in coming to terms with them.

It is thought to be important to see that the woman is given space and time to express her feelings; however, one randomised controlled trial (RCT) from Australia showed that debriefed women were more likely to be satisfied when

19 Savage, 1986a, p.160

they left the hospital but more likely to be depressed at six months. Before she leaves hospital, her midwives and doctors should ensure that she has had an opportunity to discuss the birth and ask questions. All women appreciate visits during their stay in hospital from the professionals who cared for them during labour and this is even more the case for women who have had a difficult labour or a caesarean. In some instances, it may be appropriate to offer the woman a follow-up appointment at the time of the routine six-week postnatal check or at some other time if there are still unresolved issues. Alternatively, the woman may welcome the opportunity to talk over the birth with an obstetric counsellor or member of the psychiatric staff at the hospital. After traumatic deliveries a few women feel that they lost control of their labour and report feelings akin to those of women who have been raped. Deep-rooted feelings do not respond to reassurance and women who have them may require professional psychological support beyond simply talking through the experience.

The woman's partner, if she has one, will have an important role to play, as will her family and friends. Any woman, whatever her situation, may benefit from a talk with her midwife, health visitor, GP or a social worker. For women keen to meet other local mothers with new babies, there are informal postnatal support groups as well as special caesarean support groups run by women which can be contacted through their health visitor, local branches of the NCT or through the Caesarean Support Network (see 'Further Information for Parents', p.269).

> Although I found the experience of caesarean section to be traumatic because I had a short time to prepare mentally, the pain I felt afterwards, particularly on the first night, the slower recovery time, delay in bonding and the inconvenience of being unable to drive for six weeks, I feel it is a mistake to be fixated on the birth. The most important thing to me was, and always will be, a healthy baby. For me, a natural childbirth would have been an added bonus but no more than that.

7 Women's experience of caesareans

'I felt quite let down. You read in magazines that it will be normal and natural. I never thought that this would happen.'

IT IS WOMEN WHO GIVE BIRTH AND WHO COPE WITH the after-effects but, in the past, little research has been done into their feelings and opinions about their care. We felt that it was very important to ask women about their experiences, feelings and reactions following a caesarean operation. So in the early 1990s we began collecting this information. The latest results, collected in 2004 are included in this chapter along with some information from women participating in the two previous studies. The women were contacted through hospitals randomly selected to represent the populations in different strategic and area health authority regions across the UK. Data has been collected from more than 800 women over a fifteen-year period. Almost 200 women participated in the study in 2004. A smaller sample of respondents was interviewed following their operations to provide qualitative data. Details of the methodology of the survey and tables of the results appear in Appendices B and C.

REASONS FOR CAESAREAN SECTION

The mothers were asked: 'What reason(s) did the doctors give for performing a caesarean operation? You may have been given more than one reason so please tick the answers that apply to you.' There followed a list of 'reasons' and space for women to add any explanations given to them that were not included in the list.

The results were tabulated (Table A.1, Appendix C) and show that women were told that CSs were necessary because of a combination of factors. Some women were given as many as three or four reasons and others only one. Reasons given for CSs tended to vary according to whether the operation was planned or done as an emergency.

Elective (or 'planned') caesareans

A study where the reasons given by women were checked against case notes showed that most women knew why they had had a caesarean.[1] The results of our survey show that the majority or women who had a planned caesarean had it for one or more of four main reasons: previous caesareans, size of pelvis in relation to size of the baby, breech presentation and diabetes. Almost two in five (38.5 per cent) of the operations were carried out because women had had previous caesareans. Almost one in four women (23.1% per cent) were operated on because their babies were in the breech position and one in six (15.4 per cent) were told that their babies were too big for vaginal delivery. The same number was operated on because of diabetes (15.4 per cent). Fewer women had planned caesareans because of long labours, high blood pressure, their age, the baby was small for dates or transverse lie.

Emergency caesareans

The two main reasons for emergency sections were that labour was taking a long time and that the baby was distressed. This highlights a very large difference between the planned and emergency caesarean groups in that no planned operations were done for fetal distress as compared with 40 per cent of emergency ones. But of course, planned caesareans are decided upon before labour begins. The third most common reason given for emergency sections was that the woman's blood pressure was high (12.5 per cent) followed by the 10 per cent of women who were told that their baby was too big for their pelvis. Attempts to determine antenatally whether the pelvis is too small for the baby have been unsuccessful – even when X-ray pelvimetry was used to measure the size of the bony pelvis, instead of clinical assessment. Estimating the size of the baby by ultrasound or clinical palpation is also imprecise.

Almost two in three (62.5 per cent) of the women having an emergency section were told that labour was taking too long and almost two in five (40 per cent) were told that their baby was in distress. Clearly when labour is prolonged, the woman gets tired and the baby may become distressed as its reserves of glycogen are used up, so it is not surprising that some women mentioned both reasons. Other reasons given to women for their emergency caesareans included previous caesareans (7.5 per cent), baby in breech position, bleeding before birth and cord around baby's neck (2.5 per cent each).

---

1   Hillan, 1992b

WOMEN'S REQUESTS FOR CAESAREAN SECTION

In an attempt to find out whether the use of CS was due to doctors responding to women's requests, mothers were asked: 'Did you ask to have a caesarean section?' The results show that almost one woman in five (19.7 per cent) asked for one. There were great differences in the percentage according to whether the woman was having her first baby or because of her previous experience of childbirth.

Few primigravidae request a caesarean. Of the thirty-nine women in the most recent sample who asked for the operation, only six (15.4 per cent) were first time mothers. Over two in three (69.2 per cent) of the women requesting the operation had had previous caesareans. Anecdotal evidence and media stories suggest that more women are requesting the operation as a 'lifestyle' choice. The results of our studies do not give support to such arguments. In 1991-2 we reported that 13.2 per cent of our sample requested a caesarean. By 1996 this had gone up to 21.3 per cent. There was little change in the 2004 data with 19.7 per cent of the sample asking for the operation.

Women who requested a caesarean were asked why they had done so. Many of those for whom this was not the first caesarean said that they had requested the operation because the original reasons for the previous caesarean were still valid. Others stressed their desire to pre-empt the need for an emergency caesarean. Some of the comments were as follows:

> The first was an emergency, I was induced but it did not work, after four days they did a section. With the second I chose to have a caesarean because I could not go through that again.

> I anticipated I would need one and did not want another emergency operation.

> Elective is by far preferable to emergency.

Others had requested caesareans because of concern for their babies, presumably based on their previous experiences:

> I didn't want to put baby in distress.

> I feel it's the safest option for the child.

> I had a fear of the baby being in trouble again.

One woman requested the operation because of her knowledge about her previous pregnancies:

> This is my fourth pregnancy, the first was delivered by forceps after a long labour, and the third was caesarean. They were all large. I was scanned for size at thirty-two weeks, the baby was 6lb 6oz then!

This respondent gave birth to a 10lb 11oz baby at thirty-nine weeks. Another woman elected to have a caesarean because she wanted more control over the situation compared to her previous CS:

> My previous section was a general anaesthetic emergency. I didn't want to miss out on the birth this time. Unfortunately I have.

This woman had a general anaesthetic for the operation following a failed attempt at spinal block. Her partner stayed with her until the general anaesthetic was administered, then had to leave.

Similarly those women who had previously given birth vaginally but had requested a caesarean for this birth stated reasons to do with their past experience(s), for example:

> I had a previous difficult delivery.

One woman said that her '...baby was in breech position. I decided this [the caesarean] was the safest way for him to be born. I also did not want to go through labour then have to have a section after all.'

Only a few women having their first child requested a caesarean. These were more often than not done as an emergency after a trial of labour

> I was in constant pain for hours and felt that I couldn't go on any longer.

One woman stated that she had requested the operation because of her 'very painful labour'. Another said she had asked for a caesarean because 'I was told that forceps would be necessary and I would not agree to their use'. One respondent wanted 'to avoid a vaginal breech delivery.'

It appears therefore that a small proportion of women ask for the operation because of current or previous experiences. This means that it is very important for women to understand why the operations are being performed, to be given the appropriate information to understand what is happening to them, to be aware of the relative risks and benefits and to be enabled to make informed choices.

BEING AWAKE FOR THE CAESAREAN

Women were asked: 'What type of anaesthetic were you given?' The 1991-2 data showed that almost three in five (58 per cent) women having CSs were under general anaesthetic for the birth of their babies. The highest proportion of these being in the 'emergency' category where over two out of three (70.8 per cent) were given general anaesthesia. Even though over two out of five (41.7 per cent) women receiving planned caesareans were also under general anaesthetic at the time their babies were born. However, there has been a significant change in practice since this time. The change was evident in the data from our 1996 survey and the shift in practice has continued. There has been a dramatic reduction in the use of general anaesthetic from 58 per cent of caesareans in 1991-2 to 18.2 per cent in 2004. The use of epidural anaesthetic has also declined from 23.3 per cent to 10.6 per cent over the same period. The increase has been in the use of spinal block where the number is up from 14.7 per cent to 71.2 per cent of caesarean operations. Thus 81.8 per cent of caesareans in this sample were carried out with regional anaesthesia which compares with national figures of women giving birth by CS in the UK: over 80 per cent of CSs were performed under regional anaesthesia.[2]

The huge differences found in type of anaesthetic used for emergency and planned caesareans found in the 1991-2 study are not so evident today, although slightly more of the emergency operations were performed under general anaesthetic (22.5 per cent of emergency caesareans compared to 11.5 per cent of planned operations).

Some relevant comments were as follows:

> I found a planned section with epidural a far more pleasant and positive experience than my first section which was an emergency with general anaesthetic after a very long labour. My first section was a distressing and frightening experience and one which I felt completely unprepared for.

> Although I understand that the well-being of my baby was of paramount importance, I feel very disappointed that I was not awake for the birth, and that my partner was not with me.

> With having a general I feel I missed out on the first moments.

One woman summed up her feelings very succinctly: 'One hour recovering from anaesthetic. Precious moments lost forever.'

The overwhelming majority of women who commented on the type of anaesthetic used were pleased to be awake during the birth. For example, women who had been given spinal blocks were, on the whole, particularly content:

> I found the caesarean section to be less of an ordeal than I'd anticipated.

> It avoided a long, hard labour which may have ended as a section in any case. Spinal anaesthesia has the beauty of both worlds in that you avoid labour pains and are fully alert during the operation.

> Listening to some other mothers who gave birth naturally I think I was lucky to have a spinal section with no pain and it was all over in one hour.

---

2   Pandit & Plaat, 2004

For many women the two main advantages of being awake during a caesarean were, first, that they could be aware of the birth of their babies, seeing them and even holding them immediately, and second, being able to have their partner/friend with them during the operation.

> I found the spinal block operation fascinating and was awake to see the baby delivered immediately. It was also nice to know that my husband was there to see the birth and that I was able to talk to him right through the operation.

The strength of opinion on this matter was at its highest from the women who after previous caesareans experienced a planned one. Many of these women had been given general anaesthesia the first time and so were in the best position to comment on the relative benefits of being awake or asleep. Their feelings were appropriately summed up by one woman:

> Obviously any woman would prefer a normal delivery but an elective section using a spinal or epidural anaesthetic is the next best thing. A caesarean birth can be a very positive and moving experience, and, with post-operative pain relief, can easily be coped with.

Another woman commented on the relative after-effects of the different types of anaesthetic:

> I have had two types of caesarean anaesthetic, general and spinal. I must say with the spinal the after-effects are a lot easier to deal with due to the fact that you are more alert and there are less side effects.

Obviously the women in the planned caesarean group were more likely to be prepared for the experience and to be in a situation to choose to be awake. These women appeared to have had much more satisfying experiences of CS:

> This is the second time by caesarean. The first was by general anaesthetic. Last time I felt cheated that I missed so much and did not see my baby properly until the next day. This time by spinal block was wonderful, we both saw him straight away and did not miss anything.

> Everyone was very helpful, telling me what was going on. I felt very secure about being awake. It was a lot easier after the baby was born. Epidurals are a lot better than a general as you don't seem to be in much pain. My partner was able to be there which is a very good thing as they also know what's happening. The one big plus about epidurals is that you see your baby straight away which for me was the most emotional thing that I have ever encountered.

> After having my first baby by emergency caesarean section under general anaesthetic I felt depressed and upset as I felt I had missed out a lot by not being awake during the birth. This time I had a much more pleasurable experience due to the fact that I was awake to see what was going on, I was able to see my baby

straight after he was born and my husband was allowed in this time.

I much preferred the caesarean section by spinal anaesthetic as I was able to hold the baby immediately and the after-effects of the anaesthetic were minimal.

In part the after-effects of general anaesthesia appear to be more severe and debilitating than either epidural or spinal block anaesthesia, but the main advantage to mothers about being awake is that they are able to see their babies as soon as they are born.

It's much better if you stay awake, there's no more pain and you get to see your baby straight away.

I am pleased that I was able to have this operation under epidural rather than a general anaesthetic. Thus allowing me to see the baby earlier and be part of the birth process.

A few women expressed their regret at not being awake for their first caesareans in the light of their experiences with the second:

When I had my first caesarean I was frightened to be awake but now that I know what it was like being awake with the second, I would have loved to have been awake the first time. It was a great feeling seeing baby straight away.

I found the epidural better as you can see baby straight away. The first time I lost that bond with the baby, I didn't feel he was mine.

Obviously each pregnancy and delivery must be judged according to its own specific circumstances and conditions but, given the evidence presented here, it must surely raise the question of whether it ought to be routine practice for the women to be awake in all possible cases when undergoing CS. Another important point raised by this study is the need to prepare for caesarean birth early in pregnancy, if at all possible. This is better for the woman both physically and mentally and must surely be better for the hospital staff as well as the woman's partner. This point is highlighted in the words of one respondent:

A caesarean section was queried throughout my pregnancy. An X-ray of my pelvis was taken as it is small. I feel I should have had a planned section and if I had I would have had an epidural. Instead I was made to go through full labour and then rushed to theatre for a section. My husband and I feel that we have both missed out on the birth of our son.

However, it is rare today in the United Kingdom for it to be quite certain that a woman will need a caesarean, even where feto-pelvic disproportion is suspected. The good results achieved by midwives confirm that few healthy women in fact need caesareans.[3] There are some women who would prefer a planned caesarean

---

3   Durand, 1992

rather than risk the possibility of an emergency operation. Therefore if a caesarean is needed, regional rather than general anaesthesia should be given and the partner should be present in theatre whether or not the woman is awake. This can contribute to the experience being as positive a one as possible and, if the woman can be awake, will enable her to see her baby as soon as it is born.

PARTNER'S ATTENDANCE AT A CAESAREAN

Women were asked: 'Did you have a friend/partner present for the birth?' (Table A.2, Appendix C). The results demonstrated that the majority (83.3 per cent) of the women in the sample had their friend/partner present during the delivery. This indicated a substantial increase in partners being allowed into theatre for caesarean operations from the 55 per cent found in our first survey in 1991-2. At that time, of the women who did not have their partners present, the overwhelming majority (79.4 per cent) said it was to do with hospital/doctor policy regarding CSs or the fact that the emergency situation of the operation meant that either partners were not allowed in the operating theatre or they could not have got there on time even if they were allowed in. Nine out of ten obstetricians in our survey said that the partner was invited to attend the operation, others gave conditions under which a partner might not be invited, the main one being the use of general anaesthetic. Typical comments from the women were as follows:

> Doctor didn't approve of husbands being present.
>
> We were never offered the chance due to general anaesthetic.
>
> He was not allowed to attend due to general anaesthetic.

Interestingly, this time we did not find a significant difference in partners' attendance depending on whether the operations were planned or done as emergencies as we have done in our previous studies. In 1991-2 and in 1996 more of the women in the planned category had their partner/friend present during the operation – two out of three (65.9 per cent) and three in four (76.8 per cent) respectively – whereas less than half (46.3 per cent in 1991-2) and just over half (54 per cent) of women having emergency operations in 1996 were accompanied.[4] The current data highlights a change in practice whereby the type of operation does not appear to impact upon partners' presence at the birth. Just over four in five women in both the planned and emergency categories had their partners present for their caesareans (84.6 and 82.5 per cent respectively).

The results indicate that, as in the past, the majority of women would prefer to have a friend/partner with them during the birth and occasionally it is the

---

4   Churchill, 1997

organisation of hospital services which prevents this. Our survey of 100 obstetricians in 2005 found that 90 per cent said they would invite the partner/friend to be present except when the operation was carried out under general anaesthetic. If the main reason for not allowing a partner into the operating theatre is that the woman is asleep under general anaesthetic, this is an indication that women should be given regional anaesthetic wherever possible. However, there is no reason that the partner should not be present. Clearly many obstetricians are now used to this idea, but many anaesthetists need to be made aware of the importance to the couple that at least one partner is able to see the birth.

INFORMATION GIVEN TO WOMEN

Women were asked: 'Before the operation, were you able to find out all you wanted to know about your condition and that of your nearly born baby?' The results showed (Table A.3, Appendix C) that a substantial majority (94.4 per cent) of the respondents felt that they had been kept adequately informed of their condition. This rate of response has remained constant over the fifteen years we have been collecting information from women on their experiences of caesarean birth. A small discrepancy was found on this issue between the women who had had emergency operations and those having planned caesareans. Almost one in twelve (7.5 per cent) of the women receiving emergency caesareans said that they were not able to find out all they wanted to know, compared with only 2.6 per cent of the planned caesarean group. This is probably because in the emergency situation there is not enough time to inform women adequately of all that is happening. As one respondent commented:

> I knew nothing about a caesarean birth and there wasn't enough time to explain the procedure.

It appears that much of the dissatisfaction among the emergency caesarean group stemmed from their lack of preparation for an operative delivery. This raises questions about appropriate preparation for the potential of caesarean birth during the antenatal period, given that statistically almost one in four women is likely to have a caesarean.

Information about treatment

Women were then asked: 'Were you kept informed of the treatment you were being given?' The overwhelming response was positive and 98.5 per cent answered 'yes' to this question. One respondent said 'every person involved in the delivery suite and operating theatre explained everything in detail, they were great.' Another commented:

> Yes – I had some information but I felt I had to ask. I did some reading from baby books, and I asked a friend who is a midwife.

Of the women who were not kept informed, one said she did not know 'how the pain killing treatments would have affected me.' Other comments were as follows:

> I was tired and they did explain what was happening but they did not want to worry me so they did not tell me everything, I knew something was wrong.

> They did not really say much, but I could not understand when they explained, although I agreed. My husband is a nurse and he knew a bit about it, it was still quite frightening, he had told me how the anaesthetic worked.

> I had no information, I remember consenting and the shave but there was no real discussion.

> Because I am a midwife perhaps they thought I knew enough, I was not given any specific information, I think they would have if we had asked, but we were not given any formal information, just asked 'are you happy with the decision?'

Information about the baby's condition

The next question was: 'Do you feel that you were kept fully informed about your baby's condition?' The vast majority (91.4 per cent) answered this question affirmatively. Out of the seventeen women who gave a negative response, fifteen (88.2 per cent) had an emergency caesarean, when there may not have been much time to communicate. Most of these women felt that they would have liked more information about their baby's condition. One woman said that she would have liked to have been told about the effects of the operation on her baby, for example the after-effects such as shock, anaemia and jaundice. Another said that she would have liked to have been told what risks the operation would have for her baby. A further respondent claimed that the baby's father was not told about the baby's condition even when the mother was too distressed. Other comments related to the general condition of the baby before, during and immediately after the operation.

One woman stated that her baby's condition was never discussed. Another appears to have had a particularly bad experience regarding information about her baby during the operation:

> I would have liked to have been told that the baby was okay when she was born. The doctor did not really let us know what was happening. We only knew when the baby started crying and my husband asked 'is that the baby born?'

It was not the case, however, that all the women wanted more information. For example, one mother said: 'I was glad not to be told the details until the next day.' Similarly, another implied that more information would have made her feel worse:

'I was upset and it would have bothered me more if I knew baby was distressed.'

Another mother expressed feelings of wanting to know more but also accepted that such information may have had a negative effect on her. She said: 'I would like to have been told about the baby's position in the womb, but perhaps this would have been disheartening.'

It appears from these results that overall women were satisfied with the amount of information they received from hospital staff. Among those who said that they were not kept fully informed, there were some women who did not necessarily want to know more.

DO WOMEN WHO HAVE CAESAREANS SUFFER?

Women were asked: 'Do you consider that you suffered as a result of having a caesarean?' The results (Table A.4, Appendix C) showed that the majority of women (83.3 per cent) said that they did not feel that they had suffered from the operation. This represents a decline in self-reported suffering from our 1991-2 study when three in five women (60.1 per cent) did not feel that they suffered as a result of the caesarean operation. Interestingly the gap evident in the experiences of women having planned and emergency operations in 1991-2 was not evident in 1996 and does not appear in the current data. Comments from women as to why they felt they had suffered can be analysed as follows:

Suffering caused by the pain of the operation

The overwhelming majority of comments related to the pain, although it seems that the level varies according to each woman's own physiological response, the skill of the obstetrician who performed the caesarean and the effectiveness of the post-operative pain relief. Typical comments were as follows:

> I was surprised at the pain control, only having Voltarol for analgesia, it was uncomfortable not being able to move, quite a surprise. After two days I was fine.

> I would much prefer a normal birth as the pain you have is over. But with caesarean you seem to have quite a bit of pain and discomfort for quite a while after. Also it takes you a lot longer to get back to normal which I shall find very hard.

> I had a fourteen-hour labour and have at this stage endured a further week of pain and discomfort. I cannot sit down or stand with the baby in my arms, I have to have him reached to me and it's very frustrating.

> I felt a bit anxious because moving around was so painful and I was completely dependent on the nurses' help.

Women who had experienced previous vaginal deliveries felt the pain of CS particularly worthy of comment:

Much less enjoyable and more painful than a natural birth.

My natural labour was less painful.

One respondent who had experienced a previous caesarean found that the second operation was not as painful afterwards as the first, which may indicate that she was better prepared and knew what to expect.

The first section was very painful and I was shocked at the severity of it. For the second one I was a bit wary because I knew of the pain I was in with the first. But it was nowhere near as bad.

Many women felt that the post-operative pain adversely affected their ability to cope with their newborn babies. One woman said that she had suffered 'because of not being able to see to my baby properly as I was sore and couldn't manoeuvre the same'.

Some people believe that the caesarean is a painless way of giving birth and that women who have caesareans have somehow taken the 'soft' option in not having to suffer labour pains. The fact that the mothers have undergone major abdominal surgery and have a high degree of post-operative pain may not always be fully realised by other women in the hospital. Two mothers made statements to this effect:

It is annoying that other Mums think you've had an easy time without the labour. They do not realise it is really hard getting yourself pulled together afterwards.

Myself and other women who have had babies by caesareans feel very annoyed when people who had normal deliveries think we were lucky and had an 'easy way out' as recovery is very long and painful. It is many months before you feel well again.

Unlike our earliest study, the latest data showed little differences in the experience of pain between women having planned operations and those having emergency caesareans. The number of women experiencing more pain than expected reduced over the fifteen-year period of study from just over one in four (27.3 per cent) in 1991-2 to just over one in six in 1996 and one in eight in 2004 (18.1 and 12.2 per cent respectively). This reduction is evident in both planned and emergency groups. In the past, almost one out of three (32.3 per cent) women having emergency operations felt more pain than they had expected, compared to only one in five (21.2 per cent) of women having planned sections. However, the number of women in the emergency category experiencing more pain than expected has reduced substantially over the fifteen-year period of study so that the difference between the two groups, in terms of experience of pain, has virtually disappeared. This may be attributed to women being better informed about the after effects of caesarean delivery and more women having repeat caesareans. Alternatively it may be that when the woman is awake, her partner is present and the surgery is done with regional anaesthesia the operation is done in a gentler way than when she is asleep!

Suffering caused by not being able to give birth naturally

Many women felt a severe sense of loss at not being able to give birth naturally.

One woman from the planned caesarean group said that she felt that she had suffered 'emotionally because I wanted to do it naturally by myself with little pain relief.'

Others said:

> I would have preferred a normal delivery, but the labour went on a long time and the baby was distressed. I felt guilty about not giving birth normally.

> I was really disappointed at first, I cried.

Comments from the emergency caesarean group included: 'You can't class caesarean as giving birth, I don't feel as if I have really had a baby.' Another felt disappointed that she 'didn't get the chance to deliver naturally'.

Even when understanding the necessity for the operation in their own case, some women still felt a severe sense of loss:

> It felt safer for me and baby at the time, although I am still upset that I was not able to see natural birth through.

> I would have liked to have a normal delivery. However caesarean was a life-saving operation for both myself and baby.

> I felt quite let down; you read in magazines that it will be normal and natural birth. I never thought that this would happen. But I was worried when things started to go wrong, I was relieved that he was safe.

> I was disappointed and shocked with the first, they told me in the middle of contractions. I was disappointed with the second but I wanted my daughter to be born safely.

Suffering caused by the effects on 'bonding'

In our 1991-2 survey, respondents felt that being separated from their babies immediately after the birth had a deleterious effect on their ability to bond appropriately. This was particularly true for the women who had experienced emergency caesareans, partly because this group of mothers was more likely to have been given general anaesthesia. Furthermore they were more likely to have given birth to babies who needed specialist treatment following the birth. At that time, typical comments from women were:

> Initial bonding feelings between Mum and baby seem to have taken longer to take place... I feel that caesarean takes away the vital importance of the bonding between mother and baby in the first two days.

The 1996 and 2004 data reveal a dramatic reduction in the use of general anaesthetic. The use of epidural anaesthetic has reduced slightly, the increase is in the use of spinal block. The fact that 40 per cent of planned operations were performed with the woman under general anaesthetic in 1991-2 was a cause for concern because women were missing out on the birth of their babies and reporting negative effects postnatally. It is encouraging to see a major reduction in the use of general anaesthetic for planned caesareans as well as emergency operations. This has been matched by an increase in the use of regional anaesthetic, particularly spinal block. It is also encouraging to see that spinal block is now the most common form of anaesthetic for operations as this allows women to remain conscious and take a full part in the birth of their babies. This may be attributable to the increased use of regional anaesthetic in delivery rooms generally or the growth of the speciality of obstetric anaesthesia and appointment of more anaesthetists. Therefore when the decision to perform a caesarean is made in an emergency situation, the anaesthetic is already in place.

Comments from respondents in the latest survey reflect this change. Only one woman mentioned separation (as well as her PND) as affecting her ability to bond with her baby:

> I did have postnatal depression, perhaps that did affect my relationship. He was taken away from me when he was born, he was not well and I could not breastfeed. I was put on anti-depressants. I am okay now.

Women who felt that the operation did have an effect on their ability to bond with their babies spoke of the debilitating effects of surgery rather than separation from their babies. Some respondents said that they felt bonding had suffered because of their inability to pick the baby up when needed:

> ...it is difficult to sit down and nurse them when you have had a caesarean section, putting your baby on you.

> It would have been nice to have him on my tummy and I wasn't able to cuddle him.

Another woman mentioned her 'inability to move freely due to pain and attachments'.

One respondent commented that the caesarean might have had a positive effect on bonding: 'I think that if I had had to carry on with the labour, I would never have bonded with him.'

However, it must be remembered that some mothers who have delivered vaginally find that they are unable to spend time with their baby after birth because either they or their babies need urgent treatment. Some other mothers have had a normal delivery and spent time holding their baby after birth but find that they do not form the special attachment to their baby until hours, days or even weeks later. Forming a relationship with a new baby is a unique process which every parent experiences in their own way.

Over three in five of the women in the latest sample saw their baby as soon as it was born (62.6 per cent). More than four in five (83.3 per cent) of the mothers having planned caesareans saw their babies immediately whereas only half (49.2 per cent) of the emergency caesarean group did so. This is likely to relate to type of anaesthetic used for the surgery as three in five (60 per cent) of the women in the emergency category who did not see their babies immediately after birth had been given general anaesthesia. It may also be that following complications of delivery babies were taken to special care baby units.

Suffering caused by the lengthy recovery period

Many of the women commented on the lengthy recovery period and the fact that they were not able to be up and about with their baby soon after the operation:

> The post-operative debilitation hinders your ability to respond to your baby. Pain killers etc are unfavourable during breastfeeding and I was slow to get baby skin to skin and feeding after the operation.

> I'm satisfied my caesareans were necessary for the safety of the babies in both instances. However, it must surely be the worst way to give birth as just when you need to be fit to cope with a new baby, you are coping with a major operation. I found it terribly frustrating.

> I feel relieved that such intervention is possible as it does obviously save the lives of newborn babies. However it is upsetting when for the first days or so you have to rely on the midwives and other staff so much for the care of your newborn.

> I had more attention the first time, it was better than the second. It was difficult not feeling physically well and having the baby to care for. They were short-staffed. There is a need for more after-care, need for more attention. I kept feeling a nuisance having to ask, I needed help to lift her out of the cot.

Post-operative feelings

A recurring theme on the question of how women felt they had suffered because of the CS points to women not being adequately prepared mentally for an operative delivery.

> After a trouble-free pregnancy it is difficult to accept being an 'invalid' and dependent on others.

Similarly we can see how the long recovery period following the caesarean has an adverse effect on women, especially when they have other children to think about.

> I had hoped to recover from this birth much more quickly than last time, whereas now presumably it will be as before, but harder, thanks to a two-year-old!

Some women expressed relief at not having to do all the caring for the baby in the first day or so and were pleased to have the hospital staff on hand to help out. One woman said that she felt 'okay at time, but very sore afterwards, although I miss not having baby with me. Don't know how I would have coped if they had given me baby the next day, I was very weak and tired.'

Other general comments that women made regarding how they felt they had suffered centred around conditions caused to their baby because of the operation, for example problems with breathing, and general discomfort caused to themselves in terms of headaches, wind, depression, permanent scarring to the body and infection:

> I was up and about within a day. I had problems with infection. It took six to eight weeks to clear for the last one. I had to go back to the hospital.

> For the first one I had stitches that dissolved but with the second it was a continuous stitch. It became weepy and became an open wound. It took two to three weeks to heal.

Other results showed that three in four (74.2 per cent) women having caesareans felt tired after the operation, and almost half (45.5 per cent) felt weak. To a lesser extent, one in six women felt sick (15.2 per cent) and one in twenty (5.6 per cent) felt depressed. However, women who had had emergency operations reported all of these feelings more than the women who had had planned caesareans (except for sickness which was reported equally in both groups at around 15 per cent). In the previous edition of this book we reported that, based on 1991-2 data there was a startling difference between planned and emergency caesarean women in the case of depression. Over twice as many emergency caesarean women reported feeling this post-operatively, almost one in five (19.6 per cent), compared to one in eleven (9.1 per cent) of the women who had had planned caesareans. Fewer women reported depression post-operatively in the 1996 and 2004 studies and there was little difference between the two groups.

Overall, the 2004 and 1996 data showed a reduction in the number of caesarean women reporting negative post-operative feelings compared to the 1991-2 study. This may, in part, be due to modifications to the design of the questionnaire and the addition of extra categories to map women's responses. This could have had the effect of dispersing responses among a larger number of categories thus reducing the total number in each box. However, no restriction was placed on women in terms of the number of boxes they could tick and so any difference because of design modifications is likely to be minimal. The change in perceptions is likely to be due to better experiences since 1996 in terms of women being better informed about caesarean birth and the reduced use of general anaesthetic in these samples. Even so, some differences were evident in the experiences of women who had planned operations and those having emergency sections in 2004. More planned caesarean women felt happy after the operation, over half (53.8 per cent) compared to two in five (40.0 per cent) of emergency caesarean women. Similarly, more emergency caesarean women reported feeling weak post-operatively, almost three in five (57.5 per cent) compared to just over a quarter (26.9 per cent) of women having planned operations.

Other comments that women made regarding this question reflected mostly negative feelings such as 'sore', 'shaky', 'light-headed', 'faint', 'tearful', 'confused', 'disappointed', 'cold', 'vacant', 'dizzy', 'anxious', 'cheated', 'very hot' and 'hungry!!!' One woman said that she was 'in shock and resentful towards the baby for the first day'. Some women mentioned headaches or migraine and others reported 'buzzing' or 'fuzzy sensation' in the ears. One said that she felt 'fear because of the pain, worried about the baby who was taken to SCBU and guilt because I felt no rush of love for the baby.' Others reported more positive feelings such as 'ecstatic', 'strong', 'lucky', 'fortunate', 'very grateful' and 'blessed'. One respondent expressed her gratitude saying that she felt 'extremely thankful that the staff were so competent and considerate in difficult circumstances.'

CAESAREANS AS A POSITIVE EXPERIENCE

Although many women in these studies concentrated on the negative aspect of operative birth and some suggested ways in which things could be improved for caesarean patients it is important to point out that many women were extremely happy to have had CSs, either because of their gratitude at a successful outcome for their babies or alternatively because they enjoyed the whole experience and found it to be a rewarding one. Many women emphasised their gratitude that the operation was available to help them out of what they perceived to be a very difficult situation. One woman explained how she felt after the operation:

> Painful afterwards, unable to care for baby and my other children as well as I had hoped for. Complications of wound infection are a setback. But thank goodness caesarean sections are available when one cannot deliver vaginally.

Others stressed the advantages of caesarean birth in terms of the outcome for their babies:

> If a caesarean was not done my daughter would never have been born normally, except at huge risk to her and myself.

> It was unavoidable and in the best interests of the baby. Whilst it will take a while to recover it is comforting to know the baby is now safe and well.

Some women said that they were not upset at having to have a caesarean even though they would have preferred not to:

> I had previously been given the option of caesarean section and decided against it. However, I do not regret having had a section (except for the discomfort I'm feeling) and do not feel cheated of a vaginal delivery.

> I would have preferred to have a normal delivery, it would have been a shorter recovery. But I was glad to see my baby.

Another respondent expressed her surprise that the operation was not as bad as she had expected:

> I was very reluctant to have a caesarean but decided towards the end of a sixteen-hour labour it was the sensible option. There is some discomfort but I probably would have got that anyway with a normal delivery. I am very pleased with the size and position of the scar, it is really different to what I expected.

For many women the outcome justified the means:

> As soon as they said you will have to have a section, I became very upset and cried a lot, even though I thoroughly understood the circumstances and knew it was for the very best for my baby and me. But as soon as I came round and saw my husband with my beautiful son I was glad it was all over and glad I had a section. I DON'T REGRET IT ONE BIT AND NEITHER DOES MY HUSBAND. [Emphasis in original]

Many women found the whole experience very rewarding. For some it was because they felt they had been given a reasonable trial of labour before the operation, and for others it was because they were awake during it and were therefore able to feel that they had taken part in the process and seen their babies as they were born. One woman who was awake for the operation said:

> I was very impressed by what a beautiful experience a caesarean could be. I think I would have been more disappointed if I had not been allowed such a full trial of labour but having experienced this the caesarean was a very enjoyable climax to the labour.

WOMEN'S ADVICE TO OTHER WOMEN

Some women in the studies, acknowledging the general feeling of failure among caesarean patients, offered words of advice and support to those who are to follow them onto the operating table. One woman was reassuring about the bond she felt with her baby:

I think that many women feel as though they have failed if they have to give birth by caesarean. But I definitely don't find this to be true as the love you have for your baby is just as strong with a caesarean as with a vaginal birth.

Another respondent offered very practical advice:

1   Don't try and do too much too soon in hospital. You've to be easy on yourself so you can do more later (remember that you've had a major operation).

2   Physically once you're up and walking keep your back straight.

3   Allow yourself a good cry when you want one.

CAESAREAN SECTIONS AND BREASTFEEDING

Mothers were asked: 'Did you want to breastfeed your baby?' The results revealed that two in three (68.2 per cent) of the women having CSs said that they wanted to breastfeed. One in four (27.3 per cent) of the women in this sample said that they did not want to breastfeed. This compares with national figures of women giving birth in Britain who chose to breastfeed in 2000, at 69 per cent.[5]

Those women who did not want to breastfeed were asked about their decision. Half the women in this category (50 per cent) said that their decision not to breastfeed stemmed from their wanting to share the feeding and a third (33.3 per cent) said that they prefer bottle feeding. One in four (27.8 per cent) said that they were 'not keen' on breastfeeding. This may indicate the need for more information for women about the value and convenience of breastfeeding. Once a woman has learned how to breastfeed, she may find it more convenient than bottle feeding because there are no bottles to make up and there is no formula to buy. One in six of this group (16.7 per cent) reported that their decision not to breastfeed was because the baby would not take to it and a further one in six stated previous failure of breastfeeding as the reason. Six women in the sample (11.1 per cent) said that they felt too ill to breastfeed and the same number reported that they had problems with expressing milk. Less common reasons given by women for not wanting to breastfeed were that they 'had no milk', had 'inverted nipples' or because the baby was ill. But these reasons are widespread among all women who begin to breastfeed their babies and then give up[6], and are generally the result of inadequate professional support for breastfeeding.[7]

Women's responses to the question on breastfeeding in 1991-2 raised a number of concerns over the effect that the caesarean operation had on women's ability to breastfeed. The later questionnaires were therefore amended to include a

---

5   DoH, 2003b
6   DoH, 2002
7   Royal College of Midwives, 1991

question on this. Women were asked: 'Do you feel that the caesarean has had an effect on your ability to breastfeed your baby?'

The data revealed that a substantial proportion of women delivering by caesarean feel that the operation affects their ability to breastfeed their babies. One in five (20.2 per cent) answered 'yes' to this question. In commenting on why caesareans affect breastfeeding the majority of women pointed to pain and discomfort: 'because of being so sore, it was too painful,' 'slightly more difficult to get into comfortable position for feeding,' and 'difficulty in holding him with painful belly.'

Others mentioned their lack of mobility: 'holding and lifting the baby and getting out of bed to the baby were difficult', and 'too many attachments, inadequate pain relief to enable free movement.' Some women mentioned that the milk had taken longer to 'come in.' Others blamed the difficulty on the anaesthetic: 'the first feed was difficult because of the general anaesthetic.' One respondent said: 'being a major operation it takes you a long time to recover and to cope with the demands of breastfeeding.' Another stated: 'I am in more pain so less patient with the baby.' Some respondents who had wanted to breastfeed said that they were unable to because of feeling too ill post-operatively. One said that she 'did not attempt to as I felt too ill, I could not cope with another complication.' Another said 'I was too ill to keep up with the demand.' One stated that she had 'too many emotions to continue breastfeeding.' One respondent summed up the feelings of many: 'I think I may have found it easier and been more committed if I had had a natural birth.' Only three women blamed failure to breastfeed on the effects of CS on the condition of the baby.

According to the Infant Feeding 1990 survey, having a caesarean delivery under general anaesthetic or having a low birth-weight baby were both associated with early cessation of breastfeeding. However, mothers whose babies received special care were no more likely to stop breastfeeding in the first two weeks than other mothers.[8]

Women's decisions as to whether to breastfeed and whether to continue breastfeeding are very complex and influenced by many deep-seated factors such as culture, the practice of their peer group and the attitude of their partner and other members of their family. As we have seen, when women have had a caesarean birth, the post-operative pain and the possible feelings of inadequacy from having not given birth vaginally can be added to these influences. For some women, succeeding at breastfeeding is even more important because they have not had a normal birth.

There needs to be recognition that women who have had caesareans have an

---

8   Office of Population Censuses and Surveys, 1992

increased need for support for breastfeeding, both practical and emotional. This is corroborated by the Successful Breastfeeding handbook for midwives, which states: 'There is no evidence to support the long-established belief that CS itself has any deleterious effect on the establishment of lactation. The mother will probably require more help to find a comfortable feeding position and with attaching the baby to the breast in the first few days than she would if she had been vaginally delivered.' [9]

CAESAREAN SECTION: THE WOMEN SPEAK

From the results of our surveys and the responses of women to CS it can be seen that mothers generally have a much better experience of operative delivery if they are adequately prepared for it and are supported by staff in terms of being kept informed throughout the whole process. This point is borne out by the fact that women having planned caesareans report greater satisfaction with the operation than those who have had emergency sections.

> It was a wonderful experience. Because it was elective we were able to organise for the birth, my partner was present and prepared well. He was able to organise leave to be with us, this would have been difficult under less certain circumstances.

> Being an elective section I found I was much better prepared physically and mentally than my first section. Recovery from an elective section was speedier and not as traumatic to both myself and baby.

> Having had three sections, the first being emergency by general anaesthetic, not very pleasant, second and third spinal and a great experience. I think all the information and advice you can be given by the staff helps immensely with both the operation and what the after-effects will be. This being so, there would be no great shocks. I was given brilliant advice and care, so all my experiences have been very good.

One woman explained how simply knowing that she might need another caesarean made it easier to cope:

> With the first caesarean there was great disappointment and feeling that I had suffered a labour for nothing. This time I was fairly optimistic about delivering normally but knew there was the possibility of a second caesarean. Therefore I don't feel so let down this time.

However, some women require more information and are unhappy that they did not receive the details that they required from hospital staff before the delivery. Some respondents were aware that they might have felt better if they had been

---

9   Royal College of Midwives, 1991, p.77

better prepared for the possibility of caesarean birth.

> I wished it could be explained about a caesarean birth earlier in pregnancy.

> It would have been better if I was more prepared for it.

One woman described how her lack of knowledge about caesareans made the experience worse for her:

> Caesareans should be termed as normal operations not minor operations. All along I thought a caesarean wasn't a big deal. I was told how it is done but not how you feel afterwards. [This woman made specific reference to the amount of pain encountered after the operation.]

Another respondent who had an emergency caesarean reported a traumatic experience that could have been averted by information prenatally.

> When they were finishing stitching, I started to be sick and then felt like I could not get any air into my lungs, as though someone was sitting on my chest. This lasted for three hours. When talking to the doctor a couple of days later she assured me that this was entirely clinical, to do with my blood pressure and temperature, and that this was quite common. Talking to other caesarean women on the wards later, we had all experienced this to some degree and felt that if we had been told this may happen beforehand then we would not have panicked as much at the time.

Some women from the planned caesarean group were equally dissatisfied. One said:

> I did not anticipate so much tugging and pulling. I did not know how I would be stitched up or stapled. The number of people around me was disquieting.

It therefore appears that although the majority of women in the studies were happy with the amount of information that they received from hospital staff, there are deficiencies in some areas with regards to informing women about procedures for caesarean birth and preparing them for the after-effects. Whether it is lack of time that prevents the appropriate information being imparted to women, or personnel or procedural restrictions within the hospital setting, is open to debate. It is unlikely though, that even in an emergency situation, there would not be time to inform women about the operation. Lack of time, however, does appear to have an effect on women's ability to adjust mentally and prepare for caesarean birth.

WOMEN'S ADVICE TO HOSPITAL STAFF

Some women felt able to advise medical practitioners on the use of caesareans, for example saying that it should only be used when all other options have been exhausted. One woman said that 'it is best used only in emergency cases.'

Another stated: 'Emergency section decisions should be made as early as possible as a long period in labour beforehand is very traumatic.' These two comments exemplify the significant divergence of opinion between women on whether caesareans should only be used as a last resort, when the woman has been given every chance to deliver vaginally. It is clear from our surveys that some women wish to be allowed to labour for as long as possible whereas others would prefer a caesarean to be recommended earlier to give them time to come to terms with it. The only solution is for hospital staff to get to know each woman individually, to maintain good communication in labour and to invite her to join in any decisions made about her care.

One woman gave very specific advice about caesarean birth:

1   It should be a last resort.

2   More information should be impressed on expectant mothers – so that they appreciate that it could happen to them.

This second point highlights the feelings of many women about lack of information given to expectant women. The question of what is taught at antenatal classes was a recurring theme:

I think that much more should be taught about caesareans at antenatal classes to prepare women for the after-effects as it seems commonplace nowadays.

I would have liked to know more antenatally about different kinds of pain relief given post-caesarean section. It might be helpful to consider each case individually and not just prescribe routine painkillers. Otherwise I was impressed by the standard of care and information given to me.

Many women felt that improvements in post-operative care could be made:

I think that caesarean patients should really be given more rest and not be expected to be up and around within twenty-four hours to be looking after baby.

I felt that for the first three days the baby could have been taken off me at night, and bottle fed, and then left with me when she was quiet in the day and breast fed. But the second day I was up, and doing nearly everything by the third day, which caused me stress because I couldn't quite manage because of the pain I was in. It left me feeling inadequate as a mother, and I wanted to do more.

The most important thing for recovery afterwards is sleep and you don't get any on a postnatal ward with up to ten other mums and babies. Caesarean patients should have their own rooms/side wards for recovery as I did after my first one.

I feel support for caesarean mothers is more important once they are home as depression is not always immediate and affected me several months after my previous caesarean sections.

ATTITUDE OF THE HOSPITAL STAFF

One of the most important factors affecting whether or not women had a positive experience of CS, besides being fully informed and being awake during the operation, was the attitude of the hospital staff. Not surprisingly, those women who were helped through the experience by caring and supportive staff had a much better experience overall. One woman commented on the attitude of staff on the way to the operating theatre:

> The atmosphere was very relaxed when they took me up to theatre, even managed to get me laughing. My husband and I found this a great help.

For those women who were awake during the operation the attitude of the theatre staff was equally important.

> I felt frightened but confident at the same time. The theatre staff made me feel very special, I had lots of attention. I was overwhelmed with gratitude when they delivered our baby.

> The third section was the best of the lot, much more straightforward – and went according to plan. The theatre staff were a tremendous help talking me through the operation. After, I felt on top of the world and very relaxed.

> The staff were very supportive and were always reassuring me throughout the whole birth because it was my first birth and having a hard time as well. If I have to have a caesarean again I would hope that I would be fortunate enough to have similar staff as I had for my first.

> I found the staff in the theatre very helpful and friendly which was very satisfying and made things a lot easier.

One woman pointed out how a friendly atmosphere in the theatre helps the woman and does not interfere with efficiency:

> The relaxed atmosphere of the theatre was good and should be encouraged. It did not at any time seem to interfere with its smooth and efficient running.

Of course support and understanding on the part of hospital staff is equally important post-operatively.

> I felt quite happy about this last section. The operation went fine and I have felt very well through the recovery stage. I have received very good support from the staff and this I feel is most important. They have given me the help when I have asked and have let me do things in my own time.

One woman commented on how the attitude of the staff helped her get over the shock of having to have an emergency section:

> An emergency section is very frightening because you are not prepared for it. But

if the hospital you are in has good and caring staff where nothing is too much, it makes the difference to your outlook on things.

Clearly the attitude and outlook of staff interacts with other factors such as being adequately informed and, preferably, being awake during the operation, to enable caesarean patients to have a positive experience. These thoughts are appropriately summed up in the words of one of the respondents:

Two years ago I had a 'semi-emergency' section under general anaesthetic in a different hospital. I was not offered an epidural and even had I had one my husband would not have been allowed to stay with me. So bad did I feel the experience and recovery to have been that I changed to a hospital twenty miles further away to avoid a repetition. Although the outcome was essentially the same, i.e. caesarean, the experience was completely different – everyone seemed to be 'on my side' this time. I was quite happy about the ultimate decision, hence I feel I am recovering much better. I think the two crucial factors in this are:

i)   The attitude of the staff on the labour ward, and

ii) Epidural anaesthesia, which enabled both me and my husband to be present for the birth.

SUMMING UP WOMEN'S COMMENTS

One of the most important findings that came out of our earlier studies was that women who were awake for their caesareans tended to have much better experiences of the operation and reported less suffering. There are a number of other reasons that it is preferable for women to be awake for the operation:

1   The women are conscious of all that is happening and therefore feel that they have participated in the birth.
2   The mothers are able to see their babies as soon as they are born.
3   Their partners are able to be present at the birth and to play a role.
4   The women do not have to cope with the after-effects of a general anaesthetic.

In the first edition of this book (1993) we raised the important question of whether it ought to be routine practice for women to be awake for CSs in all possible cases. At that time, of the 300 deliveries by caesarean in our study, only two in five (39.7 per cent) were performed with the woman awake. Even in the case of planned operations, only three out of five caesareans were done with the woman awake. This was the result of hospital or consultant policy rather than women's preference, as comments from women overwhelmingly suggested that they would rather be awake. There has been a change in practice since the early 1990s and now the majority of caesareans are performed under spinal block enabling women to be awake for the birth, be aware of what is going on and participate in the process.

One of the most startling observations to come out of our research over the years is the fact that many women are still relatively unprepared for operative delivery. Caesarean birth is mentioned at antenatal classes but not all women attend these classes and the philosophy of 'it'll never happen to me' may come into play, in particular when the pregnancy has been normal.

It also points to the fact that there is a lack of understanding generally about caesarean birth. Some women see it as a 'soft' option and do not realise the pain, discomfort, lack of mobility and lengthy recovery that it entails. Medical practitioners do not always realise that women who are better informed often have better experiences of operative birth. Obviously this is not always possible in an emergency situation but does indicate that all pregnant women need to have full knowledge of CS, whether they are seen to be 'at risk' in terms of possibly needing a section or not. Similarly hospital staff should be sensitive to the post-operative needs and feelings of women who have had caesareans as they will not always be able to deal with their newborns as well as they had expected and this can cause stress and depression.

From the comments made by the women in our surveys it is clear that many experience very mixed feelings about the operation. Obviously they are thankful that it is available and understand the necessity in certain circumstances. Yet because the majority of women are incapacitated by the surgery, they are unable to fulfil what they perceive to be their full maternal role with their babies. This will inevitably lead to conflict for the women concerned.

It appears that, on the whole, women are kept informed about their condition and that of their baby. However, information is often lacking in terms of the procedure for CS and the effects on women post-operatively. If women are to make informed decisions and to be empowered to take a full and rewarding part in the birth of their children, they need to realise that caesarean birth is a possibility and to be given appropriate information in order to reduce feelings of shock, disappointment and resentment. In particular, women should be made aware of the relative advantages and disadvantages of the different types of anaesthesia used for caesarean operations, and how they are likely to feel post-operatively. It should be explained that there will be reduced mobility and some pain.

At the same time, it needs to be said that in most cases where an emergency caesarean is necessary, there is time not only for the choice and administration of regional anaesthesia but also for giving all information relevant to the woman. It is only in the case of a real emergency, perhaps if the woman is bleeding heavily or having fits, that this is not the case. Also, women need to have an accurate idea of the real chances of having a caesarean.

8 The views of 100 consultants

'The ease with which this operation is performed and the general safety of spinal blocks and availability of blood in the UK prevent obstetricians from appreciating why nature intended women to deliver vaginally.'

In February 2005 we circulated a questionnaire to all 231 clinical directors in obstetrics and gynaecology listed by the Royal College of Obstetricians and Gynaecologists in the British Isles. For this chapter we analysed the responses of the first 100 consultants to reply.

Consultants' views of the rise in caesarean rates

We asked obstetricians a similar question to that asked in our 1990 survey.[1] 'The British caesarean rate has risen from 12.1 per cent in 1989 to 21.5 per cent in 2003. What do you think are the major reasons for this rise?' One answered 'No idea'. The other consultants gave 293 reasons, an average of three per consultant – see Table A.5, Appendix C.

Overall nearly ninety different reasons were suggested. Over half the consultants mentioned the fear of litigation or defensive medicine, followed by almost half who mentioned lack of skill in junior staff either generally or in dealing with operative vaginal birth. Maternal request, demand or pressure was suggested by forty-four and patient expectation by twenty-seven. Medical reasons, cited by twenty-four consultants, included a reduction in damaged babies as well as those listed in the table. The change in policy on breech birth (twenty-three consultants) was the fifth reason mentioned and repeat caesarean (often linked as a consequence of the rise in first births by CS) was mentioned by sixteen consultants and another two mentioned women's reluctance to undertake a trial of labour. It is instructive to consider some of the reasons given and the free comments on this topic, in more detail.

---

1   Francome & Savage, 1993

One consultant from a northern town listed five factors:

- Inadequate midwifery numbers and funding to promote a normal birth.

- Most consultant obstetricians/gynaecologists are not interested in or dislike practising intra-partum obstetrics.

- There are inappropriate obstetric interventions, for example, for inappropriately diagnosed 'fetal distress' and poor management of 'failure to progress'.

- There is a loss of clinical skills amongst obstetric staff. This applies to breech [birth], twin [birth], Kielland forceps – even vaginal examinations! For example, a consultant colleague last week sectioned a patient of mine who had a footling breech presentation of the second twin after the vaginal [birth] of the first!

- The Term Breech Trial results are highly suspect (e.g. extreme bias in recruitment) and yet are greatly influencing the modern management of breech presentation.

Others also expressed concern about the rising rates. One commented:

> The ease with which this operation is performed and the general safety of spinal blocks and availability of blood in the UK prevents obstetricians from appreciating why nature intended women to deliver vaginally. The art of delivering term breeches is disappearing. Even if SPRs running labour wards have a lower threshold for c-sections they should feel passionate to deliver primips vaginally and should only be performing caesareans on them if absolutely necessary.

One consultant with a 17 per cent CSR said:

> Arguably this is too high but low by Irish standards. Our section rate in spontaneous labouring primips and multips has not changed for ten years. The increase has been in repeat section (i.e. no VBAC) in women with previous section, section for breech, increased sections in multiple pregnancies etc.

Some however, take the view that the caesarean rate is the best mode of birth. One stated that 'it is a safer mode [of birth] for the baby and in the case of planned CS probably safer for the mother as well.'

Litigation, defensive medicine

This reason was mentioned by over half of the doctors compared to just under half (47 per cent) when we conducted the survey fifteen years ago. One consultant suggested it was not so simple:

> Medico-legal pressure is often blamed. I do not think it is such an important factor, it is more the pressure from women and their families for everything to go

absolutely 100 per cent and their anger at medical staff/establishment if something is not perfect. This is far more frequent and devastating than being sued, which is fairly uncommon.

The role of midwives and junior doctors

Almost half of the obstetricians mentioned the reduced skill in junior doctors especially in carrying out alternative methods such as forceps, twin or breech deliveries. One argued that 'LSCS is safer if you have inexperienced/ incompetent registrars/locums.'

Another commented 'Changes in juniors' hours means less continuity and "seeing through" of decisions made. CS becomes an easier option. The greatest thrill on the Labour Ward for me was getting a woman to deliver vaginally when the odds seemed unlikely'.

Lack of supervision of juniors was mentioned by three consultants. One consultant said 'the training of junior doctors is a major factor in the rising CSR' and two mentioned the inexperience of senior doctors and another said 'new consultants lack confidence'.

One obstetrician commented:

> Midwives, as much as obstetricians, can generate an ethos of expectation of a caesarean in many situations. It is not always doctors who are trying to do a CS. I spend more of my time trying to dissuade women than persuading them to have a caesarean.

Others felt that poor midwifery practice or a shortage of midwives so that one-to-one care was not achieved added to the rising CSR. Two commented that midwives were intolerant of long labours.

Maternal request

When we conducted our previous survey fifteen years ago this was a reason mentioned by only five of the 232 consultants surveyed. In the last decade the importance of the patient's involvement in making decisions about their care has been emphasised by the General Medical Council in *Good Medical Practice*.[2] The Winterton report[3] in 1992 and the government's response in the *Changing Childbirth*[4] report 1993 highlighted the importance of women's views and choice in childbirth so it is not surprising that in such a relatively short time it has become a leading reason given by the obstetricians in our study. It seems at

---

2   GMC, 1995
3   HoC, 1992
4   DoH, 1993

least one consultant sees maternal request as a problem and wrote 'thankfully we have not seen an increase in caesarean section for maternal request. Our unit does not grant them to primigravid women with cephalic presentation – we hope this continues.'

In contrast, another obstetrician pointed to the high caesarean rate amongst female obstetricians (erroneously – it was a survey of intentions to deliver, given various scenarios, and has some methodological flaws [5]) and went on to say:

> To be equable [sic] we should discuss the risks of normal deliveries (as well as caesarean), but do we? ... If a home [birth] in a birth pool can be demanded by patients how can we deny a caesarean section request?

Sometimes it seems that an unusual and unfortunate event can influence the obstetrician's attitude. One stated:

> I think we are compromised when patients demand a caesar and it is refused if the outcome is poor. A recent event brought this home when a lady with a breech was offered a CS and then this decision was reversed because the baby had spontaneously verted (turned round). The patient still preferred a caesarean. Sadly the baby succumbed when unanticipated vasa-praevia ruptured at the IOL (blood vessels from the placental circulation rarely cross the membranes round the baby and can bleed if torn so the baby loses blood and may die if the condition is unrecognised). Not surprisingly the parents feel that if we had acceded to their wishes the baby would still be alive – born by CS. In the face of this who are we to refuse parents requests if they feel it is the right decision for them given all the facts.

Patient expectation

Doctors commented that women were unwilling to accept any risk, the sequelae of normal labour, and were unprepared for labour. One said: 'Patients push for guaranteed [birth]'.

The unacceptability of a long labour was mentioned by six consultants and it ties in with maternal request. One consultant stated:

> I think the collective loss of society's experiences of the reality of childbirth has led women and their families to expect short, pain-free births. I would also completely support any woman's wish to have a caesarean if we have had enough opportunity to explore the reasons for her wish.

Another consultant said that it was not just the pregnant women who had changed their attitudes: 'The acceptability of a long labour or difficult vaginal

---

5   Al-Mufti et al., 1997

[birth] has diminished greatly for women, midwives and obstetricians.' A third commented:

> Our LSCS rate is greater than 25 per cent. I think the only way to reduce it is to educate/persuade women and their partners to accept the possibility of longer labour and difficult vaginal deliveries. Given the mental and physical trauma that this may cause, I doubt if it is worth it.

Informing pregnant women of the risks of a caesarean section

We wondered whether women's apparent willingness to undergo CS was due to a lack of appreciation of the risks involved. The NICE guidelines[6] suggest that all women antenatally should be given information about the risks and benefits of CS as one in five will have a CS, so it was an opportunity to see if these guidelines were followed. We asked a new question: 'What risks of caesarean, if any, do you routinely mention to women?' The results are shown in Table A.6 in Appendix C.

Only one consultant said he did not mention any risks routinely and another said 'it depends'. Two said 'as in NICE' and one 'as in RCOG guidelines'. On average they mentioned 4.2 risks so the usual risks of surgery such as haemorrhage, infection and thrombosis were mentioned by the majority. The results show that over seven out of ten consultants mentioned potential problems with infection and haemorrhage and half mentioned venous thrombo-embolism. Just under a third mentioned the fact that there would be a scar on the uterus which could cause problems in a future pregnancy, such as an adherent placenta or that the scar would dehisce. Effects on the baby were not often mentioned. Some consultants made it clear that if there was to be an emergency caesarean then they spent less time going over the risks than if a planned caesarean were to be performed.

West Suffolk Hospitals NHS Trust produced a leaflet setting out the risks which might be useful for others to copy. It is reproduced in Appendix C as Table A.7.

There is a case for the risks of a caesarean to be provided during antenatal classes in order that women are fully informed ahead of labour. The NICE guidelines suggest informing women during their antenatal care and have figures of the incidence of risks based on the literature and referenced.

Is the local caesarean rate too high?

We asked consultants 'Do you think that the caesarean rate in your hospital is too low, about right or too high?' In response over half (56) said the rate was too high, just under two in five (38) said it was 'about right' and just one in fifty (2)

6   NICE, 2004

said it was too low. One of these who said it was too low had a rate of 11 per cent, the other did not give the rate but thought an optimal rate was 40 per cent. One said he did not know and three did not reply to the question.

Reducing a caesarean rate that is 'too high'

Those who thought their caesarean rate was 'too high' were invited to comment on what steps could be taken to reduce it. The NICE guidelines[7] suggest seven ways to reduce the CSR:

- Offer ECV if breech at thirty-six weeks
- Facilitate continuous support during labour
- Offer induction of labour beyond forty-one weeks
- Use a partogram with a four-hour action line in labour
- Involve consultant obstetricians in the decision
- Do fetal blood sampling for abnormal CTG in labour
- Support women who choose VBAC.

The obstetricians cited VBAC, ECV and more consultant input, but were more likely to mention less easily measurable factors which are not on this list as shown by the responses in Table A.8 in Appendix C.

Two consultants said 'we are reducing our CSR' one from 18 per cent (from a high of 21 per cent) and one just said 21 per cent, but they did not specify how they had achieved this reduction. One who thought the caesarean rate was too high thought it was going to be very difficult to reduce it and commented: 'How do you turn round an oil tanker?' The major method of reducing the caesarean rate mentioned was to have more consultant input and thirteen of the fifty-six mentioned this reason. Two said that there should be twenty-four hour consultant care on the labour ward.

The second most frequently mentioned reason was to increase the number of vaginal births after a previous caesarean. One said 'in all cases where there has been a previous CS there should be a discussion at 12/52 in subsequent pregnancy'. Another said 'there should be a hard line on repeat sections'. Another said 'V[ery] difficult. Mx [manage] primips well to maximise vaginal [birth] will impact on CS rate.' A Scottish obstetrician commented that despite following the recommendations of the Scottish audit,[8] 'ECV, FBS pre-CS, VBAC, syntocinon augmentation, the CS rate has risen.' Despite much thought he had no other suggestions for reducing the rate.

Improved staffing and parental education were mentioned by another consultant

7   NICE, 2004
8   McIlwaine et al., 1998

as ways to reduce the rate.

Nine consultants mentioned improvements in the care provided by midwives. One stated that 'there should be different models of midwifery care to promote normality. For example the home assessment of early labour and the promotion of home birth'. Another commented 'There should be more support for newly qualified midwives'. Three consultants said we should educate, and one said encourage, women. One of these commented 'There should be a change in the public's expectation of labour and the acceptance of small risks'. Another said that if there was patient education then they would be more likely to be 'singing from the same hymn book' as the health personnel.

One stated 'no caesarean should be performed for fetal distress if FBS is possible'; another said 'should not do caesarean for fetal distress without scalp ph except for bradycardia'; and one said 'deny maternal distress'. Other comments were:

> Reduce CS just because CS before; more use of FBS in labour.
>
> There should be an experienced supportive culture and a highly experienced non-interventionist obstetrician on duty all the time.
>
> Case-note review and feedback which will be reflected in practice.

On midwifery care, one consultant said 'Midwives need to be able to practise interventionist policies efficiently e.g. induction of labour when indicated. They tend to practise low-risk protocols in high-risk patients/high-risk interventions.'

Other suggestions included 'twenty-four hour consultant presence on the labour ward' and 'more senior obstetric input to clinics and labour ward'.

Should a woman have more than three caesareans?

Anecdotally women report being told that they cannot have more than a set number of CSs and we are aware of one who was sterilised without her consent at the third operation.[9] We wondered if this was a common policy and asked the following question: 'Some women are told that they should not have more than three caesareans. Do you agree with this view?' The responses of the 100 consultants showed that only eight agreed with this view and eighty-nine disagreed with it with the others being unsure. One commented 'I know of no evidence to support this view but I believe that the risks continue to grow with increasing numbers.' Another five wrote 'No evidence'. Another commented 'Four caesareans remain statistically safe' and one said 'Always cite the Irish record of fourteen? Apocryphal'. Two of those who disagreed said: 'I would offer sterilisation at the time of the third caesarean if she wanted'. Another who

---

9   Personal correspondence – Colin Francome

opposed the three-caesarean limit nevertheless said that she would 'need to know the circumstances of the previous caesareans'. Another female consultant said that, although she opposed the three-caesarean rule, 'It depends on how difficult the last caesarean was, women do vary and if increasingly challenging I would suggest they don't have more'. The permissive approach to further surgery was surprising when compared with the conservative views about VBAC after two caesareans discussed in the next section.

Vaginal birth after two caesareans

We asked the 100 consultants the following question: 'If a woman has had two previous caesareans but wishes for a vaginal birth what would be your advice?' One said the question was too complex to answer in two lines and another asked 'Why two caesareans?'

Almost three-fifths of the consultants (56) said that they would advise another caesarean. One said that the woman 'should seek another opinion'. Another said that he would tell the women to 'be sensible' and a third said that in such a case the woman should 'find another obstetrician'. One of those who advised a repeat CS added the rider that he had never had such a request. Some were less fixed in their views and eight of them said they would support the woman if she was insistent or adamant or would agree to a trial of labour as it was her choice. One commented 'ideally she should have a caesarean again, but I have supported (successfully) a VBAC after two previous caesareans.' Another said 'The consensus is NO but it is not written in stone'. Those opposing a vaginal birth often mentioned the possibility of the rupture of the previous scar, although they had different figures for the likely risk. One said that the scar ruptures in 5 per cent of cases, others said it happens in 3 per cent of births, several said the risk was 1 per cent and another said it occurs in one in 200 births. Others did not specify the level of risk. One commented 'No, the risk of rupture is too great. Whilst I might be able to support such a decision it could only be followed through if I was available 24 hours a day'.

Forty-two said that they would support the woman's decision after reviewing the notes or with certain conditions set out. Some of the comments are set out below:

> I would advise her it is a safe thing to do but we would have a low threshold for repeat caesarean.

> As long as there is no absolute obstetric indication the patient has the choice. There is no evidence that it is unsafe.

> I would review previous decision for caesareans, advise on the possibility of risk of scar rupture and support her decision after full discussion.

> We would advise her that it is safer to have a repeat caesarean but we would support a woman if she wished a trial of labour.

> She would be allowed a vaginal birth if: 1) She laboured before, 2) She wants

spontaneous labour, and 3) She accepts the risks.

I would discuss the possible risks and document these in detail, discuss the possibility with fellow colleagues and support the patient.

I am not against it. I tell them there is a 1 per cent risk of scar rupture.

This figure is correct as recorded in the literature and is not very different from the risk of scar dehiscence after one CS which is quoted as one in 200.[10] Roberts argued persuasively in 1991 that this was a safe option.[11]

Prevalence of fetal monitoring

The RCOG guideline on electronic fetal monitoring published in 2001[12] did not recommend routine EFM for all pregnant women nor a short admission trace when they present at the labour ward. In our previous survey in 1990, 45 per cent of consultants said they used routine CEFM in labour and we wondered whether the guideline had changed this policy. We asked two questions on this subject. The first was 'Does your department monitor all women electronically in labour?' In response only 7 per cent said that they did so. However, the following question asked 'If not, does your department do a twenty-minute monitor strip on all women on admission to the labour ward?' In response the replies were evenly divided with 50 per cent saying they did so and 50 per cent saying that they did not. We know that some women will have some abnormality on an admission trace which then leads to CEFM being continued and so the 7 per cent figure may be an underestimate of its use in practice.

Use of epidurals

The respondents were asked 'What percentage of women at your hospital have an epidural?' Only five consultants seemed to have accurate data and most gave an estimated figure. However, those who had accurate figures could distinguish between rates according to whether or not the woman was a first time mother. One of these said there was a rate of 68 per cent for primips and 34 per cent for multips. For the purpose of our analysis we have grouped the figures to the nearest 5 per cent. They show that two consultants said that there were no epidurals, seven said 10 per cent, eight said 15 per cent, twenty-one said 20 per cent, seven said 25 per cent, thirteen said 30 per cent, nineteen said 40 per cent, eight said 50 per cent, and eight said 60 per cent. The other seven did not know.

---

10 NICE, 2004
11 Roberts, 1991
12 RCOG, 2001d

Agreement with NICE guidelines

We asked the respondents 'Do you accept the NICE guidelines for caesarean birth published on 27.4.04?'[13] Six did not respond to the question. One of these said 'not pragmatic in terms of time required for each detailed discussion'. Two others commented that those preparing the guidelines did not seem to have spent much time in the labour ward! A third of those responding (31), said they accepted the findings fully. One of these said 'Accept – it changed nothing'. Fifty-nine said they accepted them partially but few made comments about their reservations. One said 'Some issues do not have enough evidence so still personal practice' and another, who accepted the guidelines, disputed the HIV advice. Four said that they did not accept them. One of these said 'the evidence was evaluated very thoroughly but evidently false conclusions were drawn in many cases'. Another commented 'NICE not very helpful. Show patients the risks and then do what they want – that will not reduce the rate'. A third (who has done research in the field and shown how to reduce the CSR) commented 'I feel that they are totally inadequate/poor'.

Partner presence at the caesarean operation

The increased use of regional anaesthesia has changed the nature of the operation and led to partners being increasingly invited to watch the birth. Nine out of ten said that the partner was invited to attend and the others said that a birth partner was invited if the conditions were right, the main proviso being that the operation was not being carried out under general anaesthetic. Two also mentioned that the anaesthetist should also be happy about it. In our previous survey only 47.8 per cent of consultants said they would allow a birth partner to attend a caesarean, a slightly higher percentage (48.4) said partners were invited '*sometimes*'. So there has been a major shift in policy in the intervening fifteen years which is reflected in the results of our survey of women having caesareans. In 1991–2, 55 per cent said that their partners were permitted to attend (66 per cent at planned CS) and this rose to 83.5 per cent in 2004 (see chapter 7).

FIGO Ethics Committee recommendation

The International Federation of Gynaecology and Obstetrics published a statement in 1999 when the debate in the UK about CS on request was at its height, concluding that CS for non-medical indications was unethical. We wondered whether this had influenced British obstetricians. We asked 'Do you agree with the FIGO Ethics Committee report on "Ethical aspects regarding caesarean delivery for non-medical reasons"?'[14] Nearly nine out of ten (87)

---

13 NICE, 2004
14 FIGO, 1999

consultants had not read the report but, of those that had, nine were in agreement and three opposed to the recommendations. One did not answer the question.

Fetal distress at twenty-four weeks

We asked the respondents 'Would you perform a caesarean for fetal distress at twenty-four weeks?' Two-thirds (65) said that they would not, in contrast to 76 per cent in 1990, although several added comments such as 'never say never' or 'only if the mother is bleeding'. One in five (20) said that they would perform one compared with our last survey when only 3.5 per cent said they would perform a CS at this gestation. One commented 'I have done so occasionally'. Another said 'Only after full consultation with parents and in a hospital with intensive neonatal care'. A further one in eight (12) of consultants said that they would perform a caesarean 'occasionally' or that it 'depends'. Three did not reply and one of these said 'It's not that straightforward'.

No-fault compensation

We asked the consultants 'Do you think that we should introduce no-fault compensation for the parents of brain-damaged infants?' In response, three-quarters (76) agreed with the statement, under one in five (17) disagreed and the other seven were unsure. In 1990, 84 per cent said 'yes', 14 per cent 'no' and 2 per cent answered 'don't know' so there is no significant change.

One who said 'yes' nevertheless commented 'It will never happen because of legal impediments in our jurisdiction'. Another made the point that 'it will lower the CS rates'. A third stated that it should be introduced 'or have a society where the care package is so good for all that financial compensation needs to be minimal (dream on!!)'.

Several pointed to the drain on financial and other resources of such cases. Three typical comments were:

> The time spent (let alone the money) on such cases could be redirected into something useful.
> All brain-damaged children need good care not just those that win in litigation. It is the child that matters.
> We should stop lawyers getting rich on our behalf.

Those who disagreed made several comments. One said 'The social services support system should swing into place. Who knows whether it is intrauterine infection at the root cause?' Another commented 'I really would like trusts to have crown indemnity but this is not a realistic hope.' A third stated that she opposed no fault compensation: 'However, the government should be responsible for the needs of handicapped babies'. A fourth said ' No – it would remove the pressure to improve practice'.

Those who were unsure made a number of points. For example one said 'I think the arguments are very complicated'. Another commented 'I am uncertain – I disagree with a few getting large damages but there are some situations where aftercare is clearly at fault'.

The optimal caesarean rate

We asked the consultants: 'Given the state of medical knowledge, what would you suggest is the optimal caesarean rate for Great Britain?' We published another paper in 1993 on our survey[15] and the accompanying editorial was entitled 'What is the correct caesarean rate: how long is a piece of string?'[16] The conclusion was that there was no correct rate. However, referring to the WHO consensus statement 'Appropriate technology for birth' which stated that no WHO Region should have a CSR above 10–15 per cent,[17] we believe that it is possible to estimate a rate by looking at the indications for surgery. This was discussed by Wendy Savage in her policy report 'Is it so difficult to define an optimal caesarean rate for a population?'[18] The American Public Health doctors set targets for CS and VBAC rates in their publication *Healthy People 2000*.[19]

When we asked this question in 1990, 192 of 237 consultants answered (eighty-one per cent). A fifth of them said the optimal rate was less than 10 per cent and almost half (forty-four per cent) suggested a rate between 10 and 11.9 per cent. Seventeen per cent said between 12 per cent and 13.9 per cent. Thus only a fifth (nineteen per cent of consultants) thought the rate should be 14 per cent or above.

The replies when we asked the question in 2005 can be found in Table A.9 in Appendix C. These show that there has been a major shift in the perception of the optimal rate with over ninety per cent saying the optimal rate would be 14 per cent or more.

The results show that, of those consultants making an estimate, just over half said the optimum rate was within the range of 15-19 per cent. Some of these would give a range such as 16-18 per cent, so for the analysis we took the average, while others would plump for a single figure. The most common figure mentioned was 15 per cent, followed closely by 20 per cent. A total of thirty consultants (thirty-seven per cent) mentioned a figure of 20 per cent or above. Of these, seven proposed a figure of above 25 per cent and two even suggested 40 per cent. One consultant proposed an optimum rate of 30 per cent but then

---

15 Savage & Francome, 1993
16 Commentary, *British Journal of Obstetrics and Gynaecology*, 1993
17 WHO, 1985
18 Savage, 1997
19 DHHS, 1991

commented 'The caesarean rate will be 40 per cent in ten years – why make a fuss now the rise is inexorable.'

Nineteen of the consultants did not provide an optimal caesarean rate. One said 'too hard a question' and another said he did not have the skills to calculate this. Another simply said 'There is no answer to this' and another 'None'; three left the question blank. One argued that the research to carry out comparative safety has not been carried out:

> We do not have the evidence to prove that LSCS is less safe for the mother and baby. Until we do, all arguments are flawed. You would need huge arms with intention to treat – [planned] caesarean versus planned vaginal [birth] and then you would need to look at maternal and fetal outcomes. It will never happen.

One commented: 'There isn't one [an optimum rate]. It depends upon women's choice after being given all the information in a suitable manner.' Another suggested a rate of 22 per cent but then commented:

> Any optimal caesarean rate is arbitrary. The main thing is that the woman and her baby are healthy. A woman is more likely to complain if CS is not done and the baby dies than if the CS is done and she and her baby are well.

Discussion

In the last fifteen years the attitudes of consultants have changed. More now cited evidence in giving their answers and there is a greater awareness of the rights of women. The four medical reasons for the rise in the CSR (first enumerated in 1978 when the US Task Force[20] looked at the reasons why the rate had tripled in less than twenty years from 4.5 per cent to almost 15 per cent) are fetal distress, repeat CS, breech and 'dystocia'. However, in addition, the consultants now consider that non-medical factors are as important. Litigation, or the fear of litigation, is the leading reason, as it was in our 1990 survey; but, although some disquiet had been expressed in 1990, worries about younger doctors are now a major anxiety in 2005. Consultants seem concerned that some of the skills of the older obstetricians, for example birth using forceps , twin and breech birth are not being passed on to the younger generation.

The new factor cited is 'maternal choice' followed by 'patient expectation of a quick easy labour' or 'simple CS'. 'Empowerment of women' was given as a reason by one consultant. Others thought that women's awareness of the possibility of damage to the pelvic floor or to the baby was the reason for their choosing to deliver by CS. Demographic factors were not thought to be

---

20 US Task Force, 1978

important by the majority of consultants although the age of first birth has risen and the number of women having third and greater numbers of babies has declined.

There is a spectrum of views, from the consultant who considered the optimal CSR for Great Britain to be 9 per cent and said 'The majority of CS in Britain today could be safely avoided' by better midwifery and obstetric care, to the other extreme where 40 per cent was the optimal CSR quoted. One of these consultants considered pressure from patients 'maintained this level', referring to his own hospital.

Whether it will be possible to reduce the CSR by adherence to the NICE guidelines we doubt. What is needed is a change of philosophy on the part of obstetricians. Listening to women is important and obstetricians appeared to be doing this much more than when we did our last survey, judging from the way they framed their answers. But the way the consultant presents the risks is crucial to the way that the woman makes her decision. In a recent Appeal Court judgement where a man with a progressive neurological disorder challenged GMC guidelines about end of life decisions about care, the three judges ruled that 'a patient cannot demand that a doctor administers treatment which the doctor considers is adverse to the patient's clinical needs'. This suggests that there are limits to patient choice despite government rhetoric.[21] Although over half this small sample thought the rate was too high in their own hospital (and they had some suggestions for reducing this) it is amazing that within fifteen years the perception of what is a normal rate of CS has changed so radically. We gained the impression from reading the responses that some obstetricians felt disempowered. They appeared unable to change things in the face of factors outside their control such as doctors' hours and training, midwifery staffing and practice, and pressure from women and the public – overshadowed by the fear of litigation if something goes wrong. One obstetrician called for radical midwifery to act as a counterbalance to defensive obstetrics and several called for a re-evaluation of the Term Breech Trial. As one said in response to the question about advice after two caesareans 'To have a section – the real issue is to avoid the first section'.

Better preparation for labour, avoidance of unnecessary induction and keeping normal healthy women out of the hands of obstetricians and hospitals would be another way to reduce the CSR. To do this, we need to encourage and retain midwives and allow them to practise as they are trained to do.

---

21 Dyer, 2005, p.309

9 Vaginal birth after caesarean (VBAC)

'A planned vaginal birth after a previous caesarean section should be recommended for women whose first caesarean section was by lower segment transverse incision, and who have no other indication for caesarean section in the present pregnancy.'[1]

VBAC HAS BEEN SHOWN TO REDUCE THE CAESAREAN section rate.[2] Evidence on the appropriateness of VBAC is scant and most information comes from observational prospective cohort studies. From these, it has been concluded that VBAC is safe for the majority of women. Overall VBAC appears to be safer for mother and child than planned caesareans and VBAC mothers tend to have the same history and frequency of complications as mothers with previous vaginal births.[3] The morbidity associated with successful vaginal birth is about one-fifth that of planned caesarean.[4] Successful VBAC is associated with less postnatal morbidity including fewer blood transfusions, reduced infection rates and shorter hospital stays.[5] Further, it has been suggested that repeat caesareans offer no advantage for mother[6] or child.[7] Further, the risks associated with caesarean section rise with the number of caesareans a woman has. This means that decisions regarding VBAC versus repeat caesareans need to include consideration of the woman's future plans in terms of whether she intends to have more children. VBAC should be recommended if the woman intends to have more children as it has been suggested that each caesarean shifts some of the risks from that baby on to all the woman's future babies.[8]

1   Enkin et al., 2000, p.370
2   Walker et al., 2004; Hindawi, 2004
3   Placek & Taffel, 1988
4   Enkin et al., 2000
5   Odibo & Macones, 2003
6   NIH, 1981; Nielsen & Hökegård, 1989
7   NIH, 1981
8   www.homebirth.org, 2001

Success of VBAC

In clinical trials 70 per cent of women have been found to achieve successful VBAC. One midwifery centre in the US found that more than 98 per cent of the women who attempted VBAC with them gave birth vaginally.[9] In England and Wales, in 2000, 33 per cent of women with previous caesareans had vaginal birth and the VBAC rate ranged between the different maternity units from 6 to 64 per cent.[10] Interestingly, regions of Britain with the highest VBAC rates have lower overall caesarean section rates (Table 9.1 below). The North East region has the highest VBAC rate in Britain and the lowest rate of caesarean birth. In contrast Wales, which has one of the lowest VBAC rates in Britain, had the highest caesarean section rate in 2000. In Scotland the VBAC rate declined from 41 per cent in 1997-9 to 36 per cent in 1991-3.[11]

Table 9.1 Caesarean section and VBAC rates by region (2000)

Region	CSR %	VBAC %
England	21.5	32.6[12]
North East	19.3	38.2
North West	19.6	33.7
East Midlands	20.4	34.3
West Midlands	21.8	33.7
Eastern	21.4	32.0
London	24.2	29.6
South East	22.6	31.1
South West	19.4	34.0
Wales	23.8	26.9
Northern Ireland	23.9	23.8
Channel Islands & Isle of Man	24.8	21.8

Source: Thomas & Paranjothy, 2001

Much of the discussion on the relative benefits or disadvantages of allowing a trial of labour after a previous caesarean centres on the risks of uterine rupture (see discussion on repeat caesareans pp.43-4, 88-90). But it must be remembered that there are many more complications of pregnancy and labour that are far more likely to occur than uterine rupture. What is more, there is now a wealth of evidence to support the safety of VBAC. VBAC has been shown to

---

9   Gaskin, 2003
10   Thomas & Paranjothy, 2001
11   BirthChoiceUK, 2004
12   England & Wales

carry less risk of maternal morbidity compared to planned repeat caesareans.[13] The success of VBAC will be affected by the indications for the previous caesarean. For example non-recurrent indication such as breech or fetal distress will have a much higher VBAC success rate than recurrent conditions such as CPD (cephalo-pelvic disproportion). However, two-thirds of women with a history of CPD can achieve successful VBAC.[14]

Women with prior vaginal births (especially if the vaginal birth followed the previous caesarean) have a higher success of VBAC.[15] Vaginal birth following caesarean birth is more predictive of success than vaginal birth prior to the caesarean.[16] Fetal macrosomia and twin gestation do not preclude VBAC.[17]

Risks of VBAC

A failed trial of labour which ends in caesarean section can carry twice the risk of planned caesarean. However, only about one in five attempts at VBAC will end in this way.[18]

There is some (limited) evidence to suggest certain factors which might reduce the success of VBAC. For example, one study showed that maternal age may affect the success of VBAC. Women older than thirty-five who had not previously delivered vaginally were found to be more prone to failed trial of labour.[19] Maternal obesity may also adversely affect VBAC success[20] although there appears to be no physiological explanation for this.[21] Induction of labour using prostaglandins or misoprostol may increase the risk of uterine rupture in women with previous caesarean births[22] but induction using a transcervical Foley catheter may not.[23] Diet-controlled gestational diabetes mellitus is not a contraindication for VBAC.[24]

Some commentators in the UK and the US cautiously advise that VBAC should only be offered in hospitals equipped to care for women at high risk including twenty-four hour blood banking, electronic fetal monitoring, on-site anaesthesia coverage and the constant presence of a surgeon.[25]

---

13 Grinstead & Grobman, 2004
14 Ibid.
15 Ibid.
16 ACNM, 2004
17 Brill & Windrim, 2004
18 Enkin et al., 2000
19 Bujold et al., 2004
20 Brill & Windrim, 2004
21 Odibo & Macones, 2003
22 Aslan et al., 2004
23 Bujold et al., 2004
24 Marchiano et al., 2004
25 Bucklin, 2003

There are few absolute contraindications for successful VBAC and it should be successful in the majority of attempted cases. More research is required into VBAC as there is little quality information currently available on which to base clinical decisions and methodological deficiencies in the literature evaluating the relative safety of VBAC compared to repeat caesareans are worrying. However, the evidence on the higher risks carried by caesarean birth and repeat planned caesareans is well established. This, together with the small amount of quality information on VBAC suggests women should be encouraged to attempt trial of labour following previous caesarean(s).

Maternal request is one of the most common indications for repeat planned caesareans.[26] Thus the key to the increased use of VBAC in the future lies with an increased awareness amongst obstetricians and midwives combined with an informed public on the safety of VBAC. Women should be offered information and/or counselling which needs to be individualised and include details of both the short- and long-term risks.

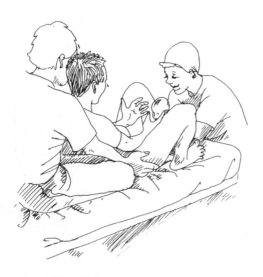

Vaginal birth after two or more caesareans

Vaginal birth after two caesareans is usually abbreviated to VBA2C, after three to VBA3C and so on.

The information on trials of labour after two or more previous caesarean sections is sparse and can be contradictory. Some researchers suggest that the rate of successful VBAC is no worse, and the risks no higher, for women with two or more prior caesareans than those with only one. Other studies have concluded that trials of labour are less successful and risks greater.[27] There is some evidence to suggest that rates of successful VBAC decrease with increasing numbers of prior caesareans, although women with two or more previous caesareans should not be discouraged from attempting VBAC. Many women have achieved successful vaginal births after two or more caesareans. However, our survey of 100 consultants showed that almost three-fifths (fifty-six) of obstetricians said they would advise another caesarean after two previous caesareans (see chapter 8).

---

26 Singh & Justin, 2004
27 Sharma & Thorpe-Beeston, 2002

WOMEN'S EXPERIENCES OF VBAC

Case study 1: A positive experience and successful VBAC in hospital

Rachel received good support from health care professionals and succeeded with a VBAC in 2004.

Rachel's VBAC story – Isaac

My first child was born in August 2001 by planned CS. My pregnancy had gone swimmingly until my thirty-six-week check when the doctor thought that the baby was breech. A scan two days later showed that she was in fact transverse, and the consultant terrified me with talk of a prolapsed cord, and made me stay in hospital. It transpired that in fact she had unstable lie, and flitted about all over the place, but very rarely head down. I found the situation so stressful, and with little apparent prospect of a natural birth, that after a week in hospital I asked for a caesarean. Physically this went quite smoothly, but I was unprepared for the psychological impact; subconsciously, I felt that since I had handed over responsibility for her birth to someone else, someone else was also responsible for her care. I didn't have a problem bonding with her, but I struggled to feel that I had the right and the ability to look after her.

Later on I realised that I felt a huge loss at having been unable to experience labour and birth. I think I might not have felt so bad about it if I'd been convinced that a caesarean was unavoidable – if I'd had the chance to labour and it hadn't worked out or if she had still been transverse when I went into labour. With hindsight I felt that I should have waited to go into labour naturally at which point she might have got into position, and if I'd had more support and encouragement rather than all the scaremongering, this might have been an option. I went round looking enviously at all the women I knew who'd had natural births, and even those who'd had an emergency CS since at least they'd had a chance to labour.

Anyway, second time around I was determined to do everything I could to get a natural birth. I'd see lots of 'real birth' programmes on TV and they filled me with horror – the poor mum, flat on her back surrounded by medical equipment and doctors telling her what to do. I really wanted and needed this birth to be my experience, not a medical event. I also didn't want to be treated like a ticking time bomb – a rupture waiting to happen. I did lots of reading and decided that medical intervention such as monitoring was unlikely to be of benefit. I did consider a home birth, but I didn't feel confident about it without a confident midwife (which really meant an independent midwife) so I kept that as a last resort. I was also concerned that this baby would have trouble engaging, given the unstable lie I'd had first time around.

Given that a hospital birth was my most likely outcome, I decided it would be better to get buy-in from the medical establishment at an early stage rather than wait until I was in labour, and run the risk of being pressurised to change my mind. I met with a registrar, who didn't mind me having a VBAC though she wasn't exactly encouraging. Hospital policy wasn't as bad as I had feared – there was no time limit on labour but she was very unhappy that I refused to have continuous monitoring and dismissive of other ways of detecting uterine rupture such as monitoring blood pressure and pulse. I went away somewhat discouraged but still determined that I would do things my way. I had lots of lengthy chats with my community midwife about what I wanted (apologies to anyone who ever had an appointment after me!) and after some initial doubts she obviously decided that I really meant it and was really supportive. She arranged for me to see the consultant midwife, who was absolutely fantastic; her attitude was that if that's what I wanted that's what I would get; no continuous monitoring, no drip, no time limits, no pain relief unless I asked for it, no ban on food and drink. We would plan for a successful natural labour. She wrote a letter to the midwifery staff, and put a copy in my notes explaining this so that I wouldn't get any hassle when the time came. She only asked that I have regular checks with a hand held sonicaid and an internal exam every three hours once I was in established labour to make sure things were progressing. My community midwife also switched me to a different consultant, whose only concern was to have me in for regular checks if I got to forty-two weeks. It just goes to show how different they can be!

The only snag at this stage (about thirty-four weeks) was that the baby was, yes, transverse! The consultant midwife gave me some tips on getting it to turn, which meant that I spent a week in the height of summer with a sarong strapped tightly around my tummy. The baby must have found this as uncomfortable as I did, because a week later he was head down and he stayed put.

The great day came when, just before midnight two days before my due date, my waters broke. Having called our friend to take care of our daughter, we duly trotted off to hospital. They confirmed that the waters had indeed gone, but the baby wasn't engaged and I wasn't dilated at all yet. On account of the lack of engagement and the previous caesarean, they were keen for us to stay in hospital, but as I was only having contractions every ten minutes and we felt that nothing would happen for ages we declined and went home. They didn't pressurise us about this decision which I felt was down to the fact that they could see from my notes that I had given my birth a great deal of thought. We arrived home at 2.30 and I sent my husband to bed to get some rest. This proved to be a bad idea because my contractions instantly speeded up to five minutes apart and, on my own, I struggled to cope. An hour later, at 3.30, I woke him up and suggested that we return to hospital, so back we went. They did an internal examination at 4.30 and I was devastated to learn that I was only 1 cm dilated, as I was finding it really hard to cope. Ironically, now that I wanted to stay, they were keen for us to go back home, or at least down to the ward to walk about. Fortunately they didn't press the point and instead offered me gas and air and a warm bath. So much for my resolve to have no pain relief – I didn't know anything could hurt so much! The next few hours were a bit of a blur. Since I wasn't, in their view, in established labour, I didn't get the fifteen-minute checks (I think they stopped by a couple of times). I was left in my husband's rather overwhelmed hands. Eventually I felt that I couldn't cope any more and sent my husband off to find a midwife and demand pethidine. The logical part of my brain knew that actually this probably wouldn't help at all, since the contractions were more or less continuous, but I was pretty desperate by now. I was even having fond thoughts of the caesarean! A midwife finally showed up and talked me through some contractions, which really helped. She opined that I was probably 3-4 cm dilated, which left me feeling that I really couldn't cope with another five hours of this. She asked me to get out of the bath so she could check what was going on and we could make a new plan; this took some time as I was waiting for a gap in the contractions before I moved, but there never was a gap – just a variation from very painful to excruciatingly painful.

I finally made it onto a bed at 8am and was heartened to find that actually I was 8 cm dilated. At this point my husband went off to go to the toilet, the midwife wandered off to find someone else and I found that I couldn't breathe. When this happened a second time it dawned on me that this was probably what pushing was, so I told the midwife when she reappeared. Another contraction and I could feel something, so I told the midwife and she had another look, at which point it was all systems go – the baby was coming very soon! My husband asked what did that mean – in the next ten minutes or so? No – it meant in the next minute! Another contraction, and out popped Isaac at 8.14am weighing 7lb 15 oz. So the notes read: Stage 1 – 3 $\frac{1}{2}$ hours (actually time from 1 cm to 8 cm), Stage 2 – 14 minutes (actually 8 cm to birth). The fly in the ointment was that the speed of the second stage meant that I tore really badly, and had to go into theatre to be stitched up under a spinal block. There was a bit of déjà vu – same place my daughter was born, drips, etc., but frankly I didn't care at this stage. I was just glad it was over and I'd done it!

I don't regret not trying for an HBAC (home birth after caesarean), although if I were to have another child I would do so; once labour got going I was fairly oblivious to my surroundings. The only thing I would have changed would have been to have a Doula (experienced birth assistant) as a bit more support would have made a big difference, and might have enabled me to avoid tearing so badly. I am also aware that I was lucky that labour progressed so quickly that there was no need for anyone to even think about intervention; if things had gone slowly then I wonder if there might have been some pressure to intervene regardless of my birth plan. I'm still really thrilled that I did it, but also sad that I didn't trust my body enough to do so first time around. I'm awestruck at my body's ability to give birth all on its own; my VBAC is the most fulfilling experience of my life.

Case study 2: A successful VBAC in hospital

Merry encountered some lack of support from some health care professionals but had a successful VBAC in hospital for her second child, followed by two more caesarean births. She wrote this VBAC story whilst pregnant with her fourth child.

Merry's VBAC story – Maddy

Having had an emergency c-section for Frances, after a traumatic twenty-four-hour labour that ended in a failed ventouse, a baby that suddenly tried to emerge conventionally after the incision had been made, the section and recovery itself, and a baby that had an unexpected cleft lip and palate, I got pregnant again eleven months later with trepidation, but I knew if I didn't do it quickly, I would never do it again.

I booked with my same midwife, and was keen to have her at the birth, although in retrospect this was a mistake as she was not terribly supportive of my anxiety for VBAC. I had an easy pregnancy although I was rather worried and apprehensive and much less well informed than I am now. It was a difficult time.

Two days before my due date, we sent Frances up to my parents for the weekend. I had had a false alarm three days before and my midwife had examined me and said she couldn't see me dilating without inducing – I was still firmly closed. In retrospect this was an odd thing to say – I had in fact dilated to a full 10 cm with my first labour but Frances had not engaged well due to a lot of extra fluid that cleft babies often have. Anyway, we couldn't decide how to spend our free evening, and ended up deciding to repaint our 24 ft living room! We worked till 1am and of course at 5am I woke up with labour pains! I also noticed that I had painted the living room matt along the bottom while my husband had used silk for the top half! So, in denial, I went for a bath to stop these 'false labour' pains and he repainted!

Anyway, things were clearly on the move, so we called the midwife, and although she was rather cross with me, she came and I was 3 cm! My contractions were mild and irregular so we went for a walk, with my tens machine on for the odd strong one, and when that didn't speed things up, we went to DFS to sit on sofas; I thought that might encourage my waters to break!

However, three hours later, the midwife came back – I was now 4cm but my BP was up and the baby's heartbeat was too. I agreed to go to hospital. Once there, the normal treadmill of monitoring and intervention started. I was very disappointed that my midwife failed to be much of an advocate for me, even though by this time everything had returned to normal. They tried to insist on a drip, and when questioned they said I was 'showing signs of toxaemia.' Fortunately my husband queried this, as everything now seemed fine again. They were very put out by his questioning and one midwife became really quite rude. She was hunting about in my arm for a vein, despite my protestations, and talking about my 'very difficult veins' over my head as if I was a difficult school child. She looked at me, strapped to my bed and said 'you have two hours, you are on a two-hour countdown to a section.' (This midwife was mentioned by name on my third birth plan as not being allowed anywhere near me!) At this point I started to cry and my wonderful husband threw them all out and told them not to come back until they had a registrar with them. I think, quite frankly, it is due to this and little else, that I got my VBAC.

After a good long time, a registrar appeared. He was wonderful. He couldn't understand the fuss and said 'Lets break your waters and give you a few hours, if that doesn't work we can try a drip and if that doesn't work we can look at a section some time tomorrow.' I was still only 4 cm and it was 8pm at this point, so all this seemed pretty reasonable. I decided, at this point, that what was most important was to keep my head and not get tired so I decided to have an epidural. Then they broke my waters. It all became very relaxed – it was a light epidural and I could feel the contractions but still cope easily. The only thing I didn't like much during this was the midwife, who sat in the corner and 'looked' at me – and I felt I wanted to hide my face for every contraction. Max did the crossword and made encouraging faces when required! The pain began to get very strong (my husband says he recalls me having two syringes of epidural with the first and only half for the second) and I had gas and air. I began to make a lot of grunting noises and the midwife said 'You CAN'T want to push – you were 4 cm less than two hours ago'. I suspect I may have muttered something less than polite – I was on quick examination '8 cm… no… just an anterior lip – oh I can feel the head.' Minutes prior to this she had been asking for names so she could write out wristbands and was most put out we didn't have a boy name!

The registrar had asked to be there at the birth as the baby's head had been very high and he was called. In these few minutes as the pain and the urge to push became overwhelming, they lost the baby's heartbeat and a panic ensued. I was bumped from my small room to a large one as I had expressed a real desperation not to have my baby removed from my room for resuscitation. Frances had been taken out and brought back several minutes later and the distress that caused me was hardly tolerable. I had dreadful nightmares for ages afterwards that she had been swapped for another baby; fortunately she looks enough like me for that not to be the case! So they moved me to a room with a resusc table. It was very unpleasant to be moved, but I appreciated that they made the effort to follow my expressed wish.

The registrar now said 'This baby has to come out now. I am putting the forceps together, if you don't want me to use them – PUSH!' And I did! With three pushes (not bad for a first birth!) out she came. I have an incredibly strong memory of visualising a bowling ball emerging out of the mechanism that delivers it back to the players during this time! I felt her crown, felt her nose and felt her swoosh out at great speed – NOTHING could have stopped me pushing! I opened my eyes just in time to see her appear on the bed, before she was grabbed, cord cut and whisked to the table. I think I knew she was fine because I didn't ask 'Is everything okay?' I asked 'Is it a girl or a boy?' and refused to believe Max who had seen it was indeed a girl!

Fortunately she was fine and came back to me quickly. I had a small tear (and kicked the registrar when he tried to stitch it without a local!) and I lost some blood, which made me faint when I tried to stand up, but after a night in hospital (she was born at 10.55pm), I was home, elated and relieved. Even afterwards, the midwife in charge was pretty rubbish really – she was shouting at a bewildered and tired Max to get things and he had no idea WHAT she was talking about. Grrrr....

My third child was born by a genuine emergency section with a presenting cord – the experience was so different to my first section and the people involved made it lovely for me. In some ways, that 3rd birth was the best of all because I was consulted, in control and respected throughout. I had planned an HBAC and that planning had made me regret bits of my VBAC that I wanted to have been better.

But in retrospect I know I was lucky to get that VBAC experience and it was a very very healing one, not least because I and we grew in power during it.

I am just pregnant again and for the first time I am not too bothered how the baby is born. It matters more to me to make my own choice and not spoil the peace I have found than to hold on desperately for a birth that might end in pain and anger again. I think some of this peace has come from knowing I really DID nearly lose my third child (and they also found a hole in my uterus when they did the section) but much of it comes from having had a VBAC, so I know I *can*.

Case study 3: a VBAC at home (HBAC)

After the birth of her first child by caesarean, Beth decided to have her second child at home, with the assistance of an independent midwife.

Beth's HBAC story – Amber

I kept waking up during the night as I had a terrible cough. At around 1:45am, my son (three years old at the time) woke up and Ian looked after him. About ten minutes later I started having contractions. They were mildly uncomfortable. I was a bit in denial as it was ten days early and I had had this horrible cough for four days. I thought that the contractions would just go away and I would fall back to sleep. About ten minutes later I called out for Ian and told him that this is it. I had a pile of pillows on the bed and I was leaning over them on all fours. I also tried leaning over a birth ball, but I found it too cold and uncomfortable. I went to the toilet with Ian and had diarrhoea. My contractions were about every five minutes lasting a minute. Ian was getting concerned and asked me if I thought we should call Melody (the midwife). I said ok. He called her at around 3.50am and told her what had been going on. Melody asked to speak to me. I was able to speak to her between the contractions. She said she was going to come over. Ian suggested we should go downstairs and have a cup of tea. I said ok, as I thought I would just try to carry on as normal. I did not know what I was thinking. I said I needed to use the toilet again. I felt as if I was going to poo again. I sat on the toilet, but nothing happened. As soon as I stood up another contraction came and I had to go on all fours, I felt my waters break. I could see that there was blood in it. Ian and I panicked for a moment. He asked me if we should call an ambulance. I said yes and then I came to my senses and realised that a bit of blood was normal. After my water broke I felt as if I was ready to push, but I did not want to do anything until Melody arrived. Ian paged her to tell her that my waters broke and there was a bit of blood. She said she would be over in thirty minutes. I asked Ian to put a stack of pillows on the floor against the wall so I could lean on them. I asked him for a pillow for under my knees. He had just bought kneepads so I could do some crawling to help the baby get into a good position. He asked me if I would like to wear the kneepads. I said 'JUST GET THE PILLOW!!!!!!' I don't know how he ever thought I could get kneepads on. I found that being on all fours was the only way I could deal with the pain. At the same time my son was calling out for Ian. Ian was looking after the two of us. My son was happy to watch TV and play with his toys. We had some new toys for him, just in case he did wake up in the night. I wanted Ian to stay with me. I found if he put his hand on my stomach during the contractions, it helped a lot.

Melody arrived at around 4.30am. I told her I needed help and that I was scared. She told me that I was doing well. I remember saying that I felt as if I was going to die and did not want to go on. She did an examination and told me I was fully dilated. Her words that I remember are 'there is no cervix there, your baby is going to be born soon'. I was so happy and wanted her to tell Ian when he came back upstairs, as he was looking after our son. The reality sunk in that I was really going to do this. I remember Melody asking Ian for certain things to prepare for the birth. She needed some lighting. He was going to get candles, but I did not want him to go. I said I did not care if they put the bedroom lights on. I did not care about anything at that point. There was nothing that distracted me. During the contraction, I would look at the plant on the floor and focus on it, or I had my head in the pillow. It is difficult to explain how I felt at that moment, at times I felt as if I was not really there.

I was on all fours for about a half an hour trying to push. Melody suggested we move to the toilet so I could be upright. During the contractions I stood up and pushed and then I would sit on the toilet and rest. Melody put a hot compress on my perineum to help avoid tearing. My son was calling Ian. He said he wanted to come upstairs. Ian asked me if I minded if he was there. I told him I did not care. My son was standing by the door of the bathroom. He was now watching it all and stayed to watch the birth. I stood up and I could feel the head coming out. I sat on the toilet again and then I stood up and this time I pushed her head out. I waited for the next contraction and I pushed and the baby was born. It was such a strange sensation when her body came out. It seemed to happen with such ease once the head was out. I looked at my husband he was crying and he said to me you did it. I sat on the toilet at this point as my legs felt like jelly. Melody put a towel around the baby and gave her to me. She left part of my baby's skin exposed and put her against my skin, so we had skin to skin contact immediately. I just could not believe it. Melody said to me that she wanted to put a bowl in the toilet to catch the placenta, as she was saying that my placenta fell out into the toilet. Ian cut the cord as the placenta stopped pulsating, as it was in the toilet. I still did not know if it was a boy or girl. I looked and saw it was a girl, but I had to check a few minutes later, just to make sure. We moved to the bedroom and sat on the bed. I put her to my breast and she latched on immediately. Melody examined me and I had no tears. Ian looked at me and said that he really saw my strength today.

I felt the whole experience very empowering and healing. It felt like some out of body experience. At times I felt as if I was a spectator at the birth. I am grateful for my husband and Melody and felt I could not have done it without them. I felt very safe with them and also being at home. I was also grateful that my son got to watch the birth. In a way I felt his presence healing for both of us, as he was born by a caesarean section. The labour was three hours and thirty-three minutes. For a while afterwards I felt as if it had all been a dream. Before I only imagined in my dreams that I would have such a straightforward and beautiful birth experience.

***

The women in the first three examples had relatively positive experiences of VBAC despite Merry encountering resistance from some health care professionals. Other women have had different experiences of vaginal birth and in the interest of balance it is instructive to include a story of a birth that did not go exactly the way we might hope.

***

Case study 4: a difficult VBAC

Amanda had a successful vaginal (ventouse) birth of her second child six years after a caesarean birth. The vaginal birth was quite traumatic with some complications but Amanda was glad she persisted and would choose VBAC again. This is her story:

Amanda's VBAC Story – Lucy Victoria

My obstetric history is by no means unusual, my first pregnancy progressed well although I did have glucose in urine on quite a few occasions but had a tolerance test which came out ok. Labour was induced at ten days over and I eventually had an emergency caesarean on day thirteen when I had 'failed to progress' further than 9 cms. Emily Louise was born weighing in at 9lbs 5ozs. From this point I was informed by most medical staff that if I was to have more children then I would of course be having a planned caesarean, this put me off as I didn't recover well from the first, until I read about VBAC. Six years later I gave birth to Lucy Victoria. Although I got my VBAC it wasn't without problems. If you are planning a VBAC because it will be easier than a CS and recovery will be quicker then do not read my story, but if you want to feel a baby being born the way it was supposed to be and you want to feel your body doing this wondrous thing called labour then yes, VBAC will be for you.

My community midwife was never anything but supportive. I had told her about my first birth as there was nothing in writing as I had given birth in Germany (Forces). I knew the problem was to do with my baby's size, a maternity nurse had told me this afterwards as Emily had 'got stuck' she had told me this in broken English. Because of the CS I was under the consultant and attended my first appointment at twenty-four weeks. I told the registrar of my concerns about baby's size as again I showed glucose in urine regularly throughout this pregnancy also. He booked me for a scan at thirty-four weeks to estimate the size and to talk about options available to me then.

At thirty-four weeks I met my consultant, I had my scan which estimated my baby's size at 6lbs 10ozs. My consultant told me this was only borderline large, and the size of the baby was not really the issue as the estimation could be as much as 15 per cent out. I had asked if I could be induced at thirty-nine weeks to give me the best chance of a vaginal birth with a smaller baby. I was told in no uncertain terms that because of my scar the only way I could try for a VBAC was if I spontaneously laboured as I was far too high risk for induction and anyway who would want to be induced at thirty-nine weeks? I had got really upset as he had indicated that I really should consider a planned caesarean section and he was quite prepared to do this at thirty-nine weeks if I wanted. I went home very upset as at no point had anybody indicated that I was such a high risk. That night I hit the Internet and found some very interesting facts from a web site called 'Radical Midwives' which then led me to the VBAC Information and Support Group. I telephoned and had a wonderful chat with one of their members, she also sent me loads of information, the name of the Radical Midwife for my area and her own personal story. This gave me the confidence to carry on with my own VBAC as I was on the verge of saying to hell with it and just do the caesarean and get it over with. Why on earth should I want to put myself through this stress when there was such an easy way out? I also called my community midwife who came for a home visit and went through the options again.

At thirty-six weeks I went back to see my consultant, this time armed with reports, tables, statistics and a lot of confidence! I told him he had treated me like a walking scar and that the information he had given me was misleading. We managed to thrash out a compromise. He was not willing to discuss the issue of baby's size and my worries on this issue as he said it was not relevant but let me have membrane sweeps and as long as I spontaneously laboured I had a reasonable chance. I wasn't happy as I didn't spontaneous labour first time, drip and gel had also failed, only ARM had worked. I could however try raspberry leaf, sex, and any other remedies within reason. At least I had got something. At thirty-seven weeks I began having contractions, five to seven minutes apart, I went up to the hospital to have them checked out, and yes, I was 1-2 cms but was sent home as it was latent first stage and could go on for hours. In fact it went on and off for four weeks.

At thirty-eight weeks I saw the consultant, still in a lot of discomfort, no change. See you again at forty weeks.

Before I attended my consultant appointment I telephoned the consultant unit to ask for advice on what was likely to be discussed at the next appointment and could I ask for a membrane sweep and what it entails etc. Sadly the midwife I spoke to wasn't at all cooperative and told me in no uncertain terms to attend the appointment and it would all be explained there. I then telephoned the midwife recommended by the VBAC support group, who rang me back that evening and went through everything and explained in detail.

At forty weeks plus three days I saw the midwife at the consultant unit and asked for a membrane sweep, she wasn't convinced it would do any good until closer to forty-one weeks but I persisted, she did it and also booked me in for another sweep at forty-one weeks and an induction at forty-one weeks plus three days. It was all happening exactly the same as first time, and all I could see was caesarean. I spent a day sobbing, I knew I wasn't going to spontaneous labour.

At forty-one weeks I went back to the hospital to have membranes swept again, although my contractions had increased in intensity they were still only seven to ten minutes apart and would fade away. My membranes were swept again and I was left on the fetal monitor for half an hour just for precaution. It was here that I felt rather damp below, and on checking I had left a rather large damp patch, but it could not be decided if my waters had been broken or just grazed. I couldn't now go back home so I was admitted to the ward to be checked again in the morning. I had a more uncomfortable night as my contractions were significantly more intense but I still did not think my waters were broken.

The next morning I met the consultant on duty, she asked me what I wanted to do, so I told her I wanted my waters broken and see if that set me off in established labour. She agreed and booked me in for 10.30am. No problems.

My waters were broken at 10.30am where a very small amount of meconium was found, and within an hour or so I was in established labour with TENS attached.

I am afraid time is sort of hazy but it was around 12-1pm that the pain got really intense and I tried the gas and air. It made me sick but I carried on using it with Marilyn Manson & Linkin Park on the MP3 player (we had brought in). By 2pm(ish) I needed something else and wanted an epidural. However, on checking I was 8-9 cms dilated and my midwife Donna thought it would not be a good idea as I didn't have long to go, but I could have Pethidine. I did and I was sick again! 4pm and pain was now getting unbearable and I again asked for an epidural. I was checked again and I was still 9 cms, my midwife went to ask about one. Unfortunately the anaesthetist was in theatre and would be at least forty-five minutes but would come to me next. The contractions were incredibly intense and I tried to get myself comfortable but being stuck on the bed and constantly monitored inhibited my movements and the insistence of a cannula in situ in case of an emergency was restrictive, I pulled it out eventually as it kept catching.

At 5pm I was ready to push, but I had a rim of cervix, and the baby was unable to come down. I couldn't stop the urge to push and was sick again. The consultant came to check me and found that when I did push the rim of cervix did go and baby was able to come down and she said she wanted to try and pull her out with a ventouse in theatre and if that failed I was set up for a caesarean. By now I had been pushing for over an hour and was completely knackered. I had somehow got into my head that it would be another hour of pushing in theatre. Donna told me it would be two or three pushes maximum, if it failed then it would be a section. I was set up in stirrups, local anaesthetics inside and around vaginal area, a theatre full of people. A midwife on each leg, one on left shoulder and hubby on right shoulder, a registrar and consultant with ventouse cap at the ready. The contraction came and I pushed for all I was worth. The consultant asked if I wanted to feel the baby's head. I was expecting a bit of head but in fact I stuck my finger up my baby's nose as the whole head was out and facing up! The second push and my baby was out and placed on my stomach to which we made a quick eye contact, and promptly wee'd on me!! We had had a little girl Lucy Victoria. Born at 18.39 hours on 19/10/03, weighing in at 9lbs 3oz.

Unfortunately Lucy didn't breathe very well and was whisked away for extra help, it did improve and her breathing was fine but she was traumatised from the birth and was taken to Special Care Baby Unit. It took forty-five minutes to sew me up, followed by three hours in recovery on a syntocinon drip as my uterus was not contracting down as it should.

I got to see Lucy in her incubator at about 10pm where I found out she had a fractured clavicle from shoulder dystocia, left arm palsy and a sore and swollen head. Although she had wee'd on me at birth, she had not wee'd for the first night so was being treated for renal failure also. I had a major tear and episiotomy. After visiting Lucy in Special Baby care I returned to the ward (in a wheelchair) and tried to get to sleep, it was about 11.30pm. The pain in my right bum cheek was immense so I called the midwife to ask about some more pain relief, she came and checked me out and told me she was going to call the doctor as the bruising and swelling was pretty severe. The pain relief did not work, the pain was more intense and still no doctor at 12.30am. I called the midwife on at least two more occasions, finally I had to put my TENS machine on my bum cheek and I was clawing the walls! Doctor came at about 1.30am and I was taken back into labour ward to be checked. I was seen by the duty consultant who advised conservative treatment which was to 'wait and see'. He didn't want to open everything back up unless it was absolutely necessary. I got a pethidine injection and was asleep by 2.15am and wheeled back to the ward. As long as the pain relief was given I was able to cope but my bum cheek was solid, black and very uncomfortable!

Although I was able to drive my car after two weeks it took over ten weeks to recover from this birth which included a severe bout of anaemia. VBAC, would I do it again? – You bet! And it just goes to show you can VBAC a traumatic ventouse birth with no problems for the scar, without spontaneously labouring. I look back now and feel desperately robbed of the vaginal birth I had planned for my first, both labours from breaking of waters were identical, quick progress to 9 cms, anterior lip of cervix and a baby in a difficult position to birth (direct OP), which is back to back with mother, yet one ends in a caesarean and one in a vaginal birth.

INFORMATION AND SUPPORT NETWORK FOR VBAC

We have seen from the academic data in this chapter and in chapter 3 that there is a great deal of concern about VBAC within the medical profession. The case histories above show that the medical attitudes to individual pregnancies have left many women feeling that they have to do battle with the profession rather than work with it. The above examples show that some obstetricians have been seen to make cutting and unhelpful comments. This is unfortunate. Childbirth is a very significant event in parents' lives and it is of the utmost importance that the quality of care, both physical and emotional, is of the highest order. Women will then have good memories of their birth and when each birthday of their child arrives, they can think back warmly to the important occasion and the support and help they received from those attending the birth.

The British groups supporting VBACs have produced an action plan for women. It reads as follows:

Vaginal Birth after Caesarean Section is not easy or straightforward for anyone. If you feel strongly about it and would like to be successful, you are well advised to make a careful and thorough assessment of your own situation.

A   Make sure you know the reason for your previous section(s).

B   Find out what your hospital's policies are, do they vary by consultant?

C   Find out what facts will adversely affect your chances of achieving a VBAC, for example:

- Continuous electronic fetal monitoring
- Restriction of food and fluid intake
- Restriction of mobility
- Acceleration of labour by ARM (artificial rupture of the membranes)
- Time limits
- Staff changes
- Induction or augmentation (acceleration of labour with oxytocin).

D   If you have, or have had, any one of the following you may find your hospital will be recommending a caesarean as routine:

- Cephalopelvic (feto-pelvic) disproportion (CPD) (see chapter 5)
- Two or more previous caesarean sections
- Twins or breech
- Postdates
- A classical or T incision.

E   Contact the lay organisations for information about achieving a VBAC next time. (See 'Further Information for Parents', p.270)

We would like to add the following points:

- Take your time over choosing your hospital and/or your consultant: do not be rushed into a hasty decision
- If you decide to change hospital from the previous time, ensure that your notes are obtained, together with the results of any X-rays taken after the caesarean
- Prepare yourself mentally and physically for a VBAC and read chapter 10 of this book, much of which is relevant to VBAC
- Contact one of the VBAC support organisations for help and advice. See details in the 'Further Information for Parents' section.

10 What choices do women have about maternity care?

Despite government rhetoric about 'choice', in many ways there is less choice now than there was forty-five years ago. Then 36.1 per cent of women gave birth at home and another 12.4 per cent in GP units.[1] A GP was free to refer to any NHS hospital in the country and District Midwives as they were called then were not managed by the Director of Midwifery Services in the hospital but worked pretty autonomously. They worked hard but had good results and provided the continuity of care and personal care that women want but frequently do not get.[2] Today a minority of GPs do full maternity care and with the 2004 contract, many have opted out of antenatal care. Most GP units have been closed and, whilst a few midwifery-led units exist, few women live near enough to one to choose to give birth there. A list of these is given in Appendix E. Women still have a right to give birth at home and midwives a legal duty to attend them.

Having your baby at home

If a woman is thinking of giving birth at home, she can discuss this with a community midwife, an independent midwife, her GP, the NCT or a local home birth support group (the local NCT branch should have details). Some GPs are very supportive of home birth and will attend women in labour at home or provide 'cover' for community midwives. Some GPs are opposed to home birth[3] and, unfortunately, have been known to strike women (and families) off their lists for requesting one. A survey by the NCT in 1995 found that only seventeen of 144 Primary Care Trusts said that most GPs offered care for a home birth with community midwives. Forty-five branches reported that women had been struck off their GP's list for requesting a home birth – although this was described as 'indefensible' by Dr Judy Gilley of the BMA's General Services Committee.[4] This behaviour is unethical as well as contrary to government policy but it is still happening.[5]

---

1   Butler & Bonham, 1963
2   Allison, 1996
3   *BMJ*, 1995; HoC, 2003b, section 3 p.34
4   *BMJ*, 1995
5   Newburn, 1993

If a woman is unable to arrange a home birth through her GP (who has the right not to provide maternity care) she can contact the local community midwives directly, or telephone or write to the director of maternity services or the supervisor of midwives (sometimes these are the same person) requesting a home birth. The supervisor of midwives has a legal duty to arrange midwifery care for a woman she knows is pregnant, and this must be provided at home if that is what the woman wishes. If a GP goes so far as to strike a woman off his/her list for requesting a home birth, the woman can complain in writing to the local Family Health Services Appeal Authority (address in telephone directory or on the internet at www.fhsaa.org.uk).

> When I told my GP I wanted a home birth and that I didn't want him to be involved in my antenatal/delivery/postnatal care, that I only wanted to be attended by the community midwives' team, he struck me off along with my three-year-old daughter who was ill at the time.[6]

A complaint to the General Medical Council might also be made (www.gmc-uk.org).

A few women who go ahead and book a home birth with community midwives are asked to go and see a consultant obstetrician in hospital. In most cases, this is more or less a courtesy visit, giving the woman and the obstetrician the opportunity to meet and to discuss the emergency back-up available from the hospital and the circumstances in which transfer to hospital might be advisable. In other cases, the appointment is used by the obstetrician to try to dissuade the woman from giving birth at home by 'shroud waving' and other unfair means. A woman invited to meet an obstetrician can usually discover from discreet enquiries what form the consultation is likely to take and may accept or decline the invitation accordingly. She does not have to go if she does not wish to. It is generally accepted that a woman should have at least one medical examination during her pregnancy to check her heart and lungs, but this can usually be done by her GP if she prefers.

However, since childbirth in Britain has become medicalised, some women do not have confidence in their ability to give birth without medical supervision and therefore feel more secure labouring in hospital. We acknowledge this need but hope that women will consider the evidence that home birth is safe and discuss with their partners and grandmothers who may well have given birth at home.[7] Despite calls by successive government committees to increase the availability of home birth, women are still reporting difficulties in arranging a home birth.

---

6   Newburn, 1993
7   Ackerman-Liebrich et al., 1996; *BMJ* editorial, 1996; Campbell & McFarlane, 1994; Johnson & Davis, 2005; NRPMSCG, 1996; Wiegers et al., 1996

The Health Select Committee in 2003 estimated that up to ten times as many women would want to give birth at home if given the choice.[8]

Continuity of carer

It seems likely that the lower rates of intervention found in the midwifery care studies referred to in chapters 5 and onwards are due to emotional/psychological factors: the more comfortable a woman feels with the place of birth and the people caring for her, the more likely it is that her birth will be straightforward. Being looked after by people with whom she has a good relationship and trusts will help her to make informed choices.

If the need for medical intervention is unexpected, the care of midwives known to the woman is of even more value than when labour progresses normally. Some GPs offer complete maternity care, including care during labour, to their patients, and usually share antenatal care with community midwives. Women usually receive a high level of continuity from this kind of arrangement, quite different from the usual pattern of 'shared care'.

One Scottish study concluded that 'routine specialist visits for women initially at low risk of pregnancy complications offer little or no clinical or consumer benefit'.[9] However, GPs have increasingly opted out of maternity care and since the new contract neither the DoH nor the BMA appear to have any statistics about the proportion of GPs providing this type of care in 2004.

Much modern maternity care is fragmented, with many women being cared for by a large number of different health professionals during pregnancy, birth and afterwards. Most midwives work in teams but the number in those teams can range from two to sixteen.[10]

Over half the women in one survey (54 per cent) said that they would prefer to see the same midwife throughout pregnancy and labour and two in five (41 per cent) said that they would prefer to see the same one or two midwives for their care.[11] In a survey in Tower Hamlets in 1991, when asked if they could choose one person to look after them who would it be, 57 per cent said a midwife, 25 per cent a GP and 13 per cent a hospital doctor. Fifty-five per cent had shared care, 16 per cent hospital care only and there was an active community scheme which involved GPs so 29 per cent never visited a hospital antenatal clinic.[12]

Often nowadays the only way to achieve continuity of carer, particularly in urban areas, is for a woman to book a home birth or domino (see Appendix A).

---

8   *BMJ*, news item, 2003
9   Tucker et al., 1996
10 DoH, 2003a
11 DoH, 2003a
12 Savage et al., 1998

In rural areas, particularly those served by small maternity units, continuity of carer is more likely to happen because there are smaller numbers of both women and midwives so it is easier for them to get to know each other. In a few areas, efforts are being made to improve continuity of carer as a result of the National Audit carried out by the Royal College of Obstetricians and Gynaecologists in 2000.[13]

In addition to the choices of place of birth, midwives and style of care, another variable a woman should take into account when choosing her care is the approach and policies of individual consultant obstetricians. As has been shown by our survey of consultants, their attitude to the management of labour can affect the chance of having a caesarean significantly. Informal sources of this information might include the senior midwife in charge of the hospital antenatal clinic and local branches of the NCT and AIMS (Association for Improvement in Maternity Services). Other more direct sources would be the senior manager of maternity services or the clinical director. These data are collected and processed at the taxpayer's expense and should therefore be available to the public. Care should be taken in interpreting data as some consultants may specialise in high-risk cases. GPs may be able to help.

Choosing the type of maternity care

It is important for the woman not to be rushed into arranging her care for pregnancy and birth until she has had time to find out all the options available and to consider which type of care she feels is best. It is very common for a woman to visit her GP after a positive pregnancy test and be expected to decide on her care there and then. GPs are not always fully aware of the options for care available to women and therefore refer women directly to consultant units, restricting their choice.[14] Women from the same GP practice can be given different choices about treatment, screening and types of maternity care.[15]

> More information on choice of places for birth should be provided by the GP earlier. I had booked into one hospital on the advice of the GP as it was our 'local' hospital. At twenty-four weeks, I requested a change so I could use a more progressive hospital. The GP respected my wishes and I was transferred. The choice of hospitals should be made after the Mum's given time to consider the options – rather than at the same time as receiving a positive pregnancy test.[16]

Many women find it hard to access services without referral from a GP.[17] Other

---

13 Thomas & Paranjothy, 2001
14 DoH, 2003b, section 3, p.3
15 DoH, 2003a
16 NCT, 1992
17 HoC, 2003b, section 2, p.1

sources of information about options for care are the local branch of the NCT, (see 'Further Information for Parents', p.270) community midwives (usually based at the nearest maternity unit), community health councils (still available in some areas, check your telephone directory or the internet), family and friends. There are a number of on-line organisations offering information and advice (see 'Further information for parents', p.270) as well as the NHS Direct (by telephone or on the internet at: www.nhsdirect.nhs.uk). The table in Appendix A shows the basic features of each type of maternity care. In addition to options provided by the NHS, some women may wish and be able to afford to use an independent midwife or a private hospital.

When looking into the local options, the woman can enquire about the approaches to care during pregnancy and birth and can also ask for up-to-date statistics as well as any other factors or facilities such as the availability of a birthing pool or special care baby unit. Caesarean rates can often be an indicator of a more or less technological approach to birth (see Appendix D), but it is important to find out at the same time whether a unit with a substantially lower caesarean rate than another unit in the same health district is only caring for women at 'low risk' of complications during labour. Caesarean rates are often also linked to forceps and/or Ventouse rates so that if one is lower, the other may be higher. If a woman has a pre-existing medical condition or a difficult obstetric history, it is probably wise for her to discuss the implications for pregnancy and birth with an obstetrician and/or other medical specialist before deciding on her care.

If a woman intends to give birth in hospital, she can arrange to visit and be given a guided tour. This will provide an idea of the atmosphere of the maternity unit and the opportunity to ask questions informally. Some units organise regular weekly tours for this purpose, often in relation to antenatal classes.

Once a woman has found out about all the local options for care and any special implications arising for her, she can consider which type feels right for her. If she has a partner, she may want to take their views into account, especially if they are going to be with her in labour. Alternatively, if the couple's attitudes to the place of birth differ, or if she prefers, the woman may ask a friend or relative to be her labour companion.

The 'booking' appointment

Once the woman has decided on her maternity care type, she will be given a 'booking appointment'. This is usually with a midwife, although in some hospitals doctors still see women for this first appointment to take a history and give a medical examination. A full medical history will be taken and the woman will be informed about the pattern of her antenatal care. The booking appointment takes place either at home, at a community clinic or at the maternity unit of her choice. There is a trend, even for women planning hospital births, to have their booking appointment at home, the idea being that a woman will feel more at ease on her own territory and that there will be a more equal exchange of information between the woman and the midwife. For some women who have booked their care without the benefit of full information about the options available, the home booking appointment gives an opportunity to fill in the gaps and they may find that they wish to change their care. In fact, a woman can change her care at any time during her pregnancy, provided that the alternative system is not fully booked. The Health Committee Ninth Report recommends that at least one 'booking appointment' should be with a community midwife who has detailed knowledge of the local services and can help you to make informed decisions about care.[18] Home births are not limited in this way because, as stated above, women have a legal right to have their babies at home and midwives have a legal duty to attend them there. However, some health professionals feel that a substantial increase in the demand for home births or dominos may put undue pressure on community midwives unless resources are shifted from hospitals into the community.

Getting the most out of antenatal care

Ideally the woman will be able to get to know the midwives who will be caring for her during labour and postnatally during her antenatal care, even if some of this is shared with a GP. If a woman has booked a home birth with NHS community midwives or an independent midwife, she will probably receive most of her care at home from a team of no more than four midwives, with one midwife being 'her' midwife, taking the lead in her care and, hopefully, being the one to deliver her. Equally with a domino, GP or midwife unit type, the team of carers should be small enough for the woman to build up a relationship with them and for her caregivers to get to know the woman. The likely result is that the woman's state of health and her preferences become well known to the team so that they are able to give her appropriate care during labour. The woman for her part feels relaxed and comfortable with people she knows so that tension is less likely to interfere with the course of her labour.

Whichever type of care a woman has chosen, it is vital that she asks questions about any part of her care which has not been explained or which she does not understand. If she has any problems at home which may affect her physical or emotional health, she should feel able to share these and to ask for professional help or support if she feels she needs it. If complications arise and she needs medical care, but does not understand what the doctor has told her or is too anxious to take it in, she can ask a midwife to give her an explanation when she feels calmer.

---

18 HoC, 2003b, section 2, p.3

Antenatal classes

I think that much more should be taught about caesareans at antenatal classes to prepare women for the after-effects of a caesarean as it seems commonplace nowadays.[19]

The take-up of antenatal classes can be low and their quality variable. But when they are good, they can be an excellent source of practical information for coping with labour and life with a new baby. They also give women and couples the opportunity to meet other people having babies at the same time and to give each other peer support which can continue after the birth. Accessibility for women who do not speak or understand English or who have physical disabilities can be a problem, as can classes held only in the daytime if women and their labour companions are at work and cannot get time off.

NHS classes are held, free of charge, both in hospitals and in community clinics. Increasingly, often in response to demand from men to be involved in antenatal classes, NHS classes are being held in the evenings and are very popular. NHS classes are usually taught by hospital or community midwives, with some input from obstetric physiotherapists and health visitors. Some hospitals arrange talks by doctors on topics such as pain relief. Every woman receiving NHS care should be offered antenatal classes and, if she wishes to attend, she should ensure a place is booked for her and, if appropriate, her labour companion.

Private classes are available, for a fee, with the following: the NCT; active birth teachers; some independent midwives as part of their type of care; some private maternity units for their clients; and independent childbirth educators including teachers of yoga and Alexander technique for pregnant women. Women often find out about private classes from friends or by contacting the NCT which sometimes has information about classes available with other teachers too, particularly if NCT classes become full very quickly. Any woman wanting NCT classes should contact her local branch at about twelve weeks of pregnancy to book them, because there are often not enough classes to meet demand (although in some rural areas classes can be difficult to get to and therefore there is not the same pressure on places). This can be difficult for women undergoing screening for fetal abnormality, but NCT teachers are trained to handle the issue sensitively.

What is covered in antenatal classes varies enormously. Some private classes such as active birth, yoga and Alexander technique concentrate mostly on physical ways of coping with labour and these can be all that a woman having her second or subsequent baby needs. The emphasis on the natural process of labour and encouraging women to develop awareness of their bodies and their

19 Churchill, 1997

ability to relax, breathe well and cope with pain, is useful for women intending to have as natural a birth as possible and to rely on their own resources for coping with pain. Teachers of these classes usually arrange occasional evening classes when labour companions can be shown how to support women using this kind of approach.

NHS and NCT classes usually have a balance of information about what to expect at the end of pregnancy, during labour and from life with a new baby; information about different methods of pain relief, hospital procedures and complications; a selection of relaxation, breathing and massage techniques for coping with labour; and opportunities for general discussion and questions. Because NCT classes are private, class sizes are smaller (an NCT teacher can only teach twelve women or eight couples in one class) and therefore it is easier for class members to get to know each other and to ask questions about the issues important to them. In addition, as NCT teachers are independent of the NHS and women attending their classes might have booked different types of maternity care, discussion about the management of labour and procedures used in different settings often shows up the wide range of possibilities and enables women to have a better idea of their preferences for care. (It has been known for women to change their care as a result of discussion in NCT classes).

Classes which teach self-help coping techniques for labour and develop a woman's confidence in her ability to give birth and in her labour companion to give support, can be very helpful. Discussing different procedures and interventions, including how to use artificial methods of pain relief well, can help a woman become aware of the sorts of things she would like to choose during her labour and those she would rather avoid.

Choosing a labour companion

As a result of campaigning by the NCT and other organisations in the 1960s, it is now generally accepted in Britain and often expected that the woman has with her in labour a birth companion, usually the father of her baby. Women often find the support of their partner invaluable during the birth and sometimes say things like 'I couldn't have done it without him'.

However, some women do not have a partner and other women are unable or unwilling to have their partner with them during labour. Equally, there are some men who do not wish to be present. In this situation, some women are happy to rely on the support of their midwives. But others find that, however sensitive and caring their midwives are, it makes a positive difference to their experience to be accompanied by someone who is not present in a professional capacity, but who is there as their friend. Some women choose to have more than one labour companion and some Trusts allow more than one companion to be present for labour and delivery. Women may invite their mother, a sister, friend, or even an acupuncturist or aromatherapist, in addition to their partner. There is evidence to suggest that having another female present to support women in birth has a positive effect on the progress of labour.[20]

The role of the labour companion will vary according to the woman's needs, but they will usually give physical as well as moral support and sometimes repeat information given to the woman by her caregivers which she was unable to take in. If a woman wishes to avoid unnecessary interventions, her labour companion can back her up. It is important for the woman's labour companion to be involved in any antenatal preparation, especially if the woman intends to use self-help coping techniques. In this way they can support the women with knowledge of what to do as well as sensitivity to her needs.

If the woman does not speak or understand English, her midwife should be able to arrange for an interpreter or link worker to accompany the woman during labour and at her antenatal check-ups. However, the woman may prefer a friend or relative to perform this function and should be encouraged to make her wishes known.

Other antenatal preparation

Women learn a vast amount from other women about birth. Hearing accounts of many different experiences can help a woman build up a picture of the range of possibilities in labour and give her some idea of what to expect. Although some women's birth stories may be rather negative, they can usually be balanced by positive ones. It is important for the woman to remember that her birth and her attitude to coping with it will be unique (and that therefore what worked well for another woman may not work so well for her). There is a wealth of books, magazines, leaflets and videos available for women wanting to learn more (see 'Further Information for Parents' on p.269 for a small selection). There can often be interesting programmes on television and radio as well. All these can help a woman add to her knowledge. If she is concerned about any of the information she comes across, she can speak to her midwife or antenatal teacher who can reassure her or put it into context.

Birth plans

The hospital also seemed more open to 'birth plans', and asked what you wanted during the birth – which is an important aspect when having a hospital delivery.

What I learnt during this time was not to make too many decisions in advance but to wait until the parameters for making them were in place.[21]

At some point during her antenatal care, perhaps during the last two or three

---

20 Hodnett, 2003; HoC, 2003b, section 4, p.8; NICE, 2004, p.41
21 Newburn, 1993

months of her pregnancy, the woman should discuss with her midwife her preferences for labour. These could include how long she wishes to stay at home in labour before going into hospital and what sort of pain relief she may choose to use. People vary and some women write a birth plan setting out exactly what they would like to happen at every stage of their labour. Others prefer to wait and see what happens, choosing to make their decisions at the time, or are content to take the advice of the midwives and doctors looking after them during labour. The latter may be a satisfactory approach if a woman's view of birth is the same as that of her caregivers, but if the hospital's approach is very 'high-tech' and the woman would prefer a 'low-tech' approach, for example, she may have a disappointing experience. Also, if a woman has strong feelings about what she would or would not like from her care, these may get lost if they are not written down.

Currently, some people have doubts about the value of birth plans. Some health professionals have been scathing about what they perceive as unrealistic, aggressively phrased birth plans insisting on no intervention, whose authors have ended up experiencing a large number of interventions, often after a change of heart. Some hospitals have short-circuited the system by producing their own form of birth plan with check-lists which may or may not correspond with an individual woman's agenda, only to ignore the plan when a woman goes into labour.

A woman should feel able to write a birth plan if she wishes but need not feel obliged to do so. In any case a woman should discuss the sort of care she would like during labour with her midwife antenatally. She may ask her partner or other labour companion to attend the appointment with her so that they are able to be present at the discussion and understand the hospital's approach to the management of labour. Alternatively, the woman may prefer to discuss different aspects of labour at different times during her pregnancy as her knowledge of what to expect and ideas for her own preferences develop. This tends to happen when a woman receives care from a small team of midwives or from an independent midwife. Another approach is for the woman and her partner each to write their own birth plans and then to compare notes.

A formal birth plan written by the woman can set the agenda for discussion with her midwife. An alternative approach is for the woman to ask about hospital policies regarding the areas of concern to her and to focus in her birth plan on those issues where her own preferences differ from hospital policy. For example, there may be a policy that every woman in labour has her waters broken by the midwife at 3 cm dilatation or on admission into hospital, whichever is the earlier. In these circumstances, the woman might ask that her waters be left to break spontaneously on the grounds that research shows that there is little benefit in breaking them early on in a normal labour. When adopting this approach, and finding that her preferences differ from hospital policy in only a few aspects, the woman may ask the midwife to record her preferences in her notes, rather than write a formal birth plan or fill in a checklist. If a woman does write a birth plan, it is advisable for it to be tactfully phrased and to take account of any professional advice about the possibilities for her birth.

Information on how to develop a birth plan and what to include is now available on-line. See for example: www.babycentre.co.uk. You can even fill in a birth plan on-line at www.amazingpregnancy.com.

If a woman has written a formal birth plan, once the final form has been agreed she should prepare two copies – one for herself and one to be kept with her notes – both of which should be signed by herself and her midwife or obstetrician. In some hospitals, a woman wishing to use a birth plan is asked to see a doctor. If this is the case, the woman should insist that the doctor is not a trainee (senior house officer), but either her consultant or a senior member of his or her team whose participation in the process of negotiating the birth plan will be meaningful.

Choosing midwifery-led care

In some parts of the country (see Appendix E) you can arrange to have your baby in a midwifery-led unit if you are assessed as healthy. Check whether the unit has a protocol which does not accept women having their first baby – though this is less common these days and, because not evidence-based, can be challenged. These units are usually small so you may be able to meet all the staff before you have your baby. Some are freestanding but others are in a hospital – though separately staffed from the consultant unit. These tend to have higher rates of intervention than the freestanding units. In the US, much lower rates of intervention are found[22] but in the UK some results are disappointing.[23] More recently the Edgware Birth Centre has achieved very good results with only a 12 per cent transfer rate in labour and 6.1 per cent CSR compared with 12.6 per cent of similar women from the district booked for hospital birth.[24] Women like these small informal units but have to fight to keep them open and rarely succeed.[25]

Independent midwives who may practice alone, in pairs or in a small group have to charge for their services but women will get continuity of care and personal attention. They charge about £2,500 which may be beyond many women but looked at another way this is a fifth to a tenth of the cost of a new car. A list can be found at www.independentmidwives.org.uk, as can their audit of results with an 82 per cent vaginal birth rate.

---

22 Rooks et al., 1992
23 MacVicar et al., 1993
24 Saunders et al., 2000
25 Bolton, 2005

Conclusion

In order to decide which kind of care is best for you, research into the local situation is needed. Whilst we are firm supporters of the NHS, the continuing inability of the maternity services to give all women the kind of services they want suggests that radical action is needed. This is despite the valiant efforts of AIMS and the NCT for almost fifty years to improve matters. For the last five years, the All Party Parliamentary Group on Maternity Care chaired by Julia Drown MP and supported by the Maternity Care Working Party (MCWP) have worked hard but achieved little. However, they did succeed in getting maternity services tacked on to the National Service Framework for Children and Young People. The MCWP is a coalition of lay activists, midwives and obstetricians who meet regularly and has been organised and chaired by the National Childbirth Trust since 1999. Some ideas about how to avoid an unnecessary CS for an individual woman and what needs to be done nationally to reduce the CSR will be found in the next chapter.

11 Avoiding unnecesary caesareans

'All women should be involved in planning their own care with information, advice and support from professionals, including choosing the place they would like to give birth...'[1]

Previous chapters have shown that caesareans are sometimes performed unnecessarily:

- There is wide variation in the caesarean rates between different maternity units which cannot be accounted for by different populations.

- Some of the indications for caesareans are relative rather than absolute. Even different obstetricians within the same maternity unit treat relative indications differently when deciding whether to advise a woman to have a caesarean.

- Although electronic fetal monitoring has become less routinely used in many units, the accuracy of its interpretation remains extremely difficult and the results are not checked by fetal blood sampling as often as they should be.

- The relative safety of the modern caesarean, particularly when performed under regional anaesthesia, has become confused with the question of a woman's choice and this, coupled with anxiety about medico-legal considerations has lowered the threshold at which a caesarean section is performed. Obstetricians appear to perform caesareans sooner rather than later.

In the first edition of this book (1993) we stated that in our opinion, the caesarean rate in Britain was too high at 13 per cent. *Changing Childbirth* (CC)[2] the government response to the Select Committee report on Maternity Services,[3] had just been published and we had high hopes that the recommended changes which focused on control and choice by women, continuity of care, communication and co-operation between professionals, and an increased role

---

1 DoH, 2004b, p.5
2 DoH, 1993
3 HoC, 1992

for midwives, would stop the rise in the CSR. However, whilst choice about having a CS seems to have been accepted by obstetricians, choice about birth at home did not materialise for the majority. Midwives, whilst showing that small teams could achieve good results in pilot projects, did not achieve the targets set by *Changing Childbirth*. The 2004 data about the CSR puts the rate at 22.7 per cent for England, 24.4 per cent for Scotland and 23.8 per cent for Wales. In 2002, Northern Ireland was 25.8 per cent. Incomplete RCOG figures give a rate of 25.3 per cent for Northern Ireland so we estimate that for the whole UK the rate is about 24.3 per cent. So the rise in the CSR continued at an average rate of about 0.8 per cent per year for the first four years of the twenty-first century, although this average masks a potential slowing down of the increase from 1.7 per cent between 2000 and 2001 to a negligible 0 or 0.1 per cent between 2003 and 2004.[4] The home birth rate rose from 1 to 2 per cent nationally. There are marked regional variations.[5]

The aim of this chapter, therefore, is to show how some caesareans could be avoided. However safe and unthreatening the operation might appear to women, the recovery after this major operation is never likely to be a positive aspect of the first few weeks of looking after a new baby. Maternity care works best when it is a team effort between each woman and her caregivers, so we suggest that women bring this chapter to the attention of those caring for them. Because a woman having her first baby is unlikely to know her way round the system, Appendix A contains a table describing the principal features of different types of maternity care.

Choosing a home birth

For low-risk women, it is clear that having a baby at home reduced the chance of having a CS by at least 50 per cent from 4.2 per cent to 2.0 per cent[6] with no difference in the outcome for the babies. The latest figures from North America from a prospective cohort study of 5,418 women found a CSR of 3.7 per cent 'substantially lower than for low-risk US women having hospital births'.[7] Having a baby at home is the surest way of achieving continuity of carer, avoiding routine procedures and intervention, and encouraging the normal progress of labour as long as one has a confident and experienced midwife. Twenty-two per cent of women in a MORI poll carried out for the Expert Maternity Group in 1993 said they would like to discuss the option of a home and 44 per cent a domino birth.[8] This was also the figure obtained by another

4 Data for N. Ireland are incomplete since 2002, so may mask a greater rise in overall CSRs.
5 www.BirthChoiceUK.org
6 Chamberlain et al., 1997
7 Johnston & Davies, 2005
8 DoH, 1993, vol.1, p.23

Select Committee on the Maternity Services in 2003. They stated that ten times as many women wanted a home birth as were obtaining one.[9]

Having a supportive companion in labour

The systematic review of RCTs done in 2003 encompassing 12,791 women[10] found that this reduced the chance of having a CS by 10 per cent. Whilst this may not sound like much, it could reduce a CSR of over 20 per cent by 2 per cent or more. If the person supporting was not a professional then the reduction was 26 per cent. This may disappoint midwives but a recent study found that 'midwives generally underestimated the ability of women to progress normally'.[11]

How antenatal teachers can help

It is clear from our study of women's experiences that they require more information about caesareans. This includes what to expect both during and after the procedure and the implications of being awake or asleep for the operation. All antenatal classes should incorporate this information as well as caesarean statistics. Thus women might realise that the experience is not as rare as one would hope and that there are choices they can make both to reduce the risk of a caesarean occurring and to make the experience (should it happen to them) and its aftermath as positive as possible. It is important that individual risks are given, not the overall, as suggested in the NICE guidelines. This is where the Robson groups[12] can be so helpful (see below).

The most valuable role of the antenatal teacher is to instil in women the confidence that they can give birth vaginally and that there are some decisions women can make to increase the likelihood of a vaginal delivery, provided that labour progresses normally. They can give advice about the steps to take to reduce the risk of ending up with an unnecessary CS. Although the current caesarean rate is high, antenatal teachers can put this figure into perspective, particularly if they obtain up-to-date caesarean rates for local hospitals and have access to midwifery-led units in their area (see Appendix E and Appendix F). They can remind women that the overwhelming chances are that they will not have a caesarean delivery. Over 95 per cent of women who start labour naturally at term should deliver vaginally. In the Home Birth study in 1994, 95 per cent[13] gave birth vaginally; in the US study the figure was 94.7 per cent.[14]

---

9   *BMJ*, 2003
10   Hodnett, 2003
11   Mead & Kornbrot, 2004
12   Robson et al., 1996
13   Chamberlain et al., 1997, p.70
14   Johnston & Davies, 2005

One of the changes that have taken place over the last fifteen years is the increasing use of protocols in the labour ward. Protocols should be evidence-based but are often designed for the least experienced member of the obstetric team and may contain matters for which there is no research evidence. These are formulated from the experiences of staff. In the late 1990s and early part of this century first the RCOG and then the National Institute for Clinical Excellence (NICE) issued evidence-based guidelines. These set a framework for what is considered acceptable practice but may be overridden by a consultant on the basis of his or her experience and locally collected data. Antenatal teachers can ask for copies of the local protocols. These can be discussed with the local branch of the NCT and, where they are felt to be unhelpful to women, can be changed.

How GPs can help

It is important that GPs give women full information about the local options for maternity care, and do not automatically assume that she will want a hospital birth in the nearest hospital. In addition, GPs need to find out from their local hospitals what their protocols and policies are about induction and time limits in labour, and what differences there are between consultants, so they can give women full information about the local options for maternity care. S/he should include how to arrange a home birth if this is a service that the GP does not offer. Sometimes, continuity of carer can be facilitated by GPs making their premises available to midwives and obstetricians wishing to take antenatal care into the community in order to make it more accessible to women. This can make GPs more confident and ensure that women are kept in the community and not referred unnecessarily to hospital: once there, women may be seen by a succession of doctors in training, whose natural reaction is to keep the woman under their supervision 'to be on the safe side'.

In Tower Hamlets, the GP was the most likely to maintain continuity of carer during the antenatal period, despite the practices having allocated midwives, because shortages of staff, sickness and leave meant that continuity of midwifery care was less than before *Changing Childbirth* and the introduction of teams. Experience in Lambeth, where Professor Ron Taylor cycled to clinics, and Tower Hamlets, where Wendy Savage worked with five practices, confirmed the benefit of this approach.[15]

How midwives can help

Midwives are generally acknowledged as the experts in normal childbirth and are trained to identify when pregnancy and birth become abnormal. It is part of their professional duty to refer women for appropriate medical assistance.

---

15 Robson et al., 1986; Savage et al., 1998

Therefore midwives were expected to give women an increasing proportion of their care, so that obstetricians could use their skills for the benefit of women experiencing complications. The experience of the South East London Midwifery Group showed how good midwifery care, with continuity and high rates of home birth, led to greater satisfaction on the part of the women, and high breast-feeding rates. However, like other innovative projects, this has been disbanded – although many of the team have gone to work in a small team at Kings College Hospital.[16] Research projects where smaller teams of midwives looked after identified caseloads of women throughout their pregnancy, birth and the postnatal period were liked by women but had no impact on the CSR[17] and were not continued after the research grants ended. When a woman ends up needing medical assistance, the fact that she continues to receive support from midwives known to her is likely to make her experience a positive one.

It is unrealistic to expect individual midwives in the NHS to rise to the challenge of working in new and flexible ways, so as to increase both women's satisfaction and their own, when the system does not allow this.

On an individual level, midwives can try to make every encounter with a woman meaningful; to ensure that the woman understands the purpose and outcome of the meeting; and that she goes away having been able to ask questions that were answered to her satisfaction. On an organisational level, midwives can try to join together to influence policies and practice, but this depends on the attitude of the Midwifery manager and the consultants towards change. Midwifery shortages bedevil such attempts. The experience of using the MIDRIS leaflets[18] suggests that midwives tailor their advice to fit in with the unit policies. If they get together to challenge the obstetricians, they could make a big difference to the way care is organised and this in itself might lead to a climate where CS is less likely to happen.

How the Royal College of Midwives (RCM) can help

The RCM could make a major contribution to improving care for women and working conditions for midwives if they were to support the idea of reorganising midwives into primary and secondary care midwives. Primary care midwives would be based in the community and work in small autonomous teams employed by the Primary Care Organisation (PCO). They would deliver women at home or in a secondary care unit, either midwifery-led or consultant-led. One of the CC targets was that midwives would be the lead carer for at least a third of women and have beds in hospital.[19] This has not happened in most places.

---

16 Robson et al., 1986; Leap, 1996
17 Flint, 1989; Page et al., 1999; Sandall 2001
18 O'Cathain et al., 2002; Stapleton et al., 2002
19 DoH, 1993, vol. 1, p.70

Secondary care midwives would work in hospital and be employed by the hospital trusts and gain expertise in the care of high-risk women and post-operative care. Student midwives would spend half their time working with primary and half with secondary care midwives. Once qualified, they could decide which sector they would like to work in. This approach would in our view stop the loss of qualified midwives who want to work with women in a non-interventionist continuous way, whilst retaining those who like the more technological approach found in hospital.[20]

Despite the efforts of the All-Party parliamentary group on Maternity, which has met regularly for five years and includes MPs, user representatives, midwives and obstetricians, women's experiences have not improved.[21] A radical re-think is needed. After CC, an implementation team was set up which disbanded in April 1997, having reported some successes in pilot studies in its quarterly newsletter. A smaller group was to take things forward in the DoH but, with the change of government in 1997, other priorities took over. Despite Select Committees in 1992 and 2003 Julia Drown, Chair of the maternity services subcommittee, expressed deep disappointment and frustration at the slow progress of change in the maternity services: 'A great many of our recommendations echo those made by our predecessor committee in 1992 which were adopted as government policy but which have not been implemented throughout the country.'[22] The National Audit Office report of 1997[23] also highlighted the problems in the Maternity services but little has changed. Midwifery shortages persist and women may be told at the last minute that they cannot have the home birth they had planned.[24]

The above suggestion should be pursued. Enabling primary care midwives to practice as they were trained could have a major impact on the CSR by keeping women out of hospital. Once women are referred to hospital, obstetricians need to adopt a less interventionist approach.

How obstetricians can help

We invite obstetricians to look critically at caesarean rates in their unit and at their own practice. The best tool for analysing CS rates is to use the Robson groups.[25] In one case, using the information from looking at the CSR in different groups of women, finding out which group made the biggest contribution (it was first pregnancies) and writing protocols for the management of dystocia enabled

20 Sandall, 1995; Savage, 2003
21 *BMJ*, 2003
22 HoC, 1992; BMJ, 2003, p.247
23 NAC, 1997
24 *BMJ*, 2003
25 Robson et al., 1996

Robson et al. to reduce the CSR from 7.5 to 2.4 per cent in spontaneously labouring women having a first baby. The groups are given below with results from England and Wales from the National Audit.[26] The third column gives the contribution of that group to the overall CSR using the CSR for that group (first column) and the proportion of women in the population who fall into that category.

Robson Group	Definition	CSR (%)	% of women	Contribution to overall CSR (%)
1	1st baby C 37 weeks natural onset of labour	12.2	24.8	14.1
2	1st baby C 37 weeks (induced) or ECS before labour	(27) 34.6	(9.7) 10.8	17.5
3	Subsequent baby C 37 weeks natural onset of labour	3.1	33	4.7
4	Subsequent baby C 37 weeks (IOL)ECS before labour	(7.8) 18.1	(9.5) 10.7	9.0
5	Subsequent baby 37 weeks uterine scar	64.4	8.0	23.9
6	1st baby breech presentation	91.7	1.9	8.1
7	Subsequent baby breech presentation	83.9	1.7	6.6
8	Multiple pregnancy including uterine scar	59.5	1.5	4.1
9	Transverse, oblique or unstable lie	99.7	0.4	1.8
10	Preterm (less than 37 weeks)	33	5.8	9.0

Taken from Table 4.5a, p.21, National Audit [27]

From this it is clear that the major contribution is from women who have a uterine scar. Therefore, if one increased the rate of VBAC to 60 per cent as Wendy Savage was able to achieve in Tower Hamlets (although she had a lower primary CSR than nationally and this included breech presentations), the CSR could be reduced by at least 10 per cent. Women having their first baby account for a third of the CS and improvement in the management of dystocia as shown by Robson et al., the use of FBS in suspected fetal distress and less frequent use of induction should be able to reduce this contribution by a third to a half. This would reduce the CSR by 10 to 15 per cent. Targeting these two groups of women with better management could reduce the CSR from 22 per cent to 17 to 18 per cent within a year. If the primary CSR falls, this reduces the number of women entering their next pregnancy with a scar and so the CSR will continue to fall. When contrasted with the present situation, where more women each year have their babies by CS, this explains why the rate rises slowly but inexorably.

26 Thomas & Paranjothy, 2001, p.107
27 Ibid.

As far as the less significant contributions are concerned, breech presentation at term contributes almost 15 per cent. Therefore a reversal of the policy of ECS for all breech presentations (to allow selected women to deliver vaginally) could reduce this contribution by at least 20 per cent, or 3 per cent of CS. Less intervention in twins and preterm births and more conservative management of unstable lie could reduce the rate by another 3 per cent making a total reduction of almost a third.

Using this tool, obstetricians could analyse their results but, although in the National Audit[28] 98 per cent said they carried out regular audit of CS in their units, usually monthly, few have used this approach. As half of the consultants in our survey put the increase in rate as due to maternal request, perhaps they need to look at the way they respond to these requests. Are women being fully informed of the disadvantages of CS? A quarter of the surveyed consultants thought that reduced skill in doctors-in-training was responsible for the rise, whilst another 13 per cent thought that reduced skill in performing assisted vaginal deliveries was to blame. About a fifth of those who gave suggestions for reducing a rate that they perceived as too high mentioned more consultant input to the labour ward, or improved consultant supervision. Is more consultant time spent training the next generation actually on the labour ward and in the theatre a way forward? Are drills and the use of models, as in the Advanced Life Support Obstetrics (ALSO) course, useful in passing on skills? Would more personal consultant involvement in supporting women having a trial of scar help? Could maternity care be organised differently so that women experiencing normal pregnancies and births were cared for entirely by midwives?

Four specific measures for reducing caesarean rates are as follows:

- VBAC should be encouraged in all suitable cases (see chapter 9 for information on the safety of VBAC)

- Induction of labour should be a consultant decision

- CTG traces and partograms should be faxed to the duty consultant to keep him/her up to date about the labour ward, thus improving decision making[29]

- Women with ruptured membranes should be left to go into labour spontaneously as this has been shown to reduce the CS rate,[30] presumably because many have hindwater leaks.

Treating women as individuals and using discretion rather than blind adherence to protocols can reduce the CSR as this example shows:

Before operating, the consultant examined me vaginally and found me sufficiently dilated to see that the placenta was not in the way and also he

---

28   Thomas & Paranjothy, 2001
29   Quinn, 1993
30   Hofmeyer & Kierse, 1990

managed to turn the baby's head down. I was therefore allowed to 'come round' [from the general anaesthetic] and delivered vaginally two hours later… he felt it right to 'let me have a go myself' in view of the problems recovering from a section would have caused my family… I felt that this was a brave decision – many consultants faced with an unconscious patient and a theatre full of staff would have carried on![31]

The audit published by the Royal College of Obstetricians and Gynaecologists in 2001[32] gathered comprehensive data about the reasons for CS and opened the doors for debate on caesarean section rates and how they might be reduced. The New Deal for doctors in the training grades and the European Working Time Directive have had an effect on the training and experience of these doctors. We concur with the House of Commons recommendation[33] that medical staff be allowed sufficient time to gain experience of normal birth in order to develop the range of skills they require and improve the quality of care they provide.

The issue of performing caesareans for medico-legal reasons rather than clinical reasons is one which needs to be dealt with as a matter of urgency. Lawyers as well as obstetricians need to take account of the research evidence and to look critically at some of the legal judgements which have been made. Our sample of consultant obstetricians showed a very positive interest in some system of no-fault compensation for all babies born handicapped and this issue needs urgent consideration.

A recent survey of obstetricians and heads of midwifery asked whether they would be prepared to take part in a randomised controlled trial and asked a variety of questions. Of 660 obstetricians, 49 per cent said that women should be able to choose their mode of delivery; 45 per cent felt such a trial was desirable; 37 per cent felt it was ethical and they would recruit women for such a trial; and 24 per cent thought it was feasible. Midwives were less likely to agree with all the statements and female obstetricians were significantly less likely than males to agree with these options. Compared with only 7 per cent of the 123 heads of midwifery who answered, 39 per cent of male and 19 per cent of female obstetricians would consider a CS for themselves or their partner.[34]

How maternity units can help

The providers of maternity care can help by publishing their caesarean and other intervention rates annually. These data are now collected and publicly available (see Appendix F). If possible, rates should also be given for each individual consultant. If particular consultants specialise in caring for women with a high

---

31 NCT, 1992
32 Thomas & Paranjothy, 2001
33 HoC, 2003a, Conclusions & Recommendations, no.26
34 Lavender et al., 2005

risk of caesarean section, this could be explained.

The maternity booklets given by every maternity unit to women should contain meaningful information about hospital policies for routine procedures and interventions for complications, options for anaesthesia during caesareans, and up-to-date intervention rates. Women using the service would be better informed and might be encouraged to express their needs more effectively than is often possible at present. Establishing schemes whereby continuity of carer can be achieved would also facilitate this process. All written information for women should be accessible in other relevant languages for the community as well as in Braille. Videos and audiotapes should also be available where appropriate.

Every provider unit should be auditing every aspect of its clinical care, including caesarean rates and women's satisfaction with their care. The results of this audit should be used to refine practice and reduce the number of unnecessary caesareans.

How Primary Care Organisations (PCOs) can help

One of the roles of PCOs (PCTs in England and Wales) when commissioning maternity care is to set quality standards. They then negotiate with different providers to what level each standard should apply, the aim being that all the providers for a Trust will eventually meet the same standards for each category of care. In practice, most PCOs will only have one hospital providing maternity care within reach and even the forthcoming merger of PCOs will not change this for most organisations. Each PCO has a director of public health and s/he should ensure that units audit their results using the Robson groups[35] so that they can see where the biggest contribution to the CSR is coming from. Standards should therefore be set, aimed at minimising the number of unnecessary caesareans, since these are an inefficient use of resources.

Secondly, PCOs should consider the possibility of running a primary care midwifery service and directly employing either NHS or independent midwives. GPs are independent contractors but in recent years have become much more managed by PCOs. There is no reason why this could not happen with midwives as was done by the SELMG for a while until the PCT management priorities changed.[36]

How Maternity Services Liaison Committees (MSLCs) can help

MSLCs still exist in some areas as forums where representatives from all the relevant professional groups as well as maternity services managers meet

---

35 Robson et al., 1996
36 Leap, 1996

together with user representatives to consider maternity services and to advise both commissioning authorities and provider units. In addition, they have carried out useful surveys of the facilities and women's experiences. MSLCs are well placed to assist GPs, midwives and obstetricians, as well as PCOs and provider units, in working together to avoid unnecessary caesareans. They can regularly review protocols.

How women can help themselves to achieve a normal birth and avoid a CS

Once pregnant, we would suggest that women read one or more of the books listed in 'Further Information for Parents' at the back of this book which will give them an idea of the range of options available. With a view to avoiding an unnecessary caesarean, the woman experiencing a normal pregnancy and anticipating a normal labour might ask about some of the following aspects of care before she books to have her baby in a hospital:

- If she is found to be in the latent phase of labour when she comes into hospital, whether she can return home until the contractions become stronger. This is a decision she can make herself.

- Whether there is a policy for listening to the baby's heartbeat using continuous electronic fetal heart monitoring, in both normal and abnormal labour. If a normal pregnancy and labour on admission, decline this even for a 'twenty minute monitor strip' – see RCOG guidelines on fetal monitoring for the evidence.[37]

- Whether fetal blood sampling is available to be used to check if abnormalities in the recording of the baby's heart rate are noted. If not, choose another unit or book a home delivery.

- Whether the waters are routinely broken artificially and if so, decline this intervention. If the hospital protocol does not 'allow' this, choose another unit or book a home delivery.

- Whether she can take up whichever position she feels most comfortable in at every stage of labour, even if it becomes necessary to monitor the baby's heart rate.

- Whether any time limits are set for the first and second stages of labour. Some flexibility is needed in watching how labour progresses: if progress is steady albeit slow and the mother and baby are in good condition then there is no need to intervene. If the hospital protocols are strictly adhered to then you might like to look at other hospitals or birth centres or having your baby at home.

- How the onset of the active phase of labour is defined, for example, when the cervix is 3 cm dilated, fully effaced and the woman is experiencing strong regular contractions.

- In what circumstances an oxytocin drip is used to accelerate labour.

- Whether, in the latent phase of the second stage of labour, the woman is allowed to wait until she has an urge to push.

- The availability of epidural or spinal anaesthesia for pain relief or an emergency caesarean.

- Whether she can eat and drink if she is hungry and thirsty throughout labour. Only 5 per cent of units in the UK are reported to allow this,[38] although it is standard practice in the Netherlands.[39] The only evidence available shows that eating a low-residue diet does increase the fluid in the stomach but whether or not this has an effect on inhaling stomach contents during general anaesthesia is unknown. Drinking isotonic drinks has been shown to be safe.

If the woman is experiencing any complications she might in addition ask about the following:

- What effect, if any, a pre-existing medical condition or disability might have on the management of her labour

- What effect a pregnancy-related illness such as gestational diabetes, raised blood pressure or pre-eclampsia might have on the management of her labour

- Whether external cephalic version is attempted to turn breech babies and, if so, when and what is the success rate and complication rate

- The management of a breech labour and who will conduct this

- The management of multiple births and what policies are available to read

- The availability of epidural or spinal anaesthesia for a planned or emergency caesarean

- Whether her labour companion can be present during all procedures.

Choosing between a planned caesarean and a trial of labour

If a woman is faced with one of the relative indications for caesarean such as suspected feto-pelvic disproportion, having had a first birth by CS for failure to progress or fetal distress when progress was slow, she may be given a choice between a planned caesarean and a trial of labour. In the National Audit, of those women who had a CS only 44 per cent had been offered a trial of labour. This ranged from 39 to 49 per cent regionally and from 8 to 90 per cent between units

---

38 O'Sullivan, 1994
39 Ludka & Roberts, 1993

– so if this is not offered, women should ask about the possibilities available to them.[40] The woman will obviously discuss her choice with her obstetrician. Although the obstetrician is likely to advise her to take one course or the other, she should feel able to choose that which feels right for her and, if necessary, to ask for a second opinion from another obstetrician. She should obtain as much information as there is about her obstetric condition, including the chances of delivering vaginally (see chapter 5). She should also ask whether an epidural or spinal anaesthetic will be available to her for a planned or an emergency caesarean.

> I desperately needed an epidural but the man who does these only comes in during the day![41]

Some women prefer the certainty of preparing for a planned caesarean – hopefully under regional anaesthesia, knowing the date on which their baby will be born and being able to make all necessary preparations – to the uncertainty of waiting for labour to begin spontaneously and then perhaps ending up with a caesarean, possibly under general anaesthetic. However, even if a repeat CS is needed, the uterine contractions may reduce the chance of the baby having breathing difficulties and the operation may be easier than if labour has not occurred as the lower part of the uterus becomes thinner. If the previous labour was long, the woman can soon feel if things are going better this time. A second labour is usually shorter than a first and she may well be able to deliver a bigger baby vaginally than the first time round.

Some women prefer to give their bodies every chance to give birth unaided and, if an emergency CS is necessary, derive satisfaction from the knowledge that they tried everything they could to avoid a caesarean. However, most women who have no need for a caesarean would prefer not to have one.[42]

One of our authors, Wendy Savage, remembers a woman who wanted to try and deliver vaginally after two previous CS, both planned, the first for breech and the second because the obstetrician thought the baby was too big for the pelvis. She had wanted to try labour but he was adamant that it was unsafe. She laboured well and reached full dilatation but the baby was occipito-posterior (see chapter 5) and the head was still above the ischial spines. This suggested that an assisted delivery would not be easy so Wendy therefore went in (it was about 11.00pm) and this is her account:

> In theatre an attempt at manual rotation was made but the head was quite a tight fit. The fetal heart went down and did not recover quickly and I judged that it would not be safe to proceed with a vaginal delivery and left the registrar to do

---

40   Thomas & Paranjothy, 2001, p.46
41   NCT, 1992
42   HoC, 2003b, section 4, p.6

the CS. The baby weighed 7lb 3oz. The mother was disappointed not to have delivered vaginally but glad to have had the chance to labour. The following year, I received a card from her to say that she had delivered her fourth baby vaginally at home weighing 6lb 13oz. I wrote to congratulate her and, although the baby was smaller, asked in what position the baby had been. He had been occipito-anterior and so the labour had proceeded more easily.

It is vital that the woman presented with such a choice thinks carefully about her decision. She may find it helpful to discuss the matter with her midwife, her partner or with a woman who has gone through a similar experience (NCT branches keep 'experiences registers' and some run caesarean support groups) as well as her obstetrician. She can then make an informed choice based on what feels right for her.

> I felt a lot of pressure to conform to the hospital policy and had to be very assertive to achieve a vaginal delivery.

> My daughter presented breech… I arrived at hospital $7^1/_2$ cm dilated and tried to convince the consultant I wanted to deliver normally… He 'talked me round' into having a section. In a way I feel cheated because I wasn't fully in control of myself and I was talked round.[43]

Coping with a normal labour or trial of labour

The same conditions apply to both if the woman is to avoid an unnecessary caesarean. In fact, the nearer the management of a trial of labour is to that of a normal labour, the more likely a woman is to be able to give birth vaginally. Ways in which a woman can be helped to deliver vaginally are as follows:

- Resisting induction of labour for non-urgent reasons if the cervix is unripe.

- Staying at home as long as possible. The woman may find that using a TENS (Transcutaneous Electrical Nerve Stimulation) machine or warm bath for pain relief at home enables her to delay going into hospital.

- Having a home assessment in labour from community midwives is usually possible on a domino or team midwifery scheme. The woman will probably find it reassuring to be given a vaginal examination to see how far her cervix has dilated and to have the baby's heart rate checked.

- If a home assessment in labour is not possible, the woman may find it reassuring to keep in touch by telephone with midwives on the hospital labour ward who will tell her whether it is advisable to remain at home.

- Being looked after by midwives she has got to know antenatally and who know her and her preferences.

43 NCT, 1992

- Procedures or interventions should not be carried out for routine reasons, but because they are necessary in the woman's labour. All procedures and interventions should be explained fully to the woman, together with the reasons for performing them.

- Not being continuously connected to an electronic fetal heart rate monitor unless there is some doubt about the baby's condition. Research shows that listening to the baby's heart rate at regular intervals is just as effective. What matters is that any doubtful results should be considered carefully and any necessary action taken quickly.

- Doubtful traces from the electronic fetal heart rate monitor should be checked using fetal blood sampling for further evidence of the baby's condition.

- Not having the waters broken artificially unless there is a good reason for doing so. Routine policy is an inadequate reason.

- Not having the labour accelerated using an oxytocin drip unless there is a good reason for doing so, since some babies become distressed as a result of their oxygen supply being reduced by the artificially strengthened contractions. Conforming to arbitrary time limits is an inadequate reason for acceleration unless there is a full active management of labour policy incorporating accurate diagnosis of the active phase of labour (see p.56), although cessation of dilatation would be a good reason for it. EFM is usually done when oxytocin is used as excessive contractions can be produced.

- Careful use of epidurals for routine pain relief. EFM is usually used if there is an epidural because blood pressure may sometimes fall, and this can affect the baby. The woman's contractions may become weaker as a result of reduced mobility and she can then be given an oxytocin drip to strengthen the contractions, which may adversely affect the baby. Sometimes a woman undergoing a trial of labour is recommended to have an epidural so that she can be awake in the event of an emergency caesarean becoming necessary. However, managing labour in this way could make a caesarean a self-fulfilling prophecy. Some women might be much more likely to deliver vaginally if able to use self-help techniques such as upright position and movement to promote the natural progress of labour and to maximise the ability of her pelvis to expand to accommodate the baby.

- Being as relaxed as possible, both during and between contractions, so as not to interfere with the natural process of labour.

- She is likely to find upright positions the most comfortable, using gravity to aid the process of labour – although RCTs have not shown clear evidence of benefit.[44] Work from the 1950s showed that contractions were stronger in the upright position.

---

44 Bloom et al., 1998

- Using a breathing technique for coping with contractions learned antenatally. One technique is to concentrate on the out-breath, letting the breaths in take care of themselves. This ensures that the woman, the baby and the uterus have enough oxygen to cope with the hard work of labour.

- Remaining mobile and changing position. Different positions will feel comfortable at different times in labour. If the woman listens to her body she will automatically take up the position most useful for labour. If the baby is in an awkward position, walking around, pelvic rocking and other rhythmic movements may help it to turn into the right position.

- Touch and massage. This is good for contractions experienced as back pain and for helping the woman feel less isolated during contractions. If the woman finds that she does not want to be touched or held in labour, she should make this known to those with her!

- Darkness promotes the release of endorphins, the body's natural painkillers produced in response to pain. Another way of helping the woman to concentrate on herself and her labour if she wears glasses or contact lenses is to remove them. But the woman may prefer to keep them on and may also appreciate eye contact to help her stay with the contractions.

- Food and drink. Essential during a long labour since a labouring woman uses 700-1,000 calories per hour. Many hospitals do not allow even women at low risk of complications to eat or drink during the active phase of labour on the grounds that they may inhale acid stomach contents during a general anaesthetic.[45] However, research shows that it is usually faulty anaesthetic technique and insufficiently experienced operators which cause this to happen. Possible ways round such a policy are to put unrestricted eating and drinking in a birth plan, to stay at home as long as possible and to eat and drink right up to the end of the latent phase of labour. However, do eat easily digestible food.

- Using large cushions, beanbags, birthing chairs, music and so on to get as comfortable as possible. A labour companion is good to lean on too!

- Using a birthing pool or warm bath can be an effective form of pain relief and may help the woman stay relaxed, particularly if she uses long baths as a way of coping with everyday life. However, the use of water for pain relief in labour has not been scientifically evaluated.

- Natural therapies such as homeopathy, acupuncture, hypnotherapy and aromatherapy can be useful in labour if the woman uses them in her normal life and if she knows a practitioner who will attend her in labour. The advantage of hypnotherapy is that the woman is usually taught self-hypnosis for labour so that the practitioner does not have to be on call. Some homeopaths suggest a kit

---

45 Ludka & Roberts, 1993

of remedies useful for labour and instruct the woman (and her labour companion) when to use them in labour, or suggest remedies over the telephone. Supporters of natural therapies believe that they can promote the normal progress of labour and thus keep interventions to a minimum.

How the government can help

The government is using 'performance management' to put pressure on PCOs to commission services which meet certain targets. The PCOs ask the hospitals to reduce waiting times for outpatient appointments or to perform a proportion of operations in a certain length of time. If they fail then in theory the PCO will move the patients elsewhere. The government could set targets (as the US government did) for the level of primary CS which is reasonable; we would suggest initially that this should be 12 per cent, accepting that most obstetricians will not share our doubts about the management of breech presentation. For VBAC, an initial target of 50 to 60 per cent should be achievable.

The second step the government could take would be to legislate to give midwives the same independent contractor status as GPs have; alternatively, the PCO could be responsible for employing them, so that they could set up in the community. The clinical governance could be via the PCO. The infrastructure would need to be provided but there is often spare capacity in health centres. We call upon the government to set up a task force to look into this suggestion: without enough midwives working, women will never get the service they need and the CSR will continue to rise. There are a probably still over 150,000 qualified midwives of whom 43,000 notified their intention to practise in 2005 but only about 24,000 are working – and not all of them fulltime. This is an enormous waste of money and skills and we need to get good midwives back working in the community where they belong.[46]

How readers of this book can help

If you care about the rise in unnecessary caesareans, you may use the information in this book to make changes at local level to reduce their number. You may be a woman who hopes to avoid a first delivery by caesarean, or a repeat caesarean; a midwife newly promoted to a management position; an antenatal teacher asked to sit on an MSLC; a GP worried about the number of women in the practice having a CS; or an obstetrician concerned enough about the issue to read this book. All of you have a role to play in keeping caesareans to the minimum necessary for the safety of women and their babies and in preventing unnecessary caesareans from blighting the first few weeks of a mother and baby's relationship.

46 NMC, 2005

Appendix A

SIX TYPES OF CARE FOR BIRTH

The table on the next page aims to explain to women the main features of the different packages of maternity care on offer in Britain. At first sight, the table may seem complex, but it is not nearly as complicated as the system which it aims to explain! By choosing one of the packages of care in the first column on the left, you can discover the main features by reading horizontally across to the right. If you are particularly interested in one feature of care such as giving birth at home for example, you can choose the column entitled 'Place of birth' and read down vertically to see which packages of care offer this option.

Package of care	Who gives antenatal care?	Where is antenatal care given?	Place of birth	Who delivers the baby?	Essential features of the package	With whom to book your care
Home birth	Community or independent midwives and/or GP	At home or in GP surgery or community clinic	At home	Community or independent midwife with cover from GP or hospital	All your care takes place at home and you have the chance to get to know the midwife or small team of midwives, one of whom will attend your birth	Community midwives or GP or via supervisor of midwives
Total hospital care	Hospital or community midwives and hospital doctors	Hospital antenatal clinic	Hospital	Hospital midwife; in a teaching hospital a student midwife or doctor under supervision; cover from obstetricians	All care conducted by hospital-based midwives and doctors directly responsible to consultant obstetricians whose (individual) policies will determine the way care is provided	GP or direct with the hospital: ring and ask for the antenatal clinic
Shared care	GP, often assisted by community midwife, and hospital midwives and doctors	GP surgery and hospital antenatal clinic	Hospital	As above	Similar to a hospital birth except that many routine antenatal appointments are with your GP or community midwives. Many women welcome this more personal form of care which may mean less travel and shorter waiting times.	Your GP or, if s/he does not offer the service, or, if you prefer, with another GP
Domino Scheme	Community midwives (can be combined with shared care from GP)	At home or GP surgery or midwives' clinic in community or in hospital	Hospital	Community midwife; cover from obstetricians	All care is given by a community midwife or small team of community midwives, so you get to know the person who will attend your delivery, provided there are flexible working patterns. An important bonus is that a community midwife assesses you in labour at home. Six-hour discharge if you want.	Your GP or with the community midwives: ring them at your local maternity unit
Team midwifery or caseload midwifery scheme	Small team of midwives working in hospital and in the community	At home or midwives' clinic in community or in hospital	At home or in hospital	Team midwife; cover as above	You receive individualised care from a small team you get to know well	The team via your GP or the local hospital
Birth centre (also known as 'midwife-led units', 'birthing centres', 'maternity hospitals' or 'GP units')	Community midwives	At home or midwives' clinic in community or in hospital	Isolated unit or unit alongside district general hospital	Community midwives; cover from GP or district general hospital	A personal form of care with a high rate of continuity of carer. A comfortable, low-tech environment. Available to women with 'low-risk' pregnancies, i.e. no potential complications. There are a number of NHS centres in the UK. There are some private birth centres run by independent midwives for those who wish to pay.	Your GP or another GP or with the community midwives

Appendix B

METHODOLOGY EMPLOYED IN THE CHAPTER 7 SURVEY OF WOMEN'S EXPERIENCES

This study utilised a survey designed to assess the experiences of women having caesarean sections. The aims of the survey were: first, to find out from women the reasons they had been given for their operations in order that a comparison could be made with the reasons given by consultants; second, to analyse women's experiences of caesarean birth in the light of current debate on medical intervention and to suggest ways in which the management of birth can best be achieved for all concerned.

The sampling procedure

A sample consisting of one hospital from each of the strategic health authorities in England, area health authorities in Wales and health boards in Scotland was randomly selected. Permission to conduct the survey of women's experiences was requested from consultant obstetricians responsible in each case. Nine hospitals, geographically spread across the country, agreed to take part in the study. The two-page questionnaires were sent out along with covering letters to the participating hospitals with the request that they be handed to fifty consecutive women having caesareans.

The questionnaire

The questionnaire asked for quantitative data about the women, the operations and the babies, as well as qualitative information regarding the women's experiences and feelings about the births.

The response rate

Completed questionnaires were received from six of the nine participating hospitals, i.e. the response rate was 66.6 per cent. The first 198 questionnaires received are analysed here. Of these, 78 (39.4 per cent) were planned caesareans and 120 (60.6 per cent) were emergency operations. The women were further divided into three categories: first births, previous vaginal births and previous births including caesareans.

The data show that almost half (47.3 per cent) of caesarean sections are being carried out on women who are giving birth for the first time. Furthermore the majority of those women (68.5 per cent) are having emergency operations. Three out of five (60.6 per cent) women having planned sections have had previous caesareans.

Appendix C

TABLES

Table A.1
Reasons women were given for their caesarean sections

	Planned		Emergency		Total	
	No.	%	No.	%	No.	%
Labour too long	3	3.8	75	62.5	78	39.4
Fetal distress	0	0	48	40.0	48	24.2
Repeat caesarean	30	38.5	9	7.5	39	19.9
Baby too big	12	15.4	12	10.0	24	12.1
Baby in breech	18	23.1	3	2.5	21	10.6
High blood pressure	3	3.8	15	12.5	18	9.0
Diabetes	12	15.4	1	0.8	13	6.6
Baby lying across womb	2	2.6	2	1.7	4	2.0
Cord around baby's neck	1	1.3	3	2.5	4	2.0
Baby small for dates	2	2.6	1	0.8	3	1.5
Bleeding before birth	0	0	3	2.5	3	1.5
Maternal age	2	2.6	1	0.8	3	1.5
Cord prolapse	1	1.3	1	0.8	2	1.0
Other reasons as specified	16	20.5	6	5.0	22	11.1
Total reasons	102		180		282	
Average no. reasons per woman	1.3		1.5		1.4	
Total women	78		120		198	

Note: percentages total more than 100 as some women were given more than one reason for their caesareans.

219

Table A.2
Partner's attendance at a caesarean

	Planned		Emergency		Total	
	No.	%	No.	%	No.	%
Partner present	66	84.6	99	82.5	165	83.3
Partner not present	12	15.4	21	17.5	33	16.7
Total	78	100	120	100	198	100

Table A.3
Did women feel that they had been adequately informed about their condition?

	Planned		Emergency		Total	
	No.	%	No.	%	No.	%
Yes	76	97.4	111	92.5	187	94.4
No	2	2.6	9	7.5	11	5.6
Total	78	100	120	100	198	100

Table A.4
Whether women having caesareans felt that they suffered

	Planned		Emergency		Total	
	No.	%	No.	%	No.	%
Yes	15	19.2	18	15.0	33	16.7
No	63	80.8	102	85.0	165	83.3
Total	78	100	120	100	198	100

Table A.5
Consultants' views on the reasons for the rise in caesarean rates

Litigation, defensive medicine	52
Reduced skill of junior & senior doctors, lack of supervision	45
Maternal request, demand or pressure	44
Patient expectation	27
Medical reasons (twins, premature babies, avoid long labour, HIV etc.)	24
Breech birth	23
Increase in repeat caesareans including reluctance to attempt VBAC (2)	18
Midwifery shortages or reduced skills	8
Poor management of normal labour, medicalisation of birth	7
Problems with fetal monitoring	5
Changed attitude/threshold for CS, long labour	4
Induction overuse	4
Smaller families (including fewer grand multiparae)	4
Premature births	3
Weight	2
Age/delayed conception	2
Babies bigger	2
Risk avoidance/management	2
Other reasons (mentioned once) *Lack of confidence in CDS, epidural pain relief, fear of failure, obstetrician doubt, mother's health worse, 'tochophobia', empowerment of women, multifactorial, confusion re advice, 'never have to say you are sorry', society gets the CSR it wants, decreased medical staff, media, no passion for vaginal birth by junior staff or midwives, reduced antenatal care, bad previous experience, evidence*	17

Table A.6
Potential risks of a caesarean

Immediate	
Haemorrhage (bleeding)	83
Infection (of wound)	72
Deep vein thrombosis (DVT)	62
Organ damage (bladder/bowel/unspecified)	58
Anaesthetic risks	9
Morbidity/risks related to major surgery	9
Death	7
Slower recovery	6
Damage to major blood vessels	4
Hysterectomy	4
Baby could have damage (e.g. respiratory complaints)	4
Those mentioned in NICE or RCOG guidelines	3
Blood transfusion	2
Post-partum haemorrhage (PPH)	2
Long term	
Placenta praevia (next pregnancy)	8
Pain, including scar pain	5
Scar on uterus (leading to repeat caesareans)	3
Other factors (mentioned once): *decreased bonding, RDS, Neonatal TTN (transient tachypnoea of the newborn), backache and headache*	

Table A.7
Risks of a caesarean section

Immediate complications after a CS	
Haemorrhage	1.3% of women will have a blood transfusion
Infection	2.2% of women will have a serious wound infection
Thrombosis	This includes DVT and pulmonary embolism
Risks of anaesthesia	
Trauma to internal organs	0.6% of women after a CS will have damage to their bladder or bowel

Long-term complications
Increased risk of placenta praevia in future pregnancies
Scar rupture in future pregnancies
Long-term bladder dysfunction from scar tissue
Increased risks associated with further caesarean sections
Reduced fertility

Rare complications
Hysterectomy
Cardiac arrest
Aspiration during anaesthesia

Risks to the baby	
Transient tachypnoea of the newborn. If a planned CS is carried out at 40 weeks, a baby will have the lowest risk of developing this complication.	
At 39 weeks	babies have 2x the risk
At 38 weeks	babies have 4x the risk
At 37 weeks	babies have 8x the risk
Scalpel injuries to the baby (approximately 1 in 500 births)	

Source: West Suffolk Hospital NHS Trust leaflet setting out potential risks of CS

Table A.8

Consultants' views on how to reduce the CSR

Bring in the obstetric team earlier/more consultant input	13
Push for VBAC, encourage trial of scar, reduce repeat CS	10
Encourage women, patient education	9
Weekly meeting, continued discussion	9
Improved training/care by midwives	9
Complete audit/review	8
More active management of labour	6
Create a culture of normality, less medical interference	4
Better explanation (highlight) risks of CS	4
Improved training of junior doctors or middle-grade staff	4
1-2-1 midwife care, increase number of midwives	3
Reduced induction of labour (IOL)	3
Increased training/use of instrumental birth	2
Reduced caesarean for fetal distress	2
Improved obstetric intra-partum care	2
ECV after 36 weeks for breech, re-evaluate breech trial	2
Other reasons (mentioned once): *Delay induction of labour until 42/40, decrease unnecessary planned sections, reduce primary CS rate, three-times-a-day consultant ward rounds, change NICE guidelines, more use of fetal blood sampling, second opinion for a request, better adherence to protocols for CS for FTP/FPD, not do CS for failure to progress without syntocinon, STAN, increase community care and close supervision of middle-grade staff*	12

Table A.9

Optimal caesarean rate: the views of 100 consultants

	Number	Percentage
Below 10%	1	1.2
10-13.9%	6	7.4
14-19.9%	44	54.3
20-24.9%	23	28.4
25-29.9%	3	3.7
30% or more	4	4.9
No estimate	19	
		Percentages exclude those who said they were 'unsure'

Appendix D

COMPARISON OF CONSULTANTS' CS RATES

The Royal London Hospital (RLH)

The Royal London Hospital is a teaching hospital in a deprived area of London with a multicultural population and, for the last twenty years, a regional neonatal intensive care unit. There are various regional specialties and so women with a range of diseases will be transferred for care at the London. One would therefore expect the hospital to have a higher CSR than the national average and, as you can see from Figure 1, this was the case for most of the 1980s. However, as the CSR rose nationally it overtook the rate at the London.

The late Peter Huntingford, who was an advocate of natural childbirth,[1] resigned in 1981 and I (Wendy Savage) was suspended from practice in April 1985.[2] Although reinstated in July 1986, I did not see a patient until November.

I had a sabbatical from September 1996 for a year and retired in September 2000. New, younger consultants have been appointed. Now Birthchoice figures suggest the RLH is approaching the national average.[3]

Figure 1

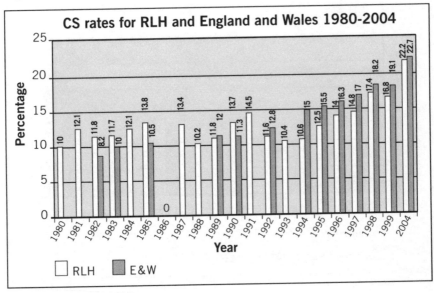

CS rates for RLH and England and Wales 1980-2004

1   Francome & Huntingford, 1980
2   Savage, 1986
3   Birthchoice.co.uk, 2005

Attitudes of the consultants at the London varied, as in most hospitals, with myself as the most prepared to support a woman wanting a vaginal birth. The colleague with whom I worked most closely on a one-in-two on-call rota for five years, after his appointment in 1991, shared many of my views and we worked together as Firm One. Firm Two was made up of three consultants who were more interventionist. One of these consultants looked after the diabetics, which would be expected to raise his CSR.

In 1991-5, amongst women who were Tower Hamlets residents and over thirty-seven weeks pregnant, there was no significant difference in the proportion of women delivering normally: 81.2% for myself, 81.8% for my close colleague and 80.6% for Firm 2.

In Figure 2, there are significant differences in assisted vaginal delivery between Firms One and Two. In this group, 7.6% of my patients had a CS whereas 11.5% of Firm Two's did so. Whether the woman is having her first baby or a subsequent one (parity) is an important factor; when I produced this analysis, it showed that I had more primigravidae (women expecting their first baby) than my colleagues and so would be expected to have a higher CSR. This was done before Robson published his paper, so I did not analyse the data using this tool.[4]

Figure 2

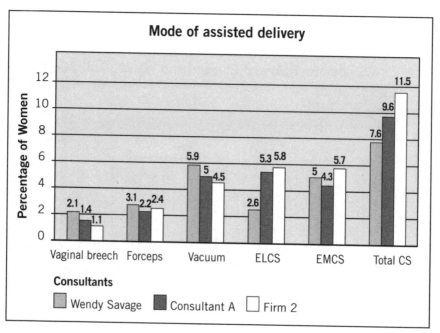

4   Robson et al., 1996

Another difference was in our approach to vaginal birth after Caesarean Section (VBAC). Figure 3 shows how women fared. Consultant A had inherited a large practice from an interventionist consultant – which explains why his proportion of women with a scar is higher than mine – and he also had more multigravidae. As the CSR rises, so does the proportion of women with a scar in the uterus. One could argue that the 11% fewer women who had a repeat CS in my patients compared with Firm Two was achieved only by having a low rate of planned CS, so that 7.2% of women laboured but ended up with another emergency CS. However, as long as the woman is prepared and supported, this seemed to me a small price to pay for achieving a 61% VBAC rate.

Figure 3

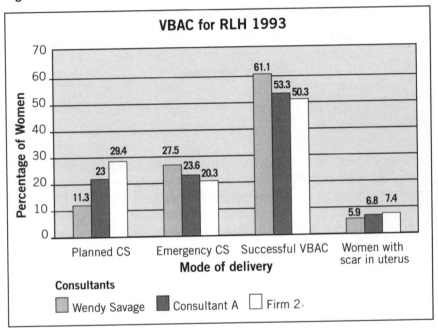

Although within the RLH my intervention rate was the lowest, compared with the other hospitals in East London our combined results showed lower rates of CS for all ethnic groups between 1991 and 1995.

Figure 4

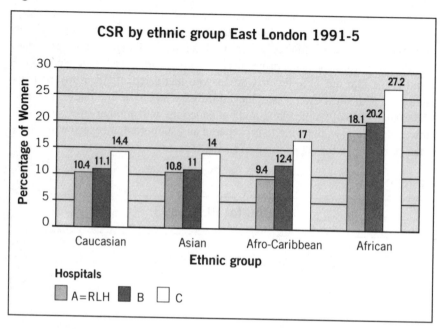

At the time I analysed these data I was unaware of the work of Robson but tried to standardize by excluding women who lived outside the area served by the hospital as they may have been referrals for difficult problems. These data appear to confirm my view that the attitude of consultants and the climate within the hospital obstetric department affect the rate at which CS is performed.

Use of Robson Groups to compare the CSR between Hospitals

The figure below shows how Robson groups can be used to compare the contribution made by different groups and the overall CSR by hospital.

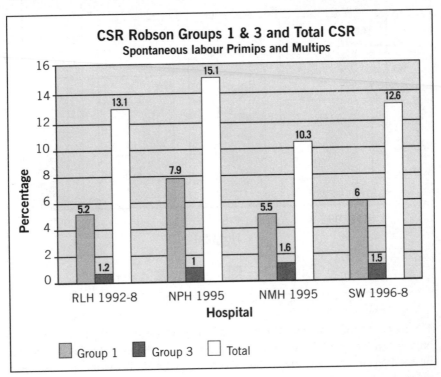

The National Maternity Hospital in Dublin had the lowest CSR in 1995 and Northwick Park the highest (figures courtesy of Harry Gordon). Despite the lowest CSR in women having their first baby (primips) and the second lowest for multips (women having subsequent babies) the overall rate was higher at the London than in Dublin or the hospital in the South West who sent me figures.

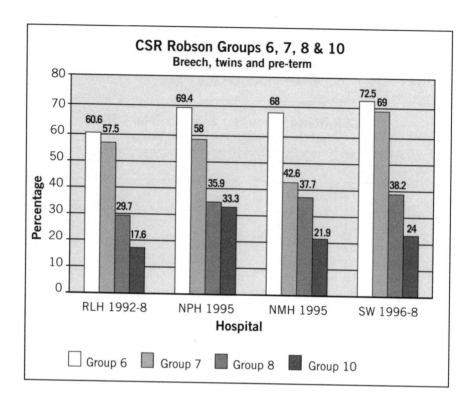

The RLH had the lowest CSR for women having their first baby presenting as a breech and the second lowest for women having subsequent babies presenting by the breech, and was lower than the other hospitals for twins and pre-term deliveries. Population differences in the proportion of primips and grand multips (women having their fifth or later child) and the incidence of gestational diabetes which is high in Asian women probably explain why the overall rate for the London is higher than the National Maternity Hospital in Dublin.

Appendix E

Midwifery-led units	GP units

England	
Calderdale Royal Hospital	St Mary's Hospital, Portsmouth
Chase Farm Hospital, Enfield	
Dewsbury and District Hospital	
East Surrey Hospital, Redhill	
Elizabeth Garrett Anderson Hospital	
Frimley Park Hospital	
Gloucestershire Royal Hospital	
Hope Hospital, Salford	
Hospital of St John and St Elizabeth (Private)	
Ipswich Hospital	
John Radcliffe Hospital, Oxford	
Kingston Hospital	
Liverpool Women's Hospital	
Newham Hospital	
North Staffordshire Hospital, Stoke-on-Trent	
Portland Hospital (Private)	
Princess Anne Hospital, Southampton	
Queen Charlotte's and Chelsea Hospital	
Queen Elizabeth Hospital, Kings Lynn	
Queen Elizabeth Hospital, Woolwich	
Royal Berkshire Hospital, Reading	
Royal Free Hospital, Hampstead	
Royal Shrewsbury Hospital	
Royal Surrey County Hospital, Guildford	
Royal United Hospital, Bath	
St George's Hospital, Tooting	
St Thomas' Hospital	
Southmead Hospital, Bristol	
Stoke Mandeville Hospital, Aylesbury	
University Hospital of North Durham	
Watford General Hospital	
Whipps Cross Hospital, Leytonstone	

* All midwifery-led units and GP units in England are attached to consultant units

Midwifery-led units	GP units
Northern Ireland	
Craigavon Area Hospital [1]	

Midwifery-led units	GP units
Scotland	
Aberdeen Maternity Hospital [2]	Balfour Hospital, Orkney
Aboyne Hospital	Campbeltown Hospital
Arbroth Infirmary	Dalrymple Hospital, Stranraer
Ayrshire Central and Maternity Hospital [3]	Dr Mackinnon Memorial Hospital, Skye
Belford Hospital, Fort William	Dunoon and District General Hospital
Chalmers Hospital, Banff	Fraserburgh Hospital
Davidson Cottage Hospital, Girvan	Gilbert Bain Memorial Hospital, Shetland
Forth Park Maternity Hospital, Kirkcaldy [3]	Islay Hospital, Bowmore
Insch and District War Memorial Hospital	Isle of Arran War Memorial Hospital
Jubilee Hospital, Huntly	Lorne and Islands District General Hospital, Oban
Mid Argyll Hospital, Lochigilphead	Portee Hospital, Skye
Montrose Royal Infirmary	
Perth Royal Infirmary	
Peterhead Cottage Hospital	
The Queen Mother's Hospital, Glasgow [3]	
Vale of Leven Hospital, Alexandria	
Victoria Hospital, Rothesay	

Midwifery-led units	GP units
Wales	
Aberdare Hospital	Dolgellau and Barmouth Community Hospital
Brecon War Memorial Hospital	
Bro Ddyfi Community Hospital, Machynlleth	
Bluith Wells Cottage Hospital	
Caerphilly Birth Centre	
Knighton Hospital	
Llandrindod Wells Hospital	
Llanidloes War Memorial Hospital	
Montgomery County Infirmary, Newtown	
Neath Port Talbot Hospital	
Victoria War Memorial Hospital, Welshpool	

Source: Birthchoiceuk.com

1   Medium-sized consultant unit with midwifery-led unit
2   Very large consultant unit with midwifery-led unit
3   Large consultant unit with midwifery-led unit

Appendix F

THE LATEST BRITISH HOSPITAL DATA

Data collected from published sources and made publicly available by www.BirthChoiceUK.com.

England, Caesarean Rates by Hospital 2004

Hospital	Caesarean Rate (%)
Airedale General Hospital	26.0
Alexandra Hospital, Redditch – data combined with Worcestershire Royal Hospital	28.0
Arrowe Park Hospital, Birkenhead	20.2
Ashington Hospital	24.7
Barnet General Hospital	24.6
Barnsley DGH	20.3
Basildon Hospital	20.1
Bassetlaw DGH, Worksop	22.3
Bedford Hospital	21.9
Birmingham Heartlands Hospital – data combined with Solihull Hospital	21.7
Birmingham Women's Hospital	23.6
Bradford Royal Infirmary	19.9
Burnley General Hospital	22.0
Calderdale Royal Hospital	22.3
Central Middlesex Hospital – data combined with Northwick Park Hospital, Harrow	28.6
Chase Farm Hospital, Enfield	24.4
Chelsea and Westminster Hospital	29.9
Cheltenham General Hospital – data combined with Gloucestershire Royal Hospital	24.1
Chesterfield & N. Derbyshire Royal Hospital	18.7
City Hospital, Birmingham	23.1
Colchester General Hospital	24.8
Conquest Hospital, St Leonards on Sea	25.2
Countess of Chester Hospital	22.8
County Hospital, Hereford	22.4

Hospital	Caesarean Rate (%)
Cumberland Infirmary, Carlisle – data combined with West Cumberland Hospital, Whitehaven	19.4
Darent Valley Hospital, Dartford	25.4
Darlington Memorial Hospital – data combined with Bishop Auckland Hospital	21.1
Derby City General Hospital	22.3
Derriford Hospital, Plymouth	19.1
Dewsbury and District Hospital	18.4
Doncaster Royal Infirmary	17.9
Dorset County Hospital	28.3
Ealing Hospital, Southall	27.3
East Surrey Hospital, Redhill	26.4
Eastbourne DGH	21.1
Elizabeth Garrett Anderson Hospital	27.1
Epsom General Hospital – data combined with St Helier Hospital, Carshalton	25.1
Fairfield General Hospital, Bury – data combined with Rochdale Infirmary, North Manchester General Hospital, The Royal Oldham Hospital	21.1
Friarage Hospital, Northallerton	14.8
Frimley Park Hospital	22.4
Furness General Hospital – data combined with Royal Lancaster Infirmary	20.7
Gloucestershire Royal Hospital – data combined with Cheltenham General Hospital	24.1
Good Hope Hospital, Sutton Coldfield	25.3
Grimsby Maternity Hospital – data combined with Scunthorpe General Hospital	18.2
Harold Wood Hospital, Romford	20.2
Harrogate District Hospital	29.0
Heatherwood Hospital, Ascot – data combined with Wexham Park Hospital, Slough	27.0
Hillingdon Hospital, Uxbridge	24.8
Hinchingbrooke Hospital, Huntingdon	25.3
Homerton Hospital	24.7
Hope Hospital, Salford	23.2
Horton Hospital, Banbury	23.7
Hospital of St John and St Elizabeth (Private)	
Huddersfield Royal Infirmary	21.2
Hull Royal Infirmary	22.0

Hospital	Caesarean Rate (%)
Ipswich Hospital	22.0
James Cook University Hospital, Middlesbrough	18.5
James Paget Hospital, Great Yarmouth	20.3
Kettering General Hospital	21.1
King George Hospital, Ilford	19.5
King's College Hospital, London	29.3
Kings Mill Centre, Sutton-in-Ashfield	17.4
Kingston Hospital	25.7
Leeds General Infirmary – data combined with St James's University Hospital, Leeds	21.2
Leicester General Hospital	19.0
Leicester Royal Infirmary	21.5
Leighton Hospital, Crewe	18.8
Lincoln County Hospital – data combined with Pilgrim Hospital, Boston	20.9
Lister Hospital, Stevenage – data combined with Queen Elizabeth II Hospital, Welwyn	23.4
Liverpool Women's Hospital	22.8
Luton & Dunstable Hospital	24.8
Macclesfield DGH	24.0
Maidstone Hospital	24.6
Manor Hospital, Walsall	22.1
Mayday Hospital, Croydon	22.7
Medway Maritime Hospital, Gillingham	25.1
Milton Keynes General Hospital	21.7
New Cross Hospital, Wolverhampton	28.5
Newham Hospital	21.6
Norfolk And Norwich University Hospital	24.4
North Devon District Hospital, Barnstaple	21.9
North Hampshire Hospital, Basingstoke	17.5
North Manchester General Hospital – data combined with Rochdale Infirmary, Fairfield General Hospital, Bury, The Royal Oldham Hospital	21.1
North Middlesex Hospital	18.2
North Staffordshire Hospital, Stoke on Trent	22.7
North Tyneside General Hospital	20.9
Northampton General Hospital	25.9
Northwick Park Hospital, Harrow – data combined with Central Middlesex Hospital	28.6

Hospital	Caesarean Rate (%)
Nottingham City Hospital	17.7
Nuneaton Maternity Hospital	22.7
Ormskirk DGH – data combined with Christiana Hartley Maternity Unit, Southport	23.3
Pembury Hospital, Tunbridge Wells	24.9
Peterborough District Hospital	22.3
Pilgrim Hospital, Boston – data combined with Lincoln County Hospital	20.9
Pontefract General Infirmary	17.2
Poole Hospital	29.3
Princess Alexandra Hospital, Harlow	27.4
Princess Anne Hospital, Southampton	21.8
Princess Royal Hospital, Haywards Heath – data combined with Royal Sussex County Hospital, Brighton	22.8
Princess Royal University Hospital, Orpington	29.7
Queen Charlotte's and Chelsea Hospital	30.1
Queen Elizabeth Hospital, Gateshead	22.0
Queen Elizabeth Hospital, Kings Lynn	23.0
Queen Elizabeth Hospital, Woolwich	23.5
Queen Elizabeth II Hospital, Welwyn – data combined with Lister Hospital, Stevenage	23.4
Queen Elizabeth the Queen Mother Hospital – data combined with Kent & Canterbury Hospital, William Harvey Hospital, Ashford	22.5
Queen Mary's Hospital, Sidcup	29.6
Queen's Hospital, Burton upon Trent	23.8
Queen's Park Hospital, Blackburn	19.7
Rochdale Infirmary – data combined with Fairfield General Hospital, Bury, North Manchester General Hospital, The Royal Oldham Hospital	21.1
Rosie Maternity Hospital	26.8
Rotherham DGH	20.6
Royal Albert Edward Infirmary, Wigan	22.4
Royal Berkshire Hospital, Reading	27.1
Royal Bolton Hospital	19.5
Royal Cornwall Hospital, Truro	15.9
Royal Devon & Exeter Hospital	24.0
Royal Free Hospital, Hampstead	27.3
Royal Hallamshire Hospital, Jessop Wing	23.1
Royal Hampshire County Hospital, Winchester	24.5
Royal Lancaster Infirmary – data combined with Furness General Hospital	20.7

Hospital	Caesarean Rate (%)
Royal London Hospital, Whitechapel	22.2
Royal Shrewsbury Hospital	14.4
Royal Surrey County Hospital, Guildford	25.7
Royal Sussex County Hospital, Brighton – data combined with Princess Royal Hospital, Haywards Heath	22.8
Royal United Hospital, Bath	20.1
Royal Victoria Infirmary, Newcastle	21.9
St George's Hospital, Tooting	22.6
St Helier Hospital, Carshalton – data combined with Epsom General Hospital	25.1
St James's University Hospital, Leeds – data combined with Leeds General Infirmary	21.2
St John's Hospital, Chelmsford	33.1
St Mary's Hospital, Isle of Wight	23.0
St Mary's Hospital, Manchester	18.8
St Mary's Hospital, Paddington	28.6
St Mary's Hospital, Portsmouth	22.6
St Michael's Hospital, Bristol	24.3
St Peter's Hospital, Chertsey	25.9
St Richard's Hospital, Chichester	26.0
St Thomas' Hospital	24.8
Salisbury District Hospital	23.3
Sandwell DGH, West Bromwich	24.8
Scarborough Hospital	17.8
Scunthorpe General Hospital – data combined with Grimsby Maternity Hospital	18.2
Sharoe Green Unit, Royal Preston Hospital	20.3
Solihull Hospital – data combined with Birmingham Heartlands Hospital	21.7
South Tyneside District Hospital	18.3
Southend Hospital	28.7
Southmead Hospital, Bristol	23.6
Staffordshire General Hospital	20.2
Stepping Hill Hospital, Stockport	23.7
Stoke Mandeville Hospital, Aylesbury	22.8
Sunderland Royal Hospital	16.5
Tameside General Hospital, Ashton-under-Lyne	16.0
Taunton and Somerset Hospital	24.0
The Great Western Hospital, Swindon	24.3

Hospital	Caesarean Rate (%)
The John Radcliffe Hospital, Oxford	19.6
The Portland Hospital (Private)	
The Royal Oldham Hospital – data combined with Rochdale Infirmary, Fairfield General Hospital, Bury, North Manchester General Hospital	21.1
Torbay Hospital	22.8
Trafford General Hospital	22.7
University Hospital of Hartlepool – data combined with University Hospital of North Tees	18.4
University Hospital of North Durham	19.9
University Hospital of North Tees – data combined with University Hospital of Hartlepool	18.4
University Hospital, Aintree	24.3
University Hospital, Lewisham	31.3
University Hospital, Nottingham	21.2
University Hospitals Coventry	26.4
Victoria Hospital, Blackpool	21.1
Warrington Hospital	26.9
Warwick Hospital	25.0
Watford General Hospital	26.0
West Cumberland Hospital, Whitehaven – data combined with Cumberland Infirmary, Carlisle	19.4
West Middlesex University Hospital, Isleworth	20.0
West Suffolk Hospital, Bury St Edmunds	31.0
Wexham Park Hospital, Slough – data combined with Heatherwood Hospital, Ascot	27.0
Whipps Cross Hospital, Leytonstone	28.7
Whiston Hospital	22.3
Whittington Hospital, Highgate	24.8
William Harvey Hospital, Ashford – data combined with Kent & Canterbury Hospital, Queen Elizabeth the Queen Mother Hospital	22.5
Worcestershire Royal Hospital – data combined with Alexandra Hospital, Redditch	28.0
Wordsley Hospital, Stourbridge	23.4
Worthing Hospital	23.6
Wycombe Hospital	22.5
Wythenshawe Hospital	26.4
Yeovil District Hospital	23.5
York District Hospital	24.0

Northern Ireland, Caesarean Rates by Hospital 2002

Hospital	Caesarean Rate (%)
Altnagelvin Area Hospital	Data unavailable
Antrim	Data unavailable
Causeway Hospital	21.9
Craigavon Area Hospital	30.1
Daisy Hill Hospital, Newry	22.6
Downpatrick Maternity Hospital	Data unavailable
Erne Hospital, Enniskillen	Data unavailable
Lagan Valley Hospital	21.5
Mater Infirmorum, Belfast	25.7
Mid Ulster Hospital, Magherafelt	Data unavailable
Royal Maternity Hospital, Belfast	Data unavailable
Ulster Hospital, Belfast	Data unavailable

Wales, Caesarean Rates by Hospital 2004

Hospital	Caesarean Rate (%)
Bronglais Hospital, Aberystwyth	26.5
Llandough Hospital & University Hospital of Wales (combined data)	25.7
Nevill Hall Hospital and Royal Gwent Hospital (combined data)	21.7
Prince Charles Hospital, Merthyr	27.1
Princess of Wales Hospital, Bridgend	19.4
Royal Glamorgan Hospital, Llantristant	26.6
Royal Gwent Hospital and Nevill Hall Hospital (combined data)	21.7
Singleton Hospital, Swansea	27.4
University Hospital of Wales and Llandough Hospital (combined data)	25.7
West Wales General Hospital, Carmarthen	25.6
Withybush Hospital, Haverfordwest	23.6
Ysbyty Glan Clwyd, Rhyl	24.9
Ysbyty Gwynedd, Bangor	18.7
Ysbyty Wrexham Maelor	21.9

Scotland, Caesarean Rates by Hospital 2004[1]

Hospital	Caesarean Rate (%)
Aberdeen Maternity Hospital	27.4
Ayrshire Central and Maternity Hospital	25.6
Balfour Hospital	25.5
Borders General Hospital	19.4
Caithness General Hospital	24.5
Cresswell Maternity Hospital, Dumfries	27.4
Dr. Gray's Hospital, Elgin	16.0
Dumfries and Galloway Royal Infirmary	27.4
Falkirk and District Royal Infirmary	16.5
Forth Park Maternity Hospital, Kirkcaldy	20.5
Gilbert Bain Memorial Hospital[2]	10.9
Inverclyde Royal Hospital	18.3
Ninewells Hospital, Dundee[3]	22.7
Perth Royal Infirmary	17.9
Princess Royal Maternity Hospital	26.1
Raigmore Hospital, Inverness	29.8
Royal Alexandra Hospital, Paisley	26.8
Royal Infirmary of Edinburgh at Little France	26.7
Southern General Hospital, Glasgow	23.3
St. John's at Howden, Livingston	23.2
Sterling Royal Infirmary	22.9
The Queen Mother's Hospital, Glasgow	31.1
Western Isles Hospital	18.7
Wishaw General Hospital	22.9

1   Excludes non-NHS hospitals
2   Emergency CS only
3   Data for Ninewells approximately 90% complete

Abbreviations

ACNM	American College of Nurse Midwives	IOL	Induction of Labour
ACOG	American College of Obstetricians and Gynecologists	IUGR	Intra-uterine growth retardation
		IVF	In-vitro fertilisation
AIMS	Association for Improvement in Maternity Services	LEDCs	Less economically developed countries
AML	Active management of labour	LSCS	Lower segment caesarean section
ARM	Artificial rupture of the membranes	MSLC	Maternity Services Liaison Committee
BMA	British Medical Association	NCT	National Childbirth Trust
CC	Changing Childbirth report	NHS	National Health Service
CDS	Central Delivery Suite	NICE	National Institute for Clinical Excellence
CEE	Central and Eastern Europe	O&G	Obstetrics and gynaecology
CEFM	Continuous electronic fetal monitoring	ONS	Office for National Statistics
		OP	Occipito-posterior
CIS	Commonwealth of Independent States	PCO	Primary Care Organisation
CPD	Cephalopelvic disproportion	PCT	Primary Care Trust
CS	Caesarean section	PET	Pre eclampsia
CSR	Caesarean section rate	PMR	Perinatal mortality rate
CTG	Cardio-tocograph	PRH	Pregnancy-related hypertension
D&C	Dilatation and curettage	RCM	Royal College of Midwives
DoH	Department of Health	RCOG	Royal College of Obstetricians and Gynaecologists
DVT	Deep vein thrombosis	RCT	Randomised controlled trial
E&W	England and Wales	RDS	Respiratory distress syndrome
ECS	Elective caesarean section	RLH	Royal London Hospital
ECV	External cephalic version	SCBU	Special Care Baby Unit
EFM	Electronic fetal monitor(ing)	SEHD	Scottish Executive Health Department
EGAMS	Expert Group on Acute Maternity Services	SELMG	South East London Midwifery Group
FIGO	International Federation of Gynaecology and Obstetrics	SGA	Small for gestational age
FBS	Fetal blood sampling	SHO	Senior House Officer
FPD	Feto-pelvic disproportion	SPR	Specialist Registrar
FTP	Failure to progress	STAN	Segment Analysis (a new method of analysing the fetal heart trace)
GA	General Anaesthetic		
GMC	General Medical Council	TED	Thromboembolic elastic (stockings)
GP	General Practitioner		
GSS	Government Statistical Service	TENS	Transcutaneous electrical nerve stimulation
HBAC	Home birth after caesarean		
HELLP	Haemolysis elevated liver enzymes & low platelet count syndrome	TTN	Transient tachypnoea
		VBAC	Vaginal birth after caesarean
HoC	House of Commons	WHO	World Health Organisation

Glossary

active birth Giving birth in positions comfortable for the mother, often using gravity and not lying down on a bed.

active phase (of labour) When contractions are strong, regular and begin to open the cervix beyond 3 cm.

Alexander technique A natural therapy in which the Alexander teacher encourages the client to use the body in accordance with its natural alignment.

amniotic fluid The sterile fluid in which the baby moves and grows within the membranes.

amniotomy Artificial rupture of the fetal membranes to induce or hasten labour.

antacids Drugs used to neutralise the stomach contents.

antepartum Before labour or childbirth.

anterior lip (of cervix) When part of the cervix remains in front of the baby's head during delivery.

areola The dark-coloured area of the nipple.

artificial rupture of the membranes Manual breaking of the waters to induce labour (amniotomy).

assisted delivery When a mother needs help with giving birth to her baby. Usually refers to forceps, Ventouse and caesarean section.

augmentation (of labour) Speeding up labour using a synthetic oxytocin drip.

bipareital diameter The diameter of the fetal head.

bradycardia A slowness of the heartbeat, as evidenced by slowing of the pulse rate to less than 60 beats per minute.

breech presentation The position of a baby who is head-up, bottom-down, before labour begins (see illustration on p.96).

cannula A tube for insertion into a duct or cavity (See *intravenous drip*).

cardiotacograph (CTG) See *electronic fetal heart monitor.*

catheter A tube inserted into the urethra to assist the passing of urine.

cauterisation Sealing blood vessels by burning to reduce bleeding.

CEE Central and Eastern Europe, currently consisting of Albania, Bosnia & Herzegovina, Bulgaria, Croatia, Czech Republic, Estonia, Hungary, Latvia, Lithuania, FYR Macedonia, Poland, Romania, Slovakia, Slovenia, Serbia & Montenegro and Turkey.

cephalic presentation The normal position for a baby before labour begins: head-down.

cephalopelvic disproportion (CPD) See *feto-pelivic disproportion.*

cerebral palsy Brain damage occurring either before or during birth resulting in physical and, less often, in mental disability.

cerebrospinal fluid The fluid which surrounds the brain and spinal cord. This can leak out if the membrane surrounding the spinal cord is accidentally punctured during the insertion of an epidural or spinal block.

cervix The neck of the uterus. Before term it is usually long, closed and firm. As pregnancy progresses it 'ripens' and becomes soft, shorter and opens up.

CIS Commonwealth of Independent States, created in December 1991, currently includes Azerbaijan, Armenia, Belarus, Georgia, Kazakhstan, Moldova, Russia, Tajikistan, Turkmenistan, Uzbekistan and Ukraine.

classical (caesarean) section or scar A vertical cut in the upper part of the uterus.

colostrum The first milk produced by the breasts during pregnancy and for the first few days after birth. It is particularly rich in anti-bodies which protect the baby against infection.

Community Health Council A statutory body set up in each district health authority to represent and safeguard the interests of users of all local health services. Can help users with information and with making complaints.

community midwives Midwives working outside hospital whose work includes attending home births and domino deliveries, seeing women antenatally and postnatally, at home, in GPs' surgeries and community clinics. (See also Appendix A.)

consultant (doctor) The most senior grade of hospital doctors who have teams of junior doctors working under them and who have considerable influence on how hospitals are run. They are often involved in research and teaching and tend to see complicated rather than normal cases. Sometimes these doctors are employed by a university as lecturers, etc., rather than a health authority, and some of them have the title 'professor' rather than 'mister' or 'ms'. The majority of NHS consultants also do private work, which is why they are not employed for NHS work full-time: some consultants work in their NHS hospital for only two half-days a week, owing to their other commitments.

cricoid An area in the neck.

dehiscence The medical term for a caesarean scar coming apart, but not rupturing the uterus.

dextrose A sterile solution of sugar and water sometimes given to newborn babies in hospital. Healthy newborn babies should never be given dextrose but should be put to the breast whenever they are hungry.

dilatation (often popularly called 'dilation') The opening of the neck of the uterus (the cervix) during labour. The cervix dilates or opens to about 10 cm diameter so that the baby can be born.

dilatation and curettage ('D & C') A minor operation carried out under general anaesthetic to gently scrape the inner walls of the uterus. Performed if any pieces of placenta or membranes remain after delivery and cause heavy bleeding or infection.

disproportion See *feto-pelvic disproportion*.

domino birth See Appendix A.

doula A woman experienced in childbirth (not necessarily medically qualified) who provides advice, information and emotional support to a mother before, during and just after childbirth.

dystocia The medical term for difficult labour or when a labour 'fails to progress'.

eclampsia The severe form of pre-eclampsia (see below) when a mother has fits or convulsions. It is also often associated with blood-clotting problems.

elective caesarean section A planned caesarean performed before labour has begun.

electronic fetal heart monitor A machine which collects information about a baby's heartbeat using ultrasound from a belt on the mother's abdomen or a clip fastened to the baby's head ('fetal scalp electrode'). The information is printed out continuously onto a strip of paper (a 'trace') which hospital staff can read during labour and which forms part of the permanent record of the birth.

emergency caesarean section A caesarean performed once labour has begun, i.e. not always in an 'emergency' situation.

endometritis Inflammation of the lining of the uterus (endometrium), often occurring as postpartum infection.

entonox A half-and-half mixture of oxygen and nitrous oxide, inhaled for pain relief during labour.

epidural (anaesthesia) A form of regional anaesthesia used to numb the abdomen for routine pain relief during labour and total pain relief during a caesarean.

episiotomy A cut made into the perineum, using surgical scissors, to enlarge the vaginal opening before delivery. It can be performed by either a midwife or a doctor.

external cephalic version The procedure whereby an obstetrician attempts to turn a breech baby into a more favourable position before labour begins.

fetal blood sampling A medical procedure performed during labour whereby a sample of blood is taken from the baby's head and tested for acid levels as a measure of how much oxygen is being transferred to the baby.

fetal distress When the baby in the uterus is short of oxygen. It can be diagnosed by changes in the baby's heart rate and sometimes from the baby passing meconium into the amniotic fluid, as well as by fetal blood sampling.

fetal hypoxia See *fetal distress*.

fetal marcosmia Defined as an estimated birth weight of more than 4,000g (8lb 13oz). Suspected fetal marcosmia may lead to caesarean section.

feto-pelvic disproportion When the baby cannot pass through the woman's pelvis, either due to the relative size of the baby's head and the size and shape of the woman's pelvis, or because of the baby's position, also known as cephalopelvic disproportion.

fetus The medical word for a baby before it is born.

fibroids Thickened muscle fibres in the uterine wall which are usually benign but which sometimes cause problems in pregnancy and labour.

firm The old-fashioned word for a consultant's 'team' of junior doctors and medical students.

foley catheter Flexible plastic tube inserted into the bladder to provide continuous urinary drainage.

forceps Medical instruments used by a doctor to help a woman deliver her baby. They are rather like a pair of salad servers which are inserted into the woman's vagina around the baby's head, locked together and then pulled and sometimes turned during contractions to help the baby out. They come in different sizes, depending on the sort of help the baby needs. An episiotomy is usually needed for a forceps delivery.

gestation The length of time needed for a baby to develop fully in the mother's body: this can be anything from thirty-seven to forty-two weeks.

gestational diabetes A condition whereby a woman's body does not produce enough insulin during pregnancy. Modern maternity care has made all forms of diabetes less hazardous for both mothers and babies.

glucose The fuel available in the blood for energy.

glycogen The stored form of energy which is broken down as needed to give glucose.

haemorrhage Heavy bleeding. Postpartum haemorrhage is defined as the loss of more than 500 ml of blood.

hellp 'Haemolysis elevated liver enzymes & low platelet count syndrome' A serious disorder of pregnancy characterised by a great reduction in the number of platelets, hemolysis, abnormal liver function tests and sometimes, hypertension. In the most severe cases, it may require delivery of the baby before term.

high risk A way of describing women who are more likely to experience complications or lose their babies.

hindwater The amniotic fluid in the uterus behind the presenting part of the fetus.

hysterectomy An operation to remove the uterus.

iatrogenic Caused (inadvertently) by medical treatment or procedures.

incision The medical term for 'cut'.

induction (of labour) Starting off labour artificially using prostaglandins, breaking the membranes and, if necessary, stimulating contractions using a synthetic oxytocin drip.

instrumental delivery Giving birth with the aid of forceps or Ventouse.

intra partum During delivery.

intra-uterine growth retardation (IUGR) When the baby appears not to be growing as it should. It is difficult to diagnose accurately, even using an ultrasound scan.

intravenous drip Fluid introduced into the body via a tube into a needle inserted into a vein in the arm (a 'cannula').

Intubation Insertion of a tube into the body e.g. the trachea.

in vitro fertilisation A process of artificial conception whereby eggs are gathered from the woman's ovaries and mixed with the man's sperm in a dish before being implanted back into the woman's womb.

Keilland forceps Used for rotational forceps delivery and have two curves instead of the usual one curve.

latent phase (of labour) The early part of labour when contractions are relatively mild, possibly irregular and have not opened the cervix beyond 3 cm.

lochia Vaginal discharge that occurs during the first week or two after birth.

lower-segment (caesarean) section Usually a horizontal cut in the lower part of the uterus.

macrosomia Large baby or babies.

Maternity Services Liaison Committee (MSLC) A committee set up by a district health authority to enable representatives from the different groups of health professionals, voluntary organisations and users to influence local policy for maternity care and to monitor the provision of services.

meconium The waste products of development retained in the baby's intestines before birth. If the baby passes meconium during labour, the amniotic fluid turns brown and this can be, but is not always, a sign of fetal distress.

membranes The tissues forming a bag around the amniotic fluid in which the baby grows in the uterus. After birth, they are usually expelled with the placenta.

membrane sweep A process of inducing labour by the doctor or midwife 'sweeping' a finger around the cervix to separate the membranes. This releases hormones (prostaglandins) which may kick-start labour.

meta-analysis Results from a collection of independent studies (investigating the same treatment) are pooled using statistical techniques to synthetise their findings into a single estimate of a treatment effect. Where studies are not compatible e.g. because of differences in the study population or in the outcomes measured, it may be statistically inappropriate to statistically pool results in this way.

midwife Usually a nurse (most are women, but a few are men) who undergoes further training in the care of women and their babies during pregnancy, labour and postnatally. In some institutions, direct-entry or 'pre-registration' training is available whereby people train solely as midwives.

morbidity The medical term for illness, disease or a physical condition other than health.

mortality The medical term for death, expressed statistically as a rate per 1000 deaths.

multip (abbreviation of multigravida) A woman having her second or subsequent baby.

neonate Newborn baby.

no-fault compensation Awarding money to people with injuries arising from medical care, without their having to prove negligence.

obstetrician A doctor specialising in pregnancy and childbirth. A gynaecologist specialises in women's medicine and may or may not have obstetric qualifications as well.

obstetric physiotherapist See *physiotherapist*.

occiput The back part of the head or skull.

Occipitoposterior position A cephalic (head-down) presentation of the fetus with the back of the head turned to the right (right occipitoposterior, ROP) or to the left (left occipitoposterior, LOP).

oedema The medical word for swelling.

ovarian cyst A growth on the ovary, usually benign, which may cause problems during labour.

oxytocin The hormone which causes the uterus to contract during labour. It is also released by the woman's body during orgasm and breastfeeding.

palpation The medical term for 'feeling' the baby within the uterus.

Partogram A visual representation of the progress of labour, cervical dilation against time.

pelvimetry Estimating the size and shape of the pelvis using X-rays and palpation.

perinatal mortality rate (PMR or PNMR) The rate (usually expressed per 1,000) of babies dying between twenty-four weeks of pregnancy and seven days after birth.

perineal massage Massaging and stretching the perineum during pregnancy so as to reduce the risk of tearing or episiotomy during labour.

perineum The area of muscle between the vagina and anus.

physiotherapist A qualified health professional who treats people by physical means, including massage, manipulation, ultrasound and heat treatment. Obstetric physiotherapists have additional qualifications for working with women having babies.

placenta The organ which grows during pregnancy to supply the baby with food and oxygen from the mother's blood and to dispose of carbon dioxide via the umbilical cord.

placental abruption An emergency condition in which the placenta separates from the wall of the uterus either before or during labour before the baby has been born. Usually necessitates an emergency caesarean if severe.

placenta praevia A placenta sited in the lower part of the uterus. If over the cervix, the woman must be delivered by caesarean. In lesser degrees she may deliver vaginally in hospital.

postpartum haemorrhage The loss of more than 500 ml of blood by a woman after birth.

poultice A bandage or compress applied to wounds.

pre-eclampsia A condition arising during pregnancy which, if left untreated, could cause fits in the mother and cut off the oxygen supply to her baby. Symptoms are increased blood pressure often accompanied by swelling of the limbs and protein in the urine. The only 'cure' is delivery of the baby, often by caesarean if the condition is severe and the cervix unfavourable.

primip (abbreviation of primigravidae) A woman having her first baby.

prognosis A medical estimate of the progress of a disease. Used to predict the ability of a woman to give birth vaginally.

prophylaxis The prevention of disease or preventative treatment.

protocol In a maternity unit, a written document specifying systems of care, such as the management of labour.

pulmonary embolism Part of a blood clot which detaches itself from a vein in the pelvis or leg and travels in the bloodstream to the lungs. A large embolus (clot which has detached itself) can cause immediate death.

randomised controlled trial A clinical trial in which subjects are randomly distributed into groups which are either subjected to the experimental procedure or not. The group that do not receive the experimental procedure or treatment are known as the 'control' group.

registrar/senior registrar (doctors) A registrar is a qualified hospital doctor specialising in one area of medicine who hopes eventually to become a consultant. Senior registrars are usually very skilled and more experienced than registrars, ready to be consultants.

respiratory distress syndrome A condition occurring mainly in premature babies and in mature babies of diabetic mothers and those born by caesarean section. Babies with this condition have difficulty breathing and have to be connected to a machine to help them breathe.

senior house officer (SHO) Qualified doctors undergoing the practical part of their training. Some will go on to be hospital doctors, others GPs after the year spent as an SHO.

sequelae A condition following as a consequence of an operation or illness.

Sonicaid A portable instrument for checking the baby's heart rate during pregnancy and labour which works by ultrasound. Easy to use, whatever the position of the mother.

special care baby unit (SCBU) Hospital department where intensive care is given to babies by specially trained doctors and nurses using sophisticated equipment and techniques. Not every hospital has one and not every SCBU is able to look after babies who are so seriously ill as to need long-term ventilation in a neonatal intensive care unit.

spinal anaesthesia A form of regional anaesthesia whereby an injection is given into the cerebrospinal fluid to numb the abdomen for a caesarean.

stages of labour First: from the beginning of labour until the cervix is 10 cm dilated. Second: the time from full dilatation to the birth of the baby. Third: the time during which the placenta is delivered.

stilette Removable centre of a needle.

supine hypertension High blood pressure when lying down.

sutures The medical word for stitches to repair a wound.

syntocinon Synthetic form of oxytocin used to make the uterus contract more strongly during induction or when spontaneous labour is thought to be progressing too slowly. Another trade name is pitocin.

syntometrine A mixture of the two drugs syntocinon and ergometrine, used routinely in most hospitals to speed up delivery of the placenta and to reduce the risk of postpartum haemorrhage.

sytstematic review A review in which evidence from scientific studies has been identified, appraised and synthesised in a methodical way according to predetermined criteria. May or may not include meta-analysis (see above).

TED (thromboembolic elastic) stockings Leg supports used to reduce risk of thrombosis.

TENS (Transcutaneous Electrical Nerve Stimulation) A low-tech form of pain relief which a woman can use on herself by means of a small, hand-held, battery-operated machine. TENS works by means of two pairs of electrodes taped to the woman's lower back, transmitting a signal which works in two ways to reduce the level of pain from contractions. The first is by interfering with the signals being transmitted to the brain; the second by promoting the production of the body's naturally occurring pain-killers, endorphins.

Term Breech Trial Refers to a study carried out by Hannah et al. (2000) comparing outcomes of breech presentation at term between planned CS and planned vaginal delivery. They found outcomes to be better in the planned vaginal delivery group.

thromboembolism Obstruction of a blood vessel with material carried by the blood stream from the site of origin to plug another vessel.

transient tachypnoea of the newborn A condition where the baby takes rapid, shallow breaths and needs admitting to a special care baby unit.

transverse lie When the baby lies across the woman's body, rather than head- or bottom-down. Sometimes associated with a shoulder or arm presentation if not recognised until labour is advanced.

trial of labour Allowing a woman to try to give birth vaginally.

trial of scar Allowing a woman to try to give birth vaginally after a previous caesarean.

ultrasound scan Sound emitted at a frequency higher than the human ear can hear which bounces off the different parts of the mother's and baby's bodies at different rates, enabling an image of the baby inside the mother's body to appear on a screen.

umbilical cord This connects the baby to the placenta and is about 50 cm long. Two umbilical arteries carry blood from the mother to the baby and one umbilical vein carries blood from the baby to the mother.

variability The way in which the fetal heart rate responds to contractions and other stimuli.

Vasa-praevia An unusual condition where one of the blood vessels from the umbilical cord crosses the membranes on its way to the placenta (normally this does not happen and the cord connects directly with the placenta).

VBAC Vaginal birth after caesarean. Vaginal birth after two or more caesareans is abbreviated to VBA2C etc.

venous thromboembolism A thromboembolism in the veins, see *thromboembolism* above.

Ventouse A method of helping a mother to deliver her baby, used by doctors. A cup is attached by a strong tube to an electric pump. The cup is put on the baby's head and a vacuum created by the pump to keep it in place. With one hand on the baby's head, the doctor pulls on the tube during a contraction to deliver the baby. If not much pulling is needed, a soft silicone cup can be used which causes less bruising to the baby's head. The mother may need a small episiotomy or none at all, depending on the position of the baby.

vitamin K A vitamin used by the liver to make the proteins needed to prevent haemorrhage. Routinely offered to most babies in the United Kingdom after birth to reduce the risks of haemorrhagic disease, a rare but often fatal disorder of the blood-clotting system.

Bibliography

ACHCEW (1992), *A Health Standards Inspectorate*, Association of Community Health Councils for England and Wales and the Association for the Victims of Medical Accidents, London

Ackerman-Leibrich, U. et al. (1996), 'Home versus hospital deliveries: follow-up study of matched pairs for procedures and outcome', *British Medical Journal*, 313: 1313-18

ACNM (American College of Nurse Midwives, 2004), 'Vaginal Birth after Previous Caesarean Section', Clinical Bulletin, 49(1): 68-74

ACOG (American College of Obstetricians and Gynaecologists, 2003), 'Surgery and Patient Choice', URL: www.acog.org/from_home/publications/ethics/ethics021.pdf, accessed 17.06.05

AIMS (1991), 'VBAC: The right to a normal birth', *AIMS Journal*, vol. 4, no. 3

Al-Mufti, R. et al. (1997), 'Survey of obstetricians' personal preference and discretionary practice', *European Journal of Obstetrics, Gynaecology and Reproductive Biology*, 73: 1-4

Al-Turki, H.A. et al. (2003), 'The outcome of pregnancy in elderly primigravidas', *Saudi Medical Journal*, 24(11): 1230-3

Allison, J. (1996), *Delivered at Home*, Chapman & Hall, London

American College of Obstetricians and Gynaecologists (1988), *Guidelines for Vaginal Delivery after a Previous Caesarean Birth*, Report by the Committee on Obstetrics, Washington DC

Amu, O. et al. (1998), 'Maternal choice alone should not determine method of delivery', *British Medical Journal*, 317: 462-465

Anderson, G. M. and J. Lomas (1984), 'Determinants of the Increasing Cesarean Birth Rate', *New England Journal of Medicine*, vol. 311, pp.887-92

Arney, W. A. (1982), in *Power and the Profession of Obstetrics*, University of Chicago Press, Chicago and London

Aslan, H. et al. (2004), 'Uterine rupture associated with misoprostol labour induction in women with previous caesarean delivery', *European Journal of Obstetrics and Gynaecology and Reproductive Biology*, 113(1): 45-8

Axten, S. (1995), 'Is active management of labour always necessary?' Modern Midwife, 5(5): 18-20

Balaskas, J. (1989), *The New Active Birth*, Cambridge University Press, Cambridge

Balen, A. H. and J. M. Smith (1992), 'The CTG in Practice', Livingstone

Baliva, R. and A. Serpierri (1886), 'Extraordinary Caesarean Section', *The Lancet*, vol. 1, pp.994-5

Barrett, J. F. R., G. J. Jarvis, H. N. MacDonald, P. C. Buchan, S. N. Tyrrell and R. J. Lilford (1990), 'Inconsistencies in Clinical Decisions in Obstetrics', *The Lancet*, vol. 330, pp.549-51

Barros, F. C. et al. (1991), 'Epidemic of caesarean section in Brazil', *The Lancet*, 338: 167-9

Baudelocque, M. (1801), *Two Memoirs on the Cesarean Operation*, trans. John Huli, Sowler and Russell, Manchester

Bell, G. (1916), 'Caesarean Section in a Pitman's Cottage', *British Medical Journal*, vol 1, pp.195-6

Bell, J. S. et al. (2001), 'Do obstetric complications explain high caesarean section rates among women over 30? A retrospective analysis', British Medical Journal, 322: 894-5

Bergholt, T. et al. (2004), 'Danish obstetricians' personal preference and general attitude to elective caesarean on maternal request: a nation-wide postal survey', *Acta Obstetrics & Gynaecology Scandinavia*, 83(3): 262-6

Berkowitz, G. S. et al, (1990), 'Delayed childbirth and the outcome of pregnancy', *New England Journal of Medicine*, 322:659-64

Beukins, P., A. Tsui, M. Kotelchuck and J. Degraft-Johnson (1991), 'An Indicator of the Content of Prenatal Care in Developing Countries', in *International Conference on Primary Care Obstetrics and Perinatal Health*, Netherlands Institute of Primary Health Care, Utrecht

Bewley, S. & Cockburn, C. (2002), 'The "unfacts" of request Caesarean Section', *British Journal of Obstetrics & Gynaecology*, 109: 597-605

BirthChoiceUK (2004), 'Historical Caesarean Rates', URL: www.birthchoiceuk.com/Professionals/ CSHistory.htm accessed 21.04.05

BirthChoiceUK (2005), 'Hospitals with Highest and Lowest Caesarean Rates', URL: www.birthchoiceuk.com/Professionals/Tables/CS_HLtables.htm accessed 21.04.05

Bloom, S.L. et al. (1998), 'Lack of effect of walking on labour and delivery', *New England Journal of Medicine*, 139: 76-9

Blumenthal, N. J., R. S. Harris, M. C. O'Connor and P. A. L. Lancaster (1984), 'Changing Caesarean Section Rates: Experience at a Sydney obstetric teaching hospital', *The Australian and New Zealand Journal of Obstetrics and Gynaecology*, vol. 24, pp.246-51

BMJ (*British Medical Journal*, News Item, 1922), 'Caesarean Section', unsigned editorial, vol. 1, pp.277-8

BMJ (*British Medical Journal*, News Item, 1936), 'Caesarean Section', unsigned editorial, vol. 2, p.1279 80

BMJ (*British Medical Journal*, News Item, 1995), 'Childbirth Trust calls for rights to home births', *British Medical Journal*, 310: 212

BMJ (*British Medical Journal*, Editorial, 1996), 'Home Birth', *British Medical Journal*, 313: 1276-77

BMJ (*British Medical Journal*, News Item, 2003), 'Commons Committee calls for more choice over home births', *British Medical Journal*, 327: 249

Bolton, T. (2005), 'Help us to save our Birthing Units', *Aims Journal*, vol. 17, no.2, p.1

Boseley, S. (2000), 'Midwife crisis over hours and workload', *Guardian*, Monday 9th October, 2000

Boyd, C. and C. Francome (1983), *One Birth in Nine*, Maternity Alliance, London

Boylan, P. C. (1989), 'Active Management of Labor: Results in Dublin, Houston, London New Brunswick, Singapore, and Valparaiso', *Birth*, vol. 16, no. 3, pp.114-18

Boylan, P. et al. (1991), 'Effect of active management of labour on the incidence of caesarean section for dystocia in nulliparas', *American Journal of Perinatology*, 8(6): 373-9

Bright Banister, J. (1935), 'Caesarean Section' *British Medical Journal*, vol. 2, pp.684-5

Brill, Y. & Windrim, R. (2004), 'Vaginal birth after caesarean section: review of antenatal predictors of success', *Journal of Obstetrics & Gynaecology*, 24(4): 275-86

Bucklin, B. A. (2003), 'Vaginal birth after caesarean delivery', *Anesthesia*, 99(6): 1444-8

Buekens, P., Curtis, S. & Alayón, S. (2003), 'Demographic and Health Surveys: caesarean section rates in sub-Saharan Africa', *British Medical Journal*, 326: 136

Bujold, E. et al. (2004), 'Trial of labour in patients with a previous caesarean section: does maternal age influence the outcome?' *American Journal of Obstetrics & Gynaecology*, 190(4): 1113-8

Burrows, L.J. et al. (2004), 'Maternal morbidity associated with vaginal versus caesarean delivery', Obstetrics & Gynaecology, 103(5,1): 907-12

Butler, N. R. & Bonham, D, G. (1963), *Perinatal Mortality*, Churchill Livingstone, Edinburgh & London

Campbell, R. & McFarlane, A. (1994), 'Where to be born: the debate and the evidence', National Perinatal Epidemiology Unit, Oxford

Canadian Conference (1986), *Final Statement of the Panel from the National Consensus Conference on Aspects of Cesarean Birth*, Planning Committee of the National Consensus Conference, Ontario

Carson, D. and C. Francome (1983), *Can We Avoid A Caesarean Crisis?* Middlesex University, London

Chalmers,I., M. Enkin and M. J. N. C. Keirse (eds.), (1989), *Effective Care in Pregnancy and Childbirth*, Oxford University Press, Oxford

Chamberlain, R. and G. Chamberlain (eds.) (1975), *British Births*, vol. 1, Heinemann Medical Books, London

Chamberlain, G. (1975), 'The First Week of Life', in Chamberlain and Chamberlain (eds.)

Chamberlain, G. and A. Peattie (1991), *Annual Report of the Department of Obstetrics and Gynaecology*, St George's Hospital, London

Chamberlain, G. et al. (1997), *Home Births: The report of the 1994 confidential enquiry by the National Birthday Trust Fund*, Parthenon Press, Carnforth

Childbirth.org (1995-1998), 'Cesarean Fact Sheet', URL: www.childbirth.org/section/CSFact.html accessed 17.03.2004

Churchill, H. (1997), *Caesarean Birth: Experience, Practice and History*, Books for Midwives Press, Manchester

Clippingdale, S. D. (1911), 'The Accouchement of Queen Jane Seymour', *Journal of Obstetrics and Gynaecology of the British Empire*, pp.109-16

Cohen, M. and B. S. Carson (1985), 'Respiratory Morbidity Benefit of Awaiting Onset of Labor after Elective Cesarean Section', *Obstetrics and Gynaecology*, vol. 65, pp.818-24

Collea, J. V., C. Chein and E. J. Quilligan (1980), 'The Randomised Management of Term Breech Presentation: A study of 208 cases', *American Journal of Obstetrics and Gynaecology*, vol. 137, pp.235-44

Coltart, T. M., J. A. Davies and M. Katesmark (1990), 'Outcome of a Second Pregnancy after a Previous Elective Caesarean Section', *British Journal of Obstetrics and Gynaecology*, vol. 97, pp.1140-3

Commentary: 'What is the correct Caesarean rate: how long is a piece of string?' *British Journal of Obstetrics and Gynaecology*, 100: 403-4

Condon, D. (2004), 'Caesarean rate jumps by 81%', URL: www.irishhealth.com/?level=4&id=6402 accessed 21.06.05

Cotgrove, S. A. and J. F. Norton (1942), 'Cesarean Section', *Journal of the American Medical Association*, vol. 118, no. 3, pp.201-4

Craigin, E. (1916), 'Conservatism in Obstetrics', *New York State Journal of Medicine*, vol. 104, pp.1-3

Cronk, M. (2005), 'Hand off that breech!' *Aims Journal*, 17, no.1: 1-3

David, S, Mamelle, N. & Riviere, O. (2001), 'Estimation of an expected caesarean section rate taking into account the case mix of a maternity hospital', *British Journal of Obstetrics and Gynaecology*, 108(9): 919-26

Davis, J. A. (1990), 'Doctors and Medical Negligence', *British Medical Journal*, vol. 300, pp.746-7

Delee, J. B. (1913), 'Principles and Practice of Obstetrics', W. B. Saunders, Philadelphia and London

Delee, J. B. (1942), 'Cesarean Section', *Journal of the American Medical Association*, vol. 118, no. 3, pp.201-9

DeMott, R. K. and H. F. Sandmire (1990), 'The Green Bay Cesarean Section Study', *American Journal of Obstetrics and Gynaecology*, vol. 162, pp.1593-602

Department of Health, DoH (1991), *Confidential Enquiries into Maternal Deaths in the United Kingdom 1985-87*, HMSO, London

Department of Health, DoH (1993), *Changing Childbirth: The Report of the Expert Maternity Group* (Cumberledge Report), HMSO, London

Department of Health, DoH (1997), Government Statistical Service, *NHS Maternity Statistics, England: 1989-90 to 1994-95,* HMSO, London

Department of Health, DoH (1998), *Why Mothers Die: Report on Confidential Enquiries into Maternal Deaths in the United Kingdom 1994-1996,* RCOG Press, London

Department of Health, DoH (2001), *Why Mothers Die 1997-1999 Executive Summary and Key Recommendations: The Confidential Enquiries into Maternal Deaths in the United Kingdom*, RCOG Press, London

Department of Health, DoH (2002), 'Infant Feeding Survey 2000: a summary report', URL: www.doh.gov.uk/assetRoot/04/08/13/98/04081398.pdf, accessed 07.04.05

Department of Health, DoH (2003a), 'Different models of maternity care: an evaluation of the roles of primary health care workers', URL: www.dh.gov.uk/PolicyAndGuidance/ResearchAndDevelopment/ResearchAnd..., accessed 12.05.05

Department of Health, DoH (2003b), 'Infant Feeding Initiative: A report Evaluating the Breastfeeding Practice Projects 1999-2002', URL: www.doh.gov/infantfeeding, accessed 25.04.05

Department of Health, DoH (2003c), 'Making Amends – A Consultation Paper Setting Out Proposals for Reforming the Approach to Clinical Negligence in the NHS, June 2003'

Department of Health, DoH (2004a), *Why mothers die 2000-2002: Report on confidential enquiries into maternal mortality in the United Kingdom*, RCOG Press, London

Department of Health (DoH), Department for Education and Skill (2004b), 'National Service Framework for Children, Young People and Maternity Services: Maternity Services, 14th September 2004'

DeRegt, R. H., H. L. Minkoff, J. Feldman and R. H. Schwarz (1986), 'Relation of Private or Clinic Care to the Cesarean Birth Rate', *New England Journal of Medicine*, vol. 315, pp.619-24

De Zuluetal, P. et al. (1999), 'Patients do not have right to impose their wishes at all costs', letters, *British Medical Journal*, 318(7176): 120

Devries et al. (2001), *Birth by Design: Pregnancy, Maternity Care, and Midwifery in North America and Europe*, Routledge, London

DHHS Department of Health and Human Services (1991), *Healthy People 2000*, DHSS Publications No. (PHS) 91-50212, Washington DC

Dickson, M.J. & Willett, M. (1999), 'Midwives would prefer a vaginal delivery', *British Medical Journal*, 319: 1008

Dillon, W. P. et al. (1992), 'Obstetric care and caesarean birth rates: A program to monitor quality of care', *Obstetrics and Gynaecology*, 80(5): 731-7

Donald, l. (1955), *Practical Obstetric Problems*, Lloyd Luke, London

Donati, S et al. (2003), 'Do Italian mothers prefer caesarean delivery?' *Birth*, 30(2): 89-93

Durand, A. M. (1992), 'The Safety of Home Birth: The Farm study', *Journal of the American Public Health Association*, vol. 82, pp.450-2

Dyer, C. (2005), 'Court rules in favour of GMC's guidance on withholding treatment', *British Medical Journal*, 331: 309

Eden, T. W. and E. Holland (1931), *Manual of Midwifery*, 7th edn., Churchill, London

EGAMS Expert Group on Acute Maternity Services (2002), Reference Report, Annex C: International Models of Maternity Care, URL: www.show.scot.nhs.uk/sehd/publications/egas/egas-25.htm, accessed 11.04.05

Eggleston, E. (1995), 'Family Planning in Brazil: Examining the role of Government', URL: www.ucis.unc.edu/resources/pubs/carolina/Family/Family2.html, accessed 21.06.05

Eisenberg, H. (1986), 'A Doctor on Trial', *New York Times*, magazine section, 20 July, pp.25-42

Engelkes, E. & van Roosmalen, J. (1992), 'The value of symphyseotomy compared with caesarean section in cases of obstructed labour', *Social Science and Medicine*, 35(6): 789-93

England, P. & Horowitz, R. (2003), 'Expectant parents face increased risks as American Obstetrics drifts towards caesarean on demand', URL: www.birthingfromwithin.com/cesarean.html accessed 17.06.05

Enkin, M. W. (1991), 'Primary Care Obstetrics and Perinatal Health: Canada', International Conference on Primary Care Obstetrics and Perinatal Health, Netherlands Institute of Primary Health Care, Utrecht

Enkin, M. et al. (2000), 'Effective care in Pregnancy and Childbirth', third edition, Oxford University Press, Oxford

Ever-Hadani P. et al. (1994), 'Breast feeding in Israel: Maternal factors associated with choice and duration', *Journal of Epidemiology and Community Health*; 48(3): 281-5

Fabri, R. H. & Murta, E.F.C. (2002), 'Socioeconomic factors and caesarean section rates', *International Journal of Gynaecology and Obstetrics*, 76(1): 87-8

Ferguson, l. L. C. (1985), 'Malpresentations and Malpositions', in J. W. Crawford (ed.), *Risks of Labour*, vol. 2, Wiley, Chichester

Ferriman, A. (1988), 'Op a Good Thing', *The Observer*, 31 July, p.36

FIGO International Federation of Gynaecology and Obstetrics (1999), 'Ethics Committee Report on Ethical aspects regarding caesarean delivery for non medical reasons', *International Journal of Obstetrics and Gynaecology*, 64: 317-22

FIGO International Federation of Gynaecology and Obstetrics (2003), 'Recommendations of Ethical Issues in Obstetrics and Gynaecology by the FIGO Committee for the Ethical Aspects of Human Reproduction and Women's Health', FIGO, London

Finney, Rev. P. A. (1935), *Moral Problems in Hospital Practice*, 5th edn., B. Herder Book Company, London

Fisk, N. & Paterson Brown, S. (2004), 'The safest method of birth is by caesarean', *The Observer*, Sunday 2nd May, 2004

Flamm, B. L. (1985), 'Vaginal Birth after Cesarean Section: Controversies old and new', *Clinics in Obstetrics and Gynaecology*, vol. 28, pp.735-44

Flamm, B. (1992), 'Should Electronic Fetal Monitoring Always be Used for Women in Labor who are Having a Vaginal Birth after a Previous Caesarean?' *Birth*, vol. 19, no. 1, pp.31-2

Flamm, B. L. et al. (1994), 'Elective repeat caesarean delivery versus trial of labour: a prospective multicenter study', *Obstetrics and Gynaecology*, 83(6): 927-32

Flint, C., Poulengeris & Grant, A. (1989), 'The "Know your Midwife Scheme"', *Midwifery*, 5: 11-16

Francome, C. (1984), *Abortion Freedom*, Unwin Hyman, London and Boston

Francome, C. (1990a), *Sane New World*, Carla Publications, London

Francome, C. (1990b), *Changing Childbirth*, Maternity Alliance, London

Francome, C. and P. J. Huntingford, 'Births by Caesarean Section in the United States of America and Britain', *Journal of Biosocial Science*, vol. 12, pp.353-62

Francome, C. et al. (1993), *Caesarean Birth in Britain: A Book for Health Professionals and Parents*, Middlesex University Press, London

Francome, C. & Savage, W. (1993), 'Caesarean Section in Britain and the United States 12% or 24%: Is either too high?' *Social Science and Medicine*, 37(10): 1199-1218

Francome, C. (1994), *Caesarean Birth in Britain (1994 Supplement)*, Middlesex University Press, London

Frigoletto, F. D., K. J. Ryan and M. Phillippe (1980), 'Maternal Mortality Rate Associated with Cesarean Section: An appraisal', *American Journal of Obstetrics and Gynaecology*, vol. 136, pp.969-70

Gaskin, I.M. (2003), 'Vaginal birth after caesarean (VBAC)', in Ina May's *Guide to Childbirth*, Bantam, New York, 294-304

Gamble, J. A. & Creedy, D. K. (2000), 'Women's request for caesarean section: a critique of the literature', *Birth*, 27(4): 256-63

Ghada, H. (1998), 'Maternal Mortality: a neglected and socially unjustifiable tragedy. Why WHO selected "Safe Motherhood" as the slogan for World Health Day 1998', *Eastern Mediterranean Health Journal*, URL: www.emro.who.int/Publications/EMHJ/0401/03.htm, accessed 21.06.05

Giesen, D. (1993), 'Legal Accountability for the Provision of Health Care: A comparative view', unpublished paper presented at the Royal Society of Medicine Forum on Quality in Health Care, 10 February

Glazerman, H. (2006), 'Five years to the term breech trial: The rise and fall of a randomized controlled trial', *American Journal of Obstetrics and Gynecology*, 194:20-5

Gleicher, N. (1984), 'Cesarean Section Rates in the United States', *Journal of the American Medical Association*, vol. 252, pp.3273-6

GMC General Medical Council (1995), *Good Medical Practice*, GMC, London

Gould, J. B., M. P. H. Becky Davey and R. S. Stafford (1989), 'Socioeconomic Differences in Rates of Cesarean Section', *New England Journal of Medicine*, vol. 321, pp.233-9

Goyert, G. L., S. F. Bottoms, M. C. Treadwell and P. C. Nehra (1989), 'The Physician Factor in Cesarean Birth Rates', *New England Journal of Medicine*, vol. 320, pp.706-9

Green, J. M., V. A. Coupland and J. V. Kitzinger (1988), *Great Expectations: A Prospective Study of Women's Expectations and Experiences of Childbirth*, unpublished report for the Health Promotion Research Trust and the Nuffield Provincial Hospital Trust

Griffin, J. (1993), *Born Too Soon*, Office of Health Economics, London

Grinstead, J. & Grobman, W.A. (2004), 'Induction of labor after one prior cesarean: predictors of vaginal delivery', Obstetrics & Gynaecology, 103(3): 534-8

Guihard, P. & Blondel, B. (2001), 'Trends in risk factors for caesarean sections in France between 1981 and 1995: lessons for reducing the rates in the future', *British Journal of Obstetrics and Gynaecology*, 108(1): 48-55

Guillimeau, J. (1612), *Childbirth*, A. Hatfield, London

Hall, M. (1999), 'Maternal mortality and mode of delivery', *The Lancet*, 354: 776

Hall, M. (2001), in Department of Health *Why Mothers Die: The Confidential Enquiries into Maternal Deaths in the United Kingdom*, RCOG Press, London

Hamilton, Alexander (1803), *Outlines of the Theory and Practice of Midwifery*, 5th edn., T. Kay, Edinburgh

Hannah, M.E. et al. (2000), 'Planned caesarean section versus planned vaginal delivery for breech presentation at term: a randomised multicentre trial', *The Lancet*, 356(9239): 1375-83

Hannah, M.E. (2004), 'Planned elective caesarean section: a reasonable choice for women?' *Canadian Medical Association Journal*, 170(5): 813-4

Hansell, R. S., K. B. McMurray and G. R. Huey (1990), 'Vaginal Birth after Two or More Cesarean Sections: A five year experience', *Birth*, vol. 17, no. 3, pp.146 50

Harris, R. P. (1880a), 'The Porro Modification of the Cesarean Operation in Continental Europe', *American Journal of Medical Science*, vol. 79, pp.335-62

Harris, R. P. (1880b), 'The Results of the First 50 Cases of Cesarean Ovaro-hysterectomy 1869-80', *American Journal of Medical Science*, vol. 80, pp.129-34

Hausknecht, R. and J. R. Heilman (1978), *Having a Cesarean Baby*, Dutton, New York

Health Committee (1992), *Maternity Services*, House of Commons, Second Report, HMSO, London

Hemminki, E., B. I. Graubard, H. J. Hoffmann, W. D. Mosher and K. Fetterly (1985), 'Cesarean and Subsequent Fertility: Results from the 1982 National Survey of Family Growth', *American Fertility Society* vol. 43, no. 4, pp.520-8

HFA (Health Funding Authority, 1999a), 'Consumer Perceptions on the 1999 National Survey'

HFA (Health Funding Authority, 1999b), 'New Zealand Mothers and Babies'

Hildingsson, I. et al. (2002) 'Few women wish to be delivered by caesarean section', *British Journal of Obstetrics & Gynaecology*, 109(6): 618-23

Hillan, E.M. (1992a), 'Maternal-Infant Attachment Following Caesarean Delivery', *Journal of Clinical Nursing*, vol. 1, no. 1 pp.33-7

Hillan, E.M. (1992b), 'Short Term Morbidity Associated with Cesarean Delivery', *Birth*, vol. 19, pp.190-4

Hillan, E.M. (1992c), 'Research and Audit, women's views of caesarean section', in Roberts, H. (ed.) *Women's Health Matters*, Routledge, London

Hillan, E.M. (1995), 'Postoperative morbidity following caesarean delivery', *Journal of Advanced Nursing*, 22(6): 1035-42

Hindawi, I.M. & Meri, Z.B. (2004), 'The Jordanian caesarean section rate', *Saudi Medical Journal*, 25(11): 1631-5

HoC House of Commons (1992), *House of Commons Select Committee Report, Health Committee Maternity Services* (Winterton Report), 'Conclusions and Recommendations', vols. 1-3, HMSO, London

HoC House of Commons (2003a), 'Select Committee on Health Fourth Report', URL: www.parliament.the-stationery-office.co.uk/pa/cm200203/cmselect/cmhealth/4... Accessed 20.04.05 (Parliamentary copyright material is reproduced with the permission of the Controller of Her Majesty's Stationery Office on behalf of Parliament)

HoC House of Commons (2003b), 'Select Committee on Health Ninth Report', URL: www.parliament.the-stationery-office.co.uk/pa/cm200203/cmselect/cmhealth/7... Accessed 19.05.05 (Parliamentary copyright material is reproduced with the permission of the Controller of Her Majesty's Stationery Office on behalf of Parliament)

Hodnett, E. D. et al. (2003), 'Continuous support for women during childbirth', *Cochrane Database System Review*

Hofmeyer, G. J. (1991), 'External Cephalic Version at Term: How high are the stakes?' *British Journal of Obstetrics and Gynaecology*, vol. 98, pp.1-3

Hofmeyer, G. J. and M. J. N. C. Keirse (1990), 'Two Ways to Reduce Caesarean Section Rates', Oxford Database of Perinatal Trials, *Newsletter*, 1-4 August

Hofmeyer, G. J. (2001), 'External version facilitation for breech presentation term', *Cochrane Database System Review*

Holland, E. (1920), 'Rupture of Caesarean Section Scar', *British Medical Journal*, vol. 1, pp.705-7

Homebirth.org (2001), 'The VBAC Pages, Vaginal Birth after Caesarean?' URL: www.homebirth.org/vbac.htm, accessed 21.04.05

Hopkins, K. (2000), 'Are Brazilian women really choosing to deliver by caesarean?' *Social Science and Medicine*, 51(5): 725-40

How, K. et al. (1995), 'Nulliparous caesarean section in the home of active management of labour', *Australian and New Zealand Journal of Obstetrics and Gynaecology*, 35(1): 12-15

Hull, John (1798), *A Defence of the Caesarean Operation*, R. & W. Dean, Manchester

Inch, S. (1989), *Birthrights*, Greenprint, London

Independent Midwives Report (2004), 'MIA statistics 31.3.2003 to 31.1.2004', URL: www.independentmidwives.org.uk accessed 22.08.05

Janowich, B., M. S. Nakamwa, L. F. Entellita, M. L. Brown and D. Clapton (1982), 'Caesarean Section in Brazil', *Social Science and Medicine*, vol. 16, pp.19-25

Janowitz, B. et al. (1985), 'Sterilization in the northeast of Brazil', *Social Science and Medicine*, 20(3): 215-221

Joffe, J. et al. (1994), 'What is the optimal caesarean section rate? An outcome based study of existing variation', *Journal of Epidemiology and Community Health*, 48: 406-11

Johnson, K.C. & Davis, B.A. (2005), 'Outcome of planned home births with certified professional midwives: large prospective study in North America', *British Medical Journal*, 330: 1416-30

Johnson, N. & Ansell, D. (1995), 'Variation in Caesarean and instrumental delivery rates in NZ hospitals', *Australian and New Zealand Journal of Obstetrics and Gynaecology*, 35: 6-11

Johnstone, R. W. (1952), *Midwifery*, 15th edn., Adam and Charles Black, London

Kambo, I. et al. (2002), 'A critical appraisal of caesarean section rates at teaching hospitals in India', *International Journal of Gynaecology and Obstetrics*, 79(2): 151-8

Kaufman, K. (1990), 'Commentary: Midwifery in Ontario', *Birth*, vol. 17, no. 3, p.144

Kennell, J., M. Klaus, S. McGrath, S. S. Robertson and C. Hinckley (1991), 'Continuous Emotional Support during Labor in a US Hospital', *Journal of the American Medical Association*, vol. 17, pp.2197-201

Kerr, J. M. M. (1937), *Operative Obstetrics*, 4th edn., Baillicre Tindall and Cox, London

Kerr, J. M. M., J. H. Ferguson, J. Young and J. Hendry (1933), *A Combined Textbook of Obstetrics and Gynaecology*, 2nd edn., Livingstone, Edinburgh

Khawaja, M, Jurdi, R. & Kabakian-Khasholian, T. (2004), 'Rising trends in caesarean section rates in Egypt', *Birth*, 31(1): 12-16

Kiwanuka, A. I. & Moore, W. M. (1987), 'The changing incidence of caesarean section in the health district of Central Manchester', *British Journal of Obstetrics and Gynaecology*, 94: 440-4

Koc, I. (2003), 'Increased caesarean section rates in Turkey', *European Journal of Contraception and Reproductive Health Care*, 8(1): 1-10

Kotaska, A. (2004), 'Inappropriate use of randomised controlled trials to evaluate complex phenomena: case study of vaginal breech delivery', *British Medical Journal*, 329: 1039-44

Krishnamurthy, S., F. Fairlie, A. D. Cameron, J. J. Walker and J. R. MacKenzie (1991), 'The Role of Postnatal X-ray Pelvimetry after Caesarean Section in the Management of Subsequent Delivery', *British Journal of Obstetrics and Gynaecology*, vol. 98, pp.716-18

Kwee, A. et al. (2004), 'Caesarean section on request: a survey in The Netherlands', *European Journal of Obstetrics and Gynaecology and Reproductive Biology*, 113(2): 186-90

Lao, T. T., B. F. H. Leung and S. S. Young (1987), 'Trial of Scar: Is it safe in developing countries?' *British Journal of Clinical Practice*, vol. 41, no. 2, pp.596-600

Lavender, T. et al. (2005), 'Could a randomised trial answer the controversy relating to elective caesarean section? National survey of consultant obstetricians and heads of midwifery', *British Medical Journal*, 331: 490-1

Lavin, J., R. Stephens, M. Miodovnik and T. Barden (1982), 'Vaginal Delivery in Patients with a Prior Caesarean Section', *Obstetrics and Gynaecology*, vol. 59, p.135

Lawrie, T. A., de Jager, M. & Hofmeyer, G. J. (2001), 'High caesarean section rates for pregnant medical practitioners in South Africa', *International Journal of Gynaecology and Obstetrics*, 72(1): 71-73

Leap, N. (1996) 'Woman-led Midwifery: The Development of a New Midwifery Philosophy in Britain', in Murray, S. (ed.) *Baby Friendly, Mother Friendly*, Mosby, London

Lee, S. et al. (2004), 'Women's attitudes toward mode of delivery in South Korea – a society with high caesarean section rates', *Birth*, 31(2): 108-16

Levene, M.I. (1986), 'Grand Multiple Pregnancies and Demand for Neonatal Intensive Care', *The Lancet*, vol. 2, pp.347-8

Lewis, G. (2004), 'Chapter 1: Introduction and Key Findings 2000-2002', in DoH (2004) *Why mothers die 2000-2002. Report on confidential enquiries into maternal mortality in the United Kingdom*, RCOG Press, London, URL: www.cmach.org.uk/publication s/WMD2000_2002/wmd-01.htm, accessed 20.07.05

Lewison, H. (1991), *Your Choices for Pregnancy and Childbirth*, Ebury Press, London

Lilford, R. J., H. A. Van Coeverden De Groot and P. J. Moore (1990), 'The Relative Risks of Caesarean Section and Vaginal Delivery', *British Journal of Obstetrics and Gynaecology*, vol. 97, pp.882-92

Lin, H.C. & Xirasagar, S. (2004), 'Institutional factors in caesarean delivery rates: policy and research implications', *Obstetrics & Gynaecology*, 103(1): 128-36

Liu, S. et al. (2004), 'Recent trends in caesarean delivery rates and indications for caesarean delivery in Canada', *Journal of Obstetrics and Gynaecology of Canada*, 26(8): 735-42

Lomas, J. (1988), 'Holding Back the Tide of Caesareans', *British Medical Journal*, vol. 297, pp.569-70

Lomas, J. (1991), 'Words Without Actions? The production, dissemination and impact of consensus recommendations', *Annual Review of Public Health*, vol. 12, pp.41-65

Lomas, J. and M. Enkin (1989), 'Variations in Operative Delivery Rates', in Chalmers, Enkin and Keirse, pp.1182-95

Lopez, I. (1998), 'One-Way Street', URL:www.brazillog.com/pages/cvrnov98.htm accessed 21.06.05

Ludka, M.M. & Roberts, C.C. (1993), 'Eating and Drinking in Labour – A literature review', *Journal of Nurse Midwifery*, 38: 199-207

Mabie, W. C., J. R. Barton and N. Wasserstrumn (1992), 'Clinical Observations on Asthma in Pregnancy', *Journal of Maternal and Fetal Medicine*, vol. 1, no. 1, pp.45-50

Macara, L.M. & Murphy, K.W. (1994), 'The contribution of dystocia to the caesarean section rate', *American Journal of Obstetrics and Gynaecology*, 171(1): 71-7

MacDonald, D. (1992), 'Should Electronic Fetal Monitoring Always be Used for Women in Labor who are Having a Vaginal Birth after a Previous Caesarean?', *Birth*, vol. 19, no. 1, p.31-2

MacDonald, D., A. Grant, M. Sheridan-Pereira, P. Boylan and I. Chalmers (1985), 'The Dublin random controlled trial of intrapartum fetal heart rate monitoring', *American Journal of Obstetrics and Gynaecology*, vol. 152, pp.524-39

Macfarlane, A. et al. (2002), *Birth Counts: Statistics of pregnancy and childbirth*, vol. 2: Tables, HMSO, London

MacLennan, A.H. et al. (2000), 'The prevalence of pelvic floor disorders and their relationship to gender, age, parity and mode of delivery', *British Journal of Obstetrics & Gynaecology*, 107: 1460-70

Macnair, P. (1992), 'Cutting both ways, the reasons behind the rising number of births by Caesarean Section', *The Guardian*, February, p.18

Maher, C. F. et al. (1994), 'Caesarean section rate reduced', *New Zealand Journal of Obstetrics & Gynaecology*, 34(4): 389-92

Mahoney, E. (2005), 'Stand and Deliver and other brilliant ways to give birth', Thorsons, London

Marchiano, D. et al. (2004), 'Diet controlled gestational diabetes mellitus does not influence the success rates for vaginal delivery after caesarean delivery', *American Journal of Obstetrics & Gynaecology*, 190(3): 790-6

Martel, M. et al. (1987), 'Maternal Age and primary caesarean section rates: a multivariate analysis', *American Journal of Obstetrics & Gynaecology*, 156: 305-8

Maternity Services (1992), *Government Response to the Second Report from the Health Select Committee*, Cmmd. 2018, HMSO, London

Mathur, G.P. et al. (1993), 'Breastfeeding in babies delivered by cesarean section', *Indian Pediatrics*, 30(11): 1285-90

McGarry, J.A. (1969), 'The management of patients previously delivered by caesarean section', *Journal of Obstetrics and Gynaecology of the British Commonwealth*; 76: 137-43

McIlroy, Dame Louise (1932), 'Indications For and Against Caesarean Section', *British Medical Journal*, vol. 2, pp.796-7

McIlwaine, G. M., S. K. Cole and M. C. Macnaughton (1985), 'The Rising Caesarean Section Rate: A matter of concern', *Health Bulletin*, vol. 43, pp.301-4

McIlwaine, G. et al. (1998), *Caesarean Section in Scotland 1994/5: National Audit. Scottish programme for Clinical effectiveness in Reproductive Health*, University of Edinburgh

McIntosh-Marshall, C. (1949), 'Modern Caesarean Section', *British Medical Journal*, vol. 2, p.147

McMahon, M. et al. (1997), 'Comparison of a Trial of Labour with an Elective Second Cesarean Section', *New England Journal of Medicine*, 335: 689-695

MacVicar, J. et al. (1993), 'Simulated home delivery in hospital: a randomised controlled trial', *British Journal of Obstetrics & Gynaecology*, 100: 316-23

Mead, M.M. & Kornbrot, D. (2004), 'The influence of maternity unit's intrapartum intervention rates and midwives' risk perception of women suitable for midwifery led care', *Midwifery*, 20: 61-71

Menacker, F. & Curtin, S.C. (2001), 'Trends in caesarean birth and vaginal birth after previous caesarean, 1991-99', *National Vital Statistics Report*, 49(13):1-16

Menghetti E. et al. (1994), *The nutrition of the nursing mother in light of a study of 200 new mothers*, Minerva Pediatrica

Minkoff, H. et al. (2004), 'Ethical dimensions of elective primary caesarean delivery', *Obstetrics & Gynaecology*, 103(2): 387-92

MoH Ministry of Health (1999), *Obstetric Procedures 1988/89 to 1997/8*, Ministry of Health, Wellington, NZ

MoH Ministry of Health (2003), 'Maternity report 2000 and 2001: Caesarean sections increasing perinatal deaths falling', URL: www.moh.gov.nz/moh.nsf accessed 14.07.05

Molina-Sosa, A. et al. (2004), 'Self-inflicted caesarean section with maternal and fetal survival', *International Journal of Gynaecology & Obstetrics*, March: 287-90

Mollison, J. et al. (2005), 'Primary mode of delivery and subsequent pregnancy', *British Journal of Obstetrics and Gynaecology*, 112(8): 1061-1065

Molloy, B. G., O. Sheil and N. M. Duignan (1987), 'Delivery after Caesarean Section: Review of 2,176 consecutive cases', *British Medical Journal*, vol. 294, pp.1645-7

Morbidity Mortality Weekly Report (MMWR), 'Vaginal birth after caesarean birth – California, 1996-2000', *MMWR* 51(44): 996-8

Murray, C.J.L. &, Lopez, A. (1997), 'Mortality by cause for eight regions of the world – Global Burden of Disease Study', *The Lancet*, 349: 1269-76

Murray, S. F. & Pradenas, F. S. (1997), 'Cesarean birth trends in Chile, 1986 to 1994', *Birth*, 24(4): 258-63

Murray, S.F. (2001), 'A cut above the rest? Private healthcare and caesarean sections in Chile', ID21 health, communicating development research, URL: www.id21.org/health/h8sm3gl.html, accessed 03.12.03

Murray-Arthur, F. and J. F. Correy (1984), 'A Review of Primary Caesarean Sections in Tasmania', *The Australian and New Zealand Journal of Obstetrics and Gynaecology*, vol. 24, p.242

Myers, S.A. & Gleicher, N. (1990), '1998 US caesarean section rate: Good news or bad?' *The New England Journal of Medicine*, 323(3): 200

NAC National Audit Commission (1997), *First Class Delivery*, Audit Commission Publications, Abingdon

National Childbirth Trust (NCT, 1992), *Maternity Services Survey*, London

National Consensus Conference on Aspects of Cesarean Birth (1986), *Final Statement of Panel*, presented by Planning Committee and Dr W. Hannah, Panel Chairman

Nationmaster.com (2000), *Births by caesarean section*, URL: www.nationmaster.com/graph-T/hea_bir_by_cae_sec, accessed 01.07.05

Newburn, M. (1993), 'NCT 1992 Maternity Services Survey', *New Generation*, vol. 12, no. 2

Newell, F. S. (1921), *Cesarean Section*, D. Appleton, New York and London

New Zealand Information Service (2004), *Report on maternity*, Maternity and Newborn Information 2002

NHS Management Executive (1993), *A Study of Midwife and GP Led Maternity Units*, London

NICE National Institute for Clinical Excellence (2004), *Caesarean Section, National Collaborating Centre for Women's and Children's Health, Clinical Guideline*, RCOG Press, London

Nielsen, T. F. & Hökegárd, K-H. (1989), 'Cesarean section and intraoperative surgical complications', *Acta Obstetrics and Gynaecology Scandanavia*, 63: 103-8

Nielsen, T. F., Olausson, P. O. & Ingemarsson, I. (1994), 'The caesarean section rate in Sweden: the end of the rise', *Birth*, 21(1): 34-8

NIH, National Institutes of Health (1982), *Cesarean Childbirth*, US Department of Health and Human Services, Public Health Service, Publication No. 82-2067, US Government Printing Office, Washington DC

NMC Nursing & Midwifery Council (2005), www.nmc-uk.org, accessed 30.09.05

NRPMSCG Northern Region Perinatal Mortality Survey Collaborating Group (1996), 'Collaborative survey of perinatal loss in planned and unplanned home births', *British Medical Journal*, 313: 1306-09

Nuttall, C. (2000), 'The caesarean culture of Brazil', letters, *British Medical Journal*, 320: 1072

O'Cathain, A. et al. (2002), 'Use of evidence based leaflets to promote informed choice in maternity care: randomised controlled trial in everyday practice', *British Medical Journal*, 324: 643

O'Driscoll, K. et al. (1970), 'Active management of labour and cephalopelvic disproportion', *Journal of Obstetrics & Gynaecology of the British Commonwealth*, 77: 385-9

O'Driscoll, K. and M. Foley (1983), 'Correlation of Decrease in Perinatal Mortality and Increase in Cesarean Section Rates', *Journal of the American College of Obstetrics and Gynaecology,* vol. 61, no. 1, pp.1-5

O'Driscoll, K. et al. (1984), 'Active management of labour as an alternative to caesarean section for dystocia', *Obstetrics & Genecology*, 63(3): 485-90

O'Sullivan, G. (1994), 'The stomach - fact and fantasy. Eating and drinking during labour', *International Anaesthesiology Clinics*, 32: 31-44

Oakley, A. and M. Richards (1990), 'Women's Experiences of Caesarean Delivery', in *The Politics of Maternity Care*, ed. J. Garcia, R. Kilpatrick and M. Richards, Oxford University Press, Oxford

Odibo, A.O. & Macones, G.A. (2003), 'Current concepts regarding vaginal birth after caesarean, delivery', *Current Opinion in Obstetrics and Gynaecology*, 15(6): 479-82

Office of Population Censuses and Surveys (1990), *Mortality Statistics - Perinatal and Infant: Social and Biological Factors in England and Wales*, HMSO, London

Office of Population Censuses and Surveys (1992), 1990 *'Infant Feeding'*, HMSO, London

Okonofua, F. (2001), 'Optimising caesarean section rates in West Africa', *The Lancet*, 358(9290): 1289

Olofsson, P. and H. Rhydstrom (1985), 'Twin Delivery: How should the second twin be delivered?' *American Journal of Obstetrics and Gynaecology*, vol. 153, pp.479-81

Omu, A. E. (1991), 'Reducing Perinatal Mortality in Nigeria through Primary Obstetric Care', International Conference on Primary Care Obstetrics and Perinatal Health, Netherlands Institute of Primary Care, Utrecht, p.70

ONS Office for National Statistics (2000), *Child Health Statistics*, 2nd edition, The Stationery Office, London

Page, L. et al. (1999), 'Clinical interventions and outcomes of One-to-One midwifery practice', *Journal of Public Health Medicine*, 21: 243-8

Pandit, V. & Plaat, F. (2004), 'Regional anaesthesia for caesarean section', *Anaesthesia and intensive care medicine*, 5(8): 269-270

Parer, J. T. & Livingstone, E. G. (1990), 'What is fetal distress?' *American Journal of Obstetrics & Gynaecology*, 162: 1421-7

Paterson-Brown, S. et al. (1998), 'Should doctors perform an elective caesarean section on request?' *British Medical Journal*, 317: 462-465

Paterson, C.M. & Saunders, N.J. St. G. (1991), 'Mode of delivery after on caesarean section: audit of current practice in a health region', *British Medical Journal*, 303: 818-20

PatientPlus (2004), 'Multiple Pregnancy', URL: www.patient.co.uk/showdoc/40000230/ accessed 16.06.05

Pattinson, R. E. (2001), 'Pelvimetry for fetal cephalic presentation at term', *Cochrane Database System Review* 13

Paul, R.H., Phelan, J.P. & Yeh, S. (1985), 'Trial of labor in the patient with prior cesarean birth', *American Journal of Obstetrics and Gynaecology*, 151: 297-304

Penna, L. & Arulkumaran, S. (2003), 'Cesarean Section for non-medical reasons', *International Journal of Obstetrics*, 82(3): 399-409

Perez, P. G. (1989), 'The Patient Observer: What really led to these cesarean births?' *Birth*, vol. 16, no. 3, pp.130-9

Phaff, J. M. L. (1986), 'The Organisation and Administration of Perinatal Services in the Netherlands', in *Perinatal Health Services in Europe*, Croom Helm, London and Sydney, pp.117-27

Phelan, J. P., M. O. Ahn and F. Diaz (1989), 'Twice a Caesarean Always a Caesarean', *Obstetrics and Gynaecology*, vol. 73, pp.161-5

Philipp, E. (1988), *Caesareans*, Sidgwick & Jackson, London

Placek, P.J. & Taffel, S.M. (1988), 'Vaginal birth after caesarean in the 1980s', *American Journal of Public Health*, 78: 512-5

Placek, P. J., S. M. Taffel and M. Moien (1988), '1986 C-sections Rise: VBACs inch upward', *American Journal of Public Health*, vol. 78, no. 5, pp.562-3

Playfair, W. S. (1886), *The Science and Practice of Midwifery*, 6th edn., Smith, Elder, London

Porreco, R. P. (1990), 'The Twice Wounded Uterus', *Birth*, vol. 17, no. 3, pp.150-1

POST Parliamentary Office of Science and Technology (2002), Postnote, Caesarean Sections, no.184

PP&BS Physician Payment & Benchmarking Strategies (2000), Ingenix Publishing Group, URL: www.obgynnetworks.com/pdf_files/Article5.pdf, accessed 23.06.05

Pradhan, P., Mohajer, M. & Deshpande, S. (2005), 'Outcome of term breech births: 10 year experience at a District General Hospital', *British Journal of Obstetrics & Gynaecology*, 112: 218-22

Quinn, M. (1993), 'Fax Transmission from the Labour Ward', *Hospital Update Plus*, April, pp.64-6

Radford, Thomas (1865), *Observations on the Caesarean Section and on Other Obstetric Operations*, T. Richards, London

RCOG Royal College of Obstetricians and Gynaecologists (2001a), Pelvimetry Guideline no. 14, RCOG, London

RCOG Royal College of Obstetricians and Gynaecologists (2001b), 'Management of Breech presentation', Guideline no. 20, RCOG, London

RCOG Royal College of Obstetricians and Gynaecologists (2001c), 'Planning for the future as consultants in obstetrics and gynaecology', A discussion document, RCOG, London

RCOG Royal College of Obstetricians and Gynaecologists (2001d), 'The use of electronic fetal monitoring',
URL: www.rcog.org.uk/resources/public/pdf/efm_guideline_final_2may2001.pdf, accessed 21.07.05

Read, A. W., W. J. Waddell, W. J. Prendiville and F. J. Stanley (1991), *Caesarean Section and Operative Vaginal Delivery in Western Australia 1981-7,* International Conference on Primary Care Obstetrics and Perinatal Health, Netherlands Institute of Primary Care, Utrecht, p.45

Redman, C. and I. Walker (1992), *Pre-eclampsia: The facts - the hidden threat to pregnancy*, Oxford University Press, Oxford

Reitberg, C.C.Th, Elferink-Stinkens, P.M. & Visser, G.H.A. (2005), 'The effect of the Term Breech Trial on medical intervention behaviour and neonatal outcome in the Netherlands: an analysis of 35,453 breech infants', *British Journal of Obstetrics & Gynaecology*, 112: 205-9

Renwick, M. Y. (1991), *The Australian and New Zealand Journal of Obstetrics and Gynaecology*, vol. 31, no. 4, pp.299-304

RHA Regional Health Authority (1997), Maternity Project, *Guidelines for referral to Obstetric and Related Specialist Medical Services*

Rhydstom, H., Ingmarrson, I. & Ohrlander, S. (1990), 'Lack of correlation between a high caesarean rate and improved prognosis for low-birthweight twins (2500g)', *British Journal of Obstetrics and Gynaecology*, 97: 229-36

Roberts, R.J. (1991), 'Elective section after two sections – where's the evidence?' *British Journal of Obstetrics and Gynaecology*, 101: 367-8

Robson, J., Boomla, K. & Savage, W. (1986), 'Reducing delay in booking for antenatal care', *Journal of the Royal College of General Practitioners*, 36: 274-5

Robson et al, (1996), 'Using the medical audit cycle to reduce caesarean section rates', *American Journal of Obstetrics & Gynaecology*, 174: 199-205

Rockenschaub, A. (1990), 'Technology-free obstetrics at the Semmelweis Clinic', *The Lancet*, 335: 977

Rosenthal, A.N. & Paterson-Brown, S. (1998), 'Is there an incremental rise in the risk of obstetric intervention with increasing maternal age?' *British Journal of Obstetrics and Gynaecology*, 105: 1064-9

Rooks, J. P., N. L. Weatherby, E. K. M. Ernst, S. Stapleton, D. Rosen and A. Rosenfield (1989), 'Outcomes of Care in Birth Centres', *New England Journal of Medicine*, vol. 321, pp.1804-11

Rooks, J.P. et al. (1992), 'The National Birth Center Study Part 3 – Intrapartum and immediate postpartum and neonatal complications and transfers, postpartum and neonatal care, outcomes and client satisfaction', *Journal of Nurse Midwifery*, 37: 361-97

Roosmalen, J. van & Roosmalen, F. (2002), 'There is still room for disagreement about vaginal delivery of breech infants at term', *British Journal of Obstetrics & Gynaecology*, 109: 967-9

Routh, A. (1911), 'On Caesarean Section in the United Kingdom', *Journal of Obstetrics and Gynaecology of the British Empire*, vol. 19, pp.1-25

Royal College of Midwives (1991), *Successful Breastfeeding*, 2nd edn. Livingstone, London

Rydhstrom, H., L. Ingemarsson and S. Ohrlander (1990), 'Lack of Correlation Between a High Caesarean Section Rate and Improved Prognosis for Low-Birthweight Twins (2500g)', *British Journal of Obstetrics and Gynaecology*, vol. 97, pp.229-36

Ryding, E. L. (1993), 'Investigation of 33 women who demanded Caesarean Section for personal reasons', *Acta Obstetrics & Gynaecology Scandinavia*, 72: 280-5

Sanchez-Ramos, L., A. M. Kaunitz, H. B. Peterson, B. Martinez-Schnell and R. J. Thompson (1990), 'Reducing Cesarean Sections at a Teaching Hospital', *American Journal of Obstetrics and Gynaecology*, vol. 163, pp.1081-8

Sandall, J. (1995), 'Choice, continuity and control: changing midwifery, towards a sociological perspective', *Midwifery*, 11(4): 201-9

Sandall, J., Davies, J., & Warwick, C. (2001), 'Evaluation of the Albany Midwifery Practice. Final Report 2001', Monograph published by Florence Nightingale School of Nursing and Midwifery, Kings College London

Sangalli, M. & Guidera A. (2004), 'Caesarean section in term nulliparous women at Wellington Hospital in 2001: a regional audit', *New Zealand Medical Journal*, 117(1206): U1184

Saporito, M. et al. (2003), 'Increase of births by caesarean section in Campania in 2000', *Epidemiol Prev*, 27(5): 291-6

Saunders et al. (2000), *Evaluation of the Edgware Birth Centre*, Barnet Health Authority, London

Savage, W. (1986a), *A Savage Enquiry: Who Controls Childbirth*, Virago, London

Savage, W. (1986b), 'Changing attitudes to intervention', *Nursing Times*, May 28, *Midwives Journal*, p.63

Savage, W. (1990), 'Technology-free Obstetrics at Semmelweis Clinic', *The Lancet*, vol. 336, p.178

Savage, W. (1992), 'The rise in caesarean section – anxiety or science?' in Chard, T. & Richards, M.P. (eds.) *Obstetrics in the 1990s: Current controversies*, Blackwell Scientific Publications Ltd, Oxford

Savage, W. (1997), 'Is it so difficult to define an optimal caesarean section rate for a population?' Health Policy report for M.Sc. in Public Health, London School of Hygiene and Tropical Medicine, London (Obtainable from the author)

Savage, W. (2003), 'New midwifery vision for the 21st century', *British Journal of Midwifery*, 2: 646

Savage, W. and C. Francome (1993), 'British Caesarean Rates: Have we reached a plateau?' *British Journal of Obstetrics and Gynaecology*, vol. 100, pp.403-6

Savage, W., Young, R. & Cochrane, R. (1998), 'Antenatal care in the community: The Tower Hamlets Antenatal Scheme and Survey', Womanschoice, London

Schroeder, C. (1873), *Manual of Midwifery*, 3rd edn., trans. C. H. Carter, Churchill, London

Schucking, B. et al. (2001), 'Cesarean section on request – a medical and psychosomatic problem', *Zentralbl Gynakol*, 123(1): 51-3

SPCERH Scottish Programme for Clinical Effectiveness in Reproductive Health (2001), *Expert Advisory Group on Caesarean Section in Scotland, Report and Recommendations to the Chief Medical Officer*, Scottish Programme for Clinical Effectiveness in Reproductive Health

Sharma, S. and Thorpe-Beeston, J.G. (2002), 'Trial of vaginal delivery following three previous caesarean sections', *British Journal of Obstetrics and Gynaecology*, 109(3): 350-1

Shearer, E. (1992), 'Should Electronic Fetal Monitoring Always be Used for Women in Labor who are Having a Vaginal Birth after a Previous Caesarean?', *Birth*, vol. 19, no. 1, pp.33-4

Shulte, A. J. (1917), quoted in *The Critic and Guide*, New York, p.52

Sibanda, J. and Beard, R.W. (1975), 'Influence on clinical practice of routine intra-partum fetal monitoring', *British Medical Journal*, 3(5979):341-3

Simkin, P. (1991), 'Just Another Day in a Woman's Life: Women's long-term perception of their first birth experience', *Birth*, vol. 18, no. 4, pp.203-10

Simmons, W. (1799), 'Reflection on the Propriety of Performing the Caesarean Operation', *The Medical and Physical Journal*, vol. 2, p.231

Singh, T. et al. (2004), 'An audit on trends of vaginal delivery after one previous caesarean section', *Journal of Obstetrics and Gynaecology*, 24(2): 135-8

Smith, G.C. et al. (2002), 'Birth order, gestational age, and risk of delivery related perinatal death in twins: retrospective cohort study', *British Medical Journal*, 325: 1004

Smith, G.C. et al. (2004), 'Combined logistic and Bayesian modelling of caesarean section risk', *American Journal of Obstetrics and Gynaecology*, 191: 2029-33

Smith, G.C. et al. (2004), 'Factors predisposing to perinatal death related to uterine rupture during attempted vaginal birth after caesarean section – A retrospective cohort study', *British Medical Journal*, 329: p.375

Smith, R. (1990), 'The Epidemiology of Malpractice', *British Medical Journal*, vol. 301, pp.621-2

Smulders, B. (1999), 'The Place of Birth, The Dutch Midwifery System', paper presented at the 'Future Birth – The Place to be Born' conference, Australia, February 1999, URL: www.acegraphics.com.au/articles/smulders02.html, accessed 21.06.05

Social Trends 33 (2001), 'Maternities with multiple births: by age of mother at childbirth', URL: www.statistics.gov.uk/StatBase/ssdataset.app?vlnk=6378&Pos=&ColRank=2&Rank =816, accessed 20.05.05

Social Trends 34 (2002), 'Caesarean deliveries in NHS Hospitals', URL: www.statistics.gov.uk/StatBase/ssdataset.app?vlnk=7412&Pos=&ColRank=2&Rank=480, accessed 12.05.04

Spastics Society (1992), *Paying for Disability: No-fault Compensation - Panacea or Pandora's Box?* London

Stapleton, H., Kirkham, M. & Thomas, G. (2002), 'Qualitative study of evidence based leaflets in maternity care', *British Medical Journal*, 324: 639

Steer, P. (1998), 'Caesarean section: An evolving procedure?' *British Journal of Obstetrics and Gynaecology*, 105: 1052-1055

Stembera, Z. (1987), 'Epidemiology of Perinatal Statistics', *Cesk-Gynekol*, vol. 52, no. 2, pp.162-4

Stembera, Z. (1992), 'Development of Indications for Cesarean Section in the Czech Republic', *Cas-lek-Cesk*, vol. 131, no. 8, pp.225-30

Stephenson, P. A. (1992), *International Difference in the Use of Obstetric Interventions*, World Health Organization, Copenhagen

Stewart, D. (1747), 'The Caesarean Operation Done with Success by a Midwife', *Medical Essays and Observations*, 3rd edn., pt. 1, pp.360-2

Sutherst, J. R. and B. D. Case (1975), 'Caesarean Section and Its Place in the Active Approach to Delivery', Clinics in Obstetrics and Gynaecology, vol. 2, no. 1, pp.241-61

Sutton, J. & Scott, P. (1996), *Understanding and teaching optimal foetal positioning*, Birth Concepts New Zealand

Taffel, S. M., P. J. Placek and C. L. Kosary (1992), 'US Cesarean Section Rates 1990: An update', *Birth*, vol. 19, no. 1, pp.21-2

Tampakoudis, P. et al. (2004), 'Cesarean section rates and indications in Greece: data from a 24-year period in a teaching hospital', *Clin Exp Obstet Gynecol*, 31(4): 289-92

Tariq, T. A. & Korejo, R. (1993), 'Evaluation of the role of craniotomy in developing countries', *Journal of the Pakistan Medical Association*, 43(2): 30-2

Tay, S. K. et al. (1992), 'The use of intradepartmental audit to contain caesarean section rate', *International Journal of Gynaecology & Obstetrics*, 39(2): 99-103

Thacker, S. B. & Stroup, D. E. (2001), 'Continuous electronic heart rate monitoring for fetal assessment during labour', *Cochrane Database System Review* (1)

Theobold, G. W. (1949), 'Modern Caesarean Section', *British Medical Journal*, vol. 2, p.147

Thivierge, B. (2002), 'Cesarean Section', URL: www.healthatoz.com/healthatoz/Atoz/cesarean_section.jsp, accessed 06.07.05

Thomas, J. & Paranjothy, S. (2001), *National Sentinel Caesarean Section Audit Report*, Royal College of Obstetricians and Gynaecologists Clinical Effectiveness Support Unit, RCOG Press

Thornton, J. G. & Lilford, R. J. (1994), 'Active management of labour: current knowledge and research issues', *British Medical Journal*, 309: 366-9

Thorpe-Beeston, J. G., Banfield, P. J. & Saunders, N. J. (1992), 'Outcome of breech delivery at term', *British Medical Journal*, 305(6856): 746-7

Treffers, P. E. and R. Laan (1986), 'Regional Perinatal Mortality and Regional Hospitalisation of Delivery in the Netherlands', *British Journal of Obstetrics and Gynaecology*, vol. 93, pp.690-3

Tucker, J.S. et al. (1996), 'Should obstetricians see women with normal pregnancies? A multicentre randomised controlled trial of routine antenatal care by general practitioners and midwives compared with shared care led by obstetricians', *British Medical Journal*, 312: 554-9

Tweedy, H. (1911), 'Caesarean Section and Its Alternatives', *British Medical Journal*, vol. 1, pp.496-8

UNICEF (2003), 'Maternal Mortality in 2000 – Estimates Developed by WHO, UMICEF and UNFPA', URL: www.childinfo.org/eddb/mat_mortal/index.htm, accessed 07.04.05

UNICEF (2005), 'Delivery Care', URL: www.childinfo.org/areas/deliverycare/, accessed 07.04.05

US Task Force (1978), 'Report on Cesarean Childbirth', US Institute of Health and Human Resources, 82(2067): 419-427

Van Alten, D., Eskes, M. & Treffers, P. E. (1989), 'Midwifery in the Netherlands: The Wormerveer study, selection, mode of delivery, perinatal mortality and infant morbidity', *British Journal of Obstetrics and Gynaecology*, 96: 656-662

Van Teijlingen, E. R. (1990), 'The Profession of Maternity Home Care Assistant and its Significance for the Dutch Midwifery Profession', *International Journal of Nursing Studies*, vol. 27, no. 4, pp.355-66

Vangen, S. et al. (2000), 'Cesarean section among immigrants in Norway', *Acta Obstetrics & Gynaecology Scandinavia*, 79(7): 553-8

Ventura S. J. et al. (1999), 'Births: Final data for 1997', *National Vital Statistics Reports*, 47: XX

Ventura S. J. et al. (2000), 'Births: Final data for 1998', *National Vital Statistics Reports*, vol. 48, no. 3, Hayattsville, MD, National Center for Health Statistics

Walker, R. et al. (2004), 'Increasing caesarean section rates: exploring the role of culture in an Australian Community', *Birth*, 31(2): 117-24

Walsh, D. (1998), 'Clinical Electronic fetal heart monitoring: revisited and reappraised', *British Journal of Midwifery*, 6(6): 400-4

Waites, B. (2003), *Breech Birth*, Free Association Books, London & New York

Warwick, C. (1995), 'Small group practices, Part 2: The midwife's perspective', *Modern Midwife*, 5(11): 22-3

Weaver, J. (2000), 'Talking about caesarean section', *Midirs Midwifery Digest*, 10(4): 487-90

Whyte, H. et al. (2004), 'Outcomes of children at 2 years after planned caesarean birth versus planned vaginal birth for breech presentation at term', *American Journal of Obstetrics and Gynaecology*, 191(3): 864-71

Whitridge, W. J. (1921), 'A Critical Analysis of 212 Years Experience with Caesarean Section', *Johns Hopkins Hospital Bulletin*, vol. 32, p.173

WHO (World Health Organisation) (1985), 'Appropriate technology for birth', *The Lancet*, 2: 436-7

WHO (World Health Organisation) (1994), 'Indicators to monitor health goals – Report of a technical working party', Geneva

Wiegers, T.A., Keirse, M.J.N.C., van der Zee, J., and Berghs G.A.H., (1996), 'Outcome of planned home and planned hospital births in low risk pregnancies in the Netherlands', *British Medical Journal*, 313: 1309-1313

Wildschut, H.U. et al. (1995), 'Planned abdominal compared with planned vaginal birth in triplet pregnancies', *British Journal of Obstetrics and Gynaecology*, 102: 292-6

Wilkinson, C., G. McIlwaine, C. Boulton-Jones and S. Cole (1998), 'Is a rising Caesarean Section rate inevitable?', *BJOG*, 105:45-52

Woodcock, H., A.W. Read, D.J. Moore, F.J. Stanley and C. Bower (1991), 'An Epidemiological Comparison of Planned Home and Hospital Births in Western Australia 1981-1987', International Conference on Primary Care Obstetrics and Perinatal Health, Netherlands Institute of Primary Health Care

World Health Organization, WHO (1985), 'Appropriate Technology for Birth', *The Lancet*, vol. 331, pp.436-7

Wright, E.A., M.M. Kapu and H.I. Onwohafua (1991), 'Perinatal Mortality and Cesarean Section in Jos University Teaching Hospital', *International Journal of Gynaecology and Obstetrics*, vol. 35, no. 4, pp.299-304

Young, G. (1987), 'Are Isolated Maternity Units run by General Practitioners Dangerous?' *British Medical Journal*, vol. 294, pp.744-7

Young, J.H. (1944), Caesarean Section: *The History and Development of the Operation from the Earliest Times*, H.K. Lewis, London

Yusamran, C. et al. (2004), 'Decision-making regarding caesarean section among Thai pregnant women', *Thai Journal of Nursing Research*, 8(2): 83-93

Zanardo, V. et al. (2004), 'Neonatal respiratory morbidity risk and mode of delivery at term: influence of timing of elective caesarean delivery', *Acta Paediatrica*, 93(5): 643-7

Zuspan, F.P., E.J. Quilligan, J.D. Lams and H.P. van Geijn (1979), 'Predictors in Intrapartum Fetal Distress: The role of electronic fetal monitoring', *American Journal of Obstetrics and Gynaecology*, vol. 135, pp.287-91

Further information for parents

Reading

Balaskas, J., *Active Birth, The new approach to giving birth naturally*, revised edition, Harvard Common Press, 1992
How to prepare for an active birth.

Chippington, D., Lowdon, G. and Barlow, F. / NCT, *Caesarean Birth, your questions answered*, NCT, 2004
Answers questions that most people commonly ask about having a baby by caesarean.

Enkin, M., Keirse, M., Neilson, J., Crowther, C., Duley, L., Hodnett, E. and Hofmeyr, J., *A Guide to Effective Care in Pregnancy and Childbirth*, Oxford University Press, 2000
A summary of research findings on all aspects of maternity care.

Inch, S., *Birthrights*, Greenprint, 1989
A critical review of hospital procedures which in many units have become routine.

Metland, D. / NCT, NCT *Pregnancy, for parents by parents*, Collins, 2000
Information covering every stage from conception through pregnancy, labour, birth and the early days with a new baby.

NCT Booklet, *Breastfeeding – A Good Start*, NCT, 2001
A straightforward, reassuring guide to breastfeeding.

Phillips, A., *Your Body, Your Baby, Your Life*, Pandora Press, 1985
'A non-patronising, non-moralising, non-sexist guide to pregnancy and childbirth.'

Thomas, P., *Every Woman's Birthrights*, Harper Collins, 1996
A practical guide to inform and empower women to get the pregnancy and birth they want.

Organisations

Association for Improvements in the Maternity Services (AIMS)
Helpline: 0870 765 1433
Website: www.aims.org
Voluntary pressure group offering support with regard to parents' rights, complaints procedures and choices for maternity care.

Association for Postnatal Illness (APNI)
145 Dawes Road, Fulham,
London, SW6 7EB
Tel: 020 7386 0868
Website: www.apni.org
Email: info@apni.org
Network of volunteers who have suffered from postnatal illness and offer information and support.

Caesarean Support Network
c/o Yvonne Williams, 55 Cool Drive, Douglas, Isle of Man IM2 2HF
Tel: 01624 661269
Offers emotional support and practical advice to women who have had or may need a caesarean.

National Childbirth Trust
Alexandra House, Oldham Terrace,
Acton, London W3 6NH
Tel: 0870 770 3236
Website:
www.nctpregnancyandbabycare.com
Email: enquiries@national-childbirth-trust.co.uk

Over 380 local branches throughout the United Kingdom with networks of informal support, including antenatal teachers, breastfeeding counsellors and postnatal support groups. Local branches will have information about what sort of service to expect from local maternity services and will have details of local support groups for home birth and for women who have had or are expecting to have a caesarean. ParentAbility provides information for parents with disabilities or medical conditions and puts them in touch with each other.

269

NCT (Maternity Sales)
Tel: 0870 112 1120
Website: www.nctms.co.uk
Supplies a wide range of books, leaflets and maternity goods, including nursing bras and the famous NCT stretch briefs, by mail order or online. Catalogue available.

Stillbirth and Neonatal Death Society (SANDS)
28 Portland Place, London W1N 4DE
Tel: 020 7436 5881
Website: www.uk-sands.org
Information and a national network of support groups for parents who have lost a baby.

VBAC Information and Support
c/o Caroline Spear, 50 Whiteways,
North Bersted, Bognor Regis,
West Sussex, PO22 9AS
Tel: 01243 868440
Network of volunteers offering information and support for women wanting a vaginal birth after a previous caesarean.

Internet Sources

www.birthchoice.org
Explains options and gives information to help you make choices about where to have your baby and who should look after you in labour.

www.caesarean.org.uk
Women's experiences, personal stories, published articles, groups and links.

www.childbirth.org
Promotes birth as a natural process. Provides links to other useful sites.

www.homebirth.org
Information about home birth for parents and professionals, including a page on VBAC.

www.nctpregnancyandbabycare.com
NCT offers support in pregnancy, childbirth and early parenthood. They aim to give every parent the chance to make informed choices.

www.vbac.org
Advice, reports and personal experiences of VBAC.

Index